Clinical Use of Blood

Cees Th. Smit Sibinga
Yetmgeta E. Abdella

Editors

Clinical Use of Blood

A Different Approach

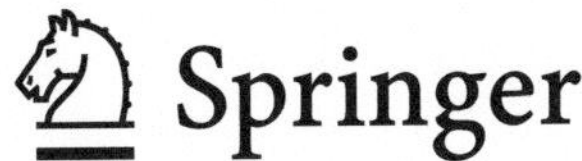

Editors
Cees Th. Smit Sibinga
IQM Consulting
Zuidhorn, The Netherlands

Yetmgeta E. Abdella
Self-employed, Freelance Consultant in
Blood and other Products of Human
Origin
Addis Ababa, Ethiopia

Section Editors
Vernon J. Louw
Department of Medicine, Clinical Hematology
Groote Schuur Hospital
Cape Town, South Africa

Arwa Z. Al-Riyami
Department of Haematology
Sultan Qaboos University Hospital
Muscat, Oman

ISBN 978-3-031-67334-4   ISBN 978-3-031-67332-0   (eBook)
https://doi.org/10.1007/978-3-031-67332-0

This Springer imprint is published by the registered company Springer Nature Switzerland AG
The registered company address is: Gewerbestrasse 11, 6330 Cham, Switzerland

If disposing of this product, please recycle the paper.

It gives me pleasure to write the foreword to this book edited by my friend and colleague Prof. Dr. Cees Smit Sibinga who served for 6 years as co-chair of the AABB Global Transfusion Forum's Education Committee and contributed to our recent book *Global Perspectives and Practices in Transfusion Medicine*. The latter book focused largely on transfusion in lower- and middle-income countries (LMICs) with 80% of the authors living in these LMICs who could thus provide contextual insights into transfusion in those settings. This book *Clinical Use of Blood: A Different Approach* hews along a different track by examining new developments in clinical blood transfusion mostly in high-income countries (HICs). The two books (that share several authors) are thus complementary and valuable additions to the compendium of global transfusion knowledge.

A good example of emerging high-end technologies entering transfusion medicine is presented in Chap. 5 by José Cancelas and co-authors who argue that AI and machine learning "…might help accelerate the bridging of the global gaps existing in the blood supply and clinical use between the more advanced world and the developing world." They explain concepts of machine learning, deep learning, and deep neural networks (DNN) to show how AI can be utilized to improve the quality of decision-making and outcomes in transfusion medicine. This chapter provides an insightful indication of future technological directions in transfusion medicine.

Along similar lines (of a "different approach"), Jerry Holmberg and Cees Smit Sibinga present compelling arguments for a "digital footprint" in transfusion medicine "supported by radio frequency identification (RFID) (to) prevent clerical errors and misidentifications…" As the authors rightly point out, introduction of any disruptive technology carries its own risks by virtue of its very disruptiveness and should therefore be well thought out and carefully monitored. This is an important cautionary note to heed as the science of transfusion medicine moves into unchartered terrains.

This book is, however, not only about disruptively different approaches to blood transfusion but also discusses emerging concepts in education that many transfusionists may not be familiar with such as the "knowledge economy" and "outcome-based education (OBE)." These concepts have as yet not gained much traction in transfusion medicine but offer important epistemic insights to the field.

Another group of chapters takes on debates that were once considered "resolved" but are now receiving renewed attention—such as presented in

Part III on "restrictive versus liberal use of blood and blood components." As new countervailing evidence emerges (often as a result of new research methods), patient safety demands that we continue to re-evaluate knowledge that we may have considered "known and settled."

The book aptly ends with a section on quality management and standard setting in transfusion medicine—a fitting reminder that every new/different approach in clinical medicine should be subjected to quality standards to ensure patient safety.

In short, this book presents several "different" approaches to the clinical use of blood ranging from potentially disruptive technologies to nuanced re-examinations of clinical evidence and new concepts in clinical education. As such it should be of great interest to a wide range of readers.

My congratulations to the editors and all the authors on the efforts in producing this book.

Vanderbilt University Medical Center   Quentin G. Eichbaum
Nashville, TN, USA

Preface

This book will not be focused on practical disciplinary or traditional "how to do's" in clinical transfusion medicine, but highlight more important issues like restricted versus liberal prescription and use of blood and blood components, implementation and use of artificial intelligence (machine learning and deep learning), and a digital footprint including radiofrequency identification (RFID) in clinical transfusion prescription and practice, education of clinicians in transfusion medicine at the bedside based on educational environment and expected outcomes. The approach of the clinical use of blood will be different, more fundamental, and more based on knowledge economy.

The book will contribute to the stewardship development of clinical use of blood and blood components highlighting patient-focused blood management (PBM), evidence-based decision-making supported by big data, prescription behavior, and bedside practice of well-educated professionals (clinicians, nurses, and laboratory professionals), and the necessary education climate and environment, knowledge economy, and quality management. The implementation and use of artificial intelligence with its big data principles, robotics, and education algorithms in clinical transfusion medicine, machine and deep learning manifold of applications and future extensions are recognized.

This book will serve as a source of knowledge to improve on patient-oriented and individualized clinical transfusion practices, clinical indication setting and decision making in transfusion medicine, and patient comfort and welfare reducing unnecessary harm and risks with deep learning and RFID.

As a unique book of reference, it will enlighten the conditions and requirements needed to come to an optimal, individualized, and supportive transfusion practice that will positively influence the procurement process (manufacturing of blood products or components) in an evidence-based and economic way, which will support the necessary developments needed in the low- and middle-income country (LMIC) world, home to 84% of the global population.

This book is edited in 4 parts and 11 chapters:

Part I—Education of Clinicians in Bedside Transfusion Medicine

   Chapter 1—The Importance of Educational Environment and Climate in Transfusion Medicine

   Chapter 2—Outcomes-Based Clinical Transfusion Medicine Education

Chapter 3—The Role of Knowledge Economy in Clinical Transfusion Practice

Part II—Artificial Intelligence and a Digital Footprint in Clinical Transfusion Medicine

Chapter 4—Documentation and Data Collection: Tools for Improvement

Chapter 5—Clinical Blood Transfusion and Artificial Intelligence

Chapter 6—The Importance of Digital Footprinting in Clinical Transfusion Medicine

Part III—Clinical Practice: Restrictive Versus Liberal Use of Blood and Blood Components

Chapter 7—Patient Blood Management

Chapter 8—Platelet Transfusion

Chapter 9—Red Blood Cell Transfusion

Part IV—Quality Management in Clinical Transfusion Medicine

Chapter 10—The Need for a Quality System and Quality System Management in Clinical Transfusion Medicine

Chapter 11—The Effect of Standards and Guidelines in Clinical Transfusion Practice

The different approach underpins the importance of understanding and owning the clinical transfusion processes from bedside to laboratory to bedside.

Zuidhorn, The Netherlands
Addis Ababa, Ethiopia Cees Th. Smit Sibinga
Yetmgeta E. Abdella

Contents

Abbreviations

AABB	Association for the Advancement of Blood and Biotherapies
AATM	Asian Association of Transfusion Medicine
ACGME	Accreditation Council for Graduate Medical Education
ADP	Adenosine di-phosphate
AE	Adverse event
AFR	Africa Region (WHO)
AfSBT	African Society of Blood Transfusion
AGM	Aorta/gonad/mesonephros
AI	Artificial intelligence
AI/ML	Artificial intelligence/machine learning
AIDC	Automatic information and data capture
AIHA	Auto immune hemolytic anemia
AKI	Acute kidney injury
AMEE	Association for Medical Education in Europe
AML`	Acute myeloid leukemia
ANH	Acute normovolemic hemodilution
ANN	Artificial neural network
ARDS	Acute respiratory distress syndrome
AS	Additive solution
BFU-E	Burst-forming unit—erythroid
ISQua	International Society for Quality in Health Care
BLL	Blood lead level
BPA	Best practice advisor
BSA	Body surface area
BUR	Blood utilization rate
CAGR	Compound annual growth rate
CBD	Competent by design
CCI	Corrected count increment
CCP	Critical control point
CDS	Clinical decision support
CEO	Chief Executive Officer
CFU-E	Colony-forming unit—erythroid
cGCP	Current good clinical practice
cGMP	Current good manufacturing practice
CI	Confidence interval
CIA	Central Intelligence Agent
CMV	Cytomegalo virus

CoP	Community of Practice
COVID-19	Corona Virus Disease-2019
CPD	Citrate phosphate dextrose
CPD	Continuous professional development
CPDA-1	Citrate phosphate dextrose adenine-1
CPG	Clinical practice guidelines
CPOE	Computerized provider order entry
CRISP	Clustered regularly interspaced short palindromic repeats
DIC	Diffuse intravascular coagulation
DL	Deep learning
DNN	Deep neural network
DTT	Dithiothreitol
EDQM	European Directorate for Quality of Medicine and Healthcare
EFQM	European Foundation for Quality Management
ELBW	Extreme low body weight
EMR	Eastern Mediterranean Region (WHO)
EOP	Equipment operating procedure
EPA	Entrustable professional activities
Epo/rEpo	Erythropoietin/recombinant erythropoietin
ESA	Erythropoietin-stimulating agent
ETTNO	Effects of transfusion thresholds on neurocognitive outcomes
EU	European Union
EUR	European Region (WHO)
FAIR	Findable, accessible, interoperable, reusable
FDA	Food and Drug Administration
FDP	Fibrinogen degradation product
FNAIT	Fetal and neonatal alloimmune thrombocytopenia
GCP	Good clinical practice
GDBS	Global Database on Blood Safety
GDPR	General Data Protection Regulation
GLP	Good laboratory practice
GMC	General Medical Council
GMP	Good manufacturing practice
GP	Glycoprotein
GTP	Good transfusion practice
GxD	Good practices
HAS	Haute Authorité Santé
HDFN	Hemolytic disease of the fetus and the newborn
HDI	Human development index
HE	Higher education
HF	High frequency
Hgb	Hemoglobin
HLA	Human leukocyte antigen
HMISS	Healthcare Information and Management Systems Society
HPA	Human platelet antigen
HPC	Hematopoietic proliferative cell

HR	Hazard ratio
HSC	Hematopoietic stem cell
HSCT	Hematopoietic stem cell transplantation
HTC	Hospital Transfusion Committee
HTM	Human resource management
ICCBBA	International Committee for Commonality in Blood Bank Automation
ICH	Intracranial hemorrhage
ICT	Information and communication technology
ICU	Intensive care unit
IE	Ineffective erythropoiesis
IEEA	International External Evaluation Association
IOM	Institute of Medicine
IoT	Internet of things
IPC	Immature platelet count
ISBT	International Society of Blood Transfusion
ISH	International Society of Hematology
ISO	International Organization for Standardization
ITP	Immune thrombocytopenia
IUT	Intrauterine transfusion
IVIg	Intravenous immunoglobulin
JD	Job description
KPI	Key performance indicator
LF	Low frequency
LMIC	Low- and Middle-Income Country
M&E	Monitoring and evaluation
MATISS	Management of thrombocytopenia in special subgroup
MCI	Medical Council of India
MIABIS	Minimum information about biobank-data sharing
ML	Machine learning
MM	Multiple myeloma
MPP	Multipotent progenitor
NATO	North Atlantic Treaty Organization
NEC	Necrotizing enterocolitis
NET	Neonatal exchange transfusion
NGC	National Guideline Clearinghouse
NICE	National Institute for Health and Care Excellence
NIMO-Rad	Near Infrared Spectroscopy for Monitoring Brain Oxygenation
NK	Natural killer
NLD	Natural language processing
NO	Nitrogen oxide
OBE	Outcome-based education
OPD	Out-patient department
OR	Operation room, odd ratio
OTS	Off the shelf
PAI-1	Plasminogen activator inhibitor-1
PAS	Platelet additive solution

PBM	Patient blood management
PD	Process description
PD-BO-BT	Process description-blood ordering-blood transfusion
PICC	Peripherally inserted central catheter
PINT	Premature infants in need of transfusion
PLADO	Platelet dose (study)
Planet=2	Platelets for neonatal thrombocytopenia (study)
POCT	Point-of-care testing
PROMMIT	Prospective, Observational, Multicenter, Major Trauma Transfusion (study)
PROPPR	Pragmatic, Randomized Optimal Platelet and Plasma Ratio (study)
PT	Prothrombin time
PTR	Platelet transfusion refractoriness
QA	Quality assurance
QC	Quality control
QMS	Quality management system
QS	Quality system
QSM	Quality system management
RBC	Red blood cell
RBCT	Red blood cell transfusion
RCE	Red cell exchange
RCT	Randomized controlled trial
RFID	Radio frequency identification
ROTEM	Rotational thromboelastography
RTTI	Relevant transfusion transmissible infection
RTTIA	Relevant transfusion transmissible agent
SAGM	Saline adenine glucose mannitol
SC	Synthetic cannabinoid
SCD	Sickle cell disease
SCM	Supply chain management
SD	Standard deviation
SDG	Sustainable Development Goals
SEAR	South East Asia Region (WHO)
SMART	Specific, measurable, acceptable, realistic, timely
SOP	Standard operating procedure
SPC	Statistical process control
SToP	Strategies for Transfusion of Platelets
T&S	Type and screen
T&T	Traceability and trackability
TA-GvHD	Transfusion-associated graft-versus-host disease
TAH	Transfusion-associated hyperkalemia
TARA	Tasks, authority, responsibility, accountability
TDT	Transfusion-dependent therapy
TEG	Thromboelastography
TF	Tissue factor
TFPI	Tissue factor pathway inhibitor
THC	Tetra hydrocannabinoid

TM	Transfusion medicine
TOPPS	Trial of prophylactic platelets study
tPA	Tissue plasminogen activator
Tpo	Thrombopoietin
TRALI	Transfusion-related lung injury
TRICC	Transfusion requirement in clinical care (study)
TRT	Testosterone replacement therapy
Tsat	Transferrin saturation
TTIA	Transfusion transmissible infectious agent
TXA2	Thromboxane A2
UGI	Upper gastrointestinal
UHC	Universal health coverage
UHF	Ultra high frequency
UK	United Kingdom
UNDP	United Nations Development Programme
USA	United States of America
USD	US dollar
USMLE	United States Medical Licensing Examination
V2V	Vein-to-vein
VLBW	Very low birth weight
VMI	Vendor-managed inventory
Vv/va ECMO	Venovenous/venoarterial extracorporeal membrane oxygenation
vWF	Von Willebrand Factor
WBC	White blood cell
WBIT	Wrong blood in tube
WEF	World Economic Forum
WHO	World Health Organization
WNOT	Wrong name on tube
WOMAN	World Maternal Antifibrinolytic
WPR	Western Pacific Region (WHO)

Part I

Education of Clinicians in Bedside Transfusion Medicine

Vernon J. Louw

The Importance of Educational Environment and Climate in Transfusion Medicine Education

Vernon J. Louw, Claire L. Barrett, and Vanitha Rambiritch

1.1 Introduction

History is filled with the names of famous writers, artists, musicians and scientists, who were to a large extent self-taught in the fields in which they excelled. Some names that come to mind include Leonardo da Vinci, William Blake, Charles Dickens, and Albert Einstein, as well as several Nobel laureates, including Hermann Hesse, Knut Hamsun, Camilo José Cela, Eugene O'Neill, José Saramago, William Faulkner, George Bernard Shaw, Rabindranath Tagore, and Ernest Hemingway. Still, these self-made scholars remain the exception rather than the rule. Over the centuries, the way in which we learn, for better or for worse, has undergone many changes, and is still changing [1, 2]. It has been recognized that, in an increasingly complex world, where strict regulatory frameworks abound and knowledge is exponentially increasing in all fields, specialization and often subspecialization have become the norm for many individuals. This is especially so in the field of medicine, and more specifically, in the case of transfusion medicine. To optimize learning in such a world, it is key to understand the context within which students learn, the pressures they are under, and competencies expected from them.

The focus of this chapter is to look at the role the learning environment plays and how it can be optimized to ensure that the needs and requirements of all stakeholders are met.

1.2 Defining the Learning Environment

A learning environment for training medical doctors in clinical transfusion medicine is a multifaceted, integrative milieu consisting of various physical, virtual, social, and psychological contexts and conditions that impact learning processes and outcomes [3]. It includes the physical spaces (e.g., lecture halls, laboratories, and clinical settings such as hospitals and clinics), simulation environments, and digital platforms where instruction takes place (e.g. smart classrooms) [3, 4]. It also includes the relationships with instructors, mentors, peers, and patients, as well as the medical and scientific content, practical skills

V. J. Louw (✉)
Division of Clinical Haematology, Department of Medicine, Groote Schuur Hospital, University of Cape Town, Cape Town, South Africa
e-mail: vernon.louw@uct.ac.za

C. L. Barrett
School of Medicine, University of the Free State, Bloemfontein, South Africa

V. Rambiritch
South Africa National Blood Service (SANBS), Roodepoort, South Africa
e-mail: vanitha.rambiritch@sanbs.org.za

training, problem-solving activities, research opportunities, and ethical considerations related to transfusion medicine [5].

The learning environment should be conducive to promoting hands-on experiences, knowledge acquisition and application, critical thinking, professional competencies, and ethical decision-making skills that are transferrable and pertinent to transfusion medicine [6]. Given the serious implications of errors in this field, the learning environment should prioritize patient safety, with a culture that encourages questions, creating a safe space where the student can make errors and learn from these errors, and fosters ongoing self-reflection and improvement. The environment should furthermore be adaptive and responsive to changes and new developments in medical science, educational approaches, technology (including artificial intelligence, augmented reality, and eLearning), healthcare policy, and societal needs, and be inclusive and respectful of diverse learners and patients [7]. It must also offer avenues for reflective practice, formative feedback, and continuous learning, and foster a commitment to lifelong learning and professional development. This environment would not only involve learning the technical aspects of transfusion medicine, such as blood typing, cross-matching, blood component therapy, and managing adverse reactions to transfusions, but also incorporate holistic medical practices, patient communication, and ethical considerations related to blood component use. The foundation of knowledge economy is intricately tied to the learning environment.

1.3　The Components Required for a Learning Environment Conducive to the Study of Transfusion Medicine (A Walled Garden)

A learning environment conducive to the study of transfusion medicine is multifaceted, comprising several key components that together cultivate a thriving educational experience. It can be online (eLearning) or in person [8]. In this discussion we use a garden with a protective wall as a metaphor for the elements required in a learning environment and how each of these fit together. A garden is a space where seeds, plants, and trees, all different, are planted, tended, weeded, watered, and protected, to ensure that the produce (e.g., fruit, vegetables, herbs, wood) is of the highest quality. We can think of the learning environment as a walled garden, with an entrance and exit gate, with gardeners that tend, weed, and water, of plants that are grown and developed, and produce that can be delivered to society. With the teacher as gardener and the student as the plant, let us explore the garden and see what an ideal learning environment should look like.

When a student enters the learning environment, it is important that the student has a strong sense of trust from the beginning. Not only should the student trust that the training institution is an established, recognized and accredited training facility, but the training programs must be recognized with a good track record of student throughput and success. First impressions are important in all spheres of life, also here. Students who are welcomed, acknowledged, and who sense that they will become part of an enthusiastic safe and engaging environment are much more likely to invest themselves fully in the learning process and eventually succeed. Aiming to understand students' expectations, career goals, and the environment within which they will eventually practice and having an environment that can be adapted to accommodate these needs, will greatly empower successful learning. At the same time, a learning environment should be such that it makes provision for the individual needs of students, who may be diverse in terms of culture, race, ethnicity, gender, language, socio-economic status, physical abilities, and mental health status. Additionally, the learning environment should accommodate international students, adult learners, as well as first-generation students, acknowledging that there is not an "ideal student." These elements together should create a safe learning environment; where the student feels safe to make mistakes and grow.

One of the foundational elements of any quality learning experience is a curriculum that is standardized, and benchmarked against international best practice, with adequate time, focus, and access to resources [9]. This encompasses textbooks, journals, guidelines, online resources, digital tools (e.g., podcasts, social media applications used as education platforms, webinars) and the physical spaces (e.g., traditional or smart classrooms, simulation facilities, hospitals, clinics, and blood establishments) to apply what has been learned in a real-world setting [4, 10]. The role of skilled, approachable, and knowledgeable instructors cannot be overstated. Instructors who are well-versed in transfusion medicine, both on the clinical and laboratory side and who are adept at simplifying complex concepts and providing examples from real-world and personal experience, serve to enhance students' comprehension and spur their interest. Instructors who are themselves engaged in continuous learning and research in transfusion medicine, may add to the richness of the learning environment. It should be noted though that it is not just the quality of teachers that is important here, but also having adequate teacher-to-trainee ratios to avoid burnout on the instructor side, while simultaneously ensuring that teaching staff have enough time available to meet student needs [11].

The essence of teaching is not only imparting theoretical knowledge (teaching), but also providing practical skills (training). Practical, hands-on learning experiences play a crucial role in cementing theoretical knowledge. Offering students opportunities to practice skills and procedures in controlled settings, such as laboratories or simulations, fosters a deeper understanding of transfusion medicine and cultivates confidence in their learning. Simulation and role-play provide an opportunity to train on rare but important transfusion events that may not be readily witnessed in the clinical environment—for example, the management of an acute hemolytic transfusion reaction. Additionally, working with actual patients and being part of the work done in real-life settings, whether in blood establishments or in the clinical environment, will add to the students' experience of learning in a way that brings the whole of their learning to bear on their activities, not just their academic knowledge, but also

the real-life experience of the emotional and responsibility-bearing elements of transfusion medicine practice. Real-world exposure is integral for bridging the gap between theory and practice [3]. Allowing students to observe or participate in transfusion medicine practice in clinical settings illuminates practical applications and contextualizes their theoretical knowledge.

A good learning environment should encourage active, student-centered learning, but also stimulate self-directed learning. This fosters ownership over the educational journey and cultivates a proactive learning spirit in an environment that values student engagement. Ensuring variety in the styles and methods of teaching may increase student engagement, as different students learn best in different ways (e.g., visual versus auditory learning, doing versus studying, flipped classroom versus classic didactic teaching). It is important that the environment encourages students to engage dynamically with the material provided and learn how to apply it, especially in a field such as transfusion medicine.

Professionalism is a pivotal trait students must imbibe to deliver safe and effective transfusion medicine. By participating in an environment that advocates and models professional behaviors, students can cultivate necessary skills and uphold ethical standards of patient care. Given that clinical transfusion medicine necessitates collaboration with other healthcare professionals, instilling the values of teamwork and interprofessional communication is paramount. Offering opportunities for interprofessional practice fosters a deeper understanding of clinical transfusion medicine, as well as developing critical problem-solving and communication skills. Fostering positive interpersonal interactions, which stimulate questioning, curiosity, and critical thinking, are essential. An inclusive, diverse, and welcoming environment that allows students to comfortably seek clarification, question assumptions, and request assistance augments their learning experience. Creating a Community of Practice (CoP) promotes a supportive network where students/peers can ask questions, share relevant experiences, exchange information and best practices. Such a setting nurtures a sense of community, belonging, capacity building, knowledge sharing, networking, collaborations, and mentorship, further enriching the learning experience.

Furthermore, with increasing globalization and mobility of the workforce, the learning process (curriculum, outcomes, assessment, etc.) should align with international best practices, while also being tailored to suit the local environment. Local needs as well as the availability of human and other resources may vary greatly from one setting to another [1]. Education, therefore, needs to cater to the specific requirements, capacities, and resources of the community served, ensuring both accessibility and relevance.

Consistent teaching and learning practices should be underpinned by appropriate institutional policies and procedures, which include policies on important elements of the training [e.g., assessment, plagiarism, use of technology such as artificial intelligence, eLearning, digital foot printing, Radio Frequency Identification (RFID, see also Chap. 6), and recognition of prior learning]. These policies should support best practices and ensure continuity in the education process, resulting in consistently high-quality learning experiences and competent student outcomes. The institution should also have established student support procedures in place, these may include mentorship programs, academic advising, counselling and mental health services, healthcare, financial aid offices, support for international students and students with disabilities, and in many resource-limited environments, access to food and nutritional support is important.

This section would be incomplete without mentioning the importance of digital learning environments. We live in a time and age where students, as digital natives, increasingly make use of digital tools, online learning platforms, big data, machine learning, simulation, augmented reality, and artificial intelligence [1]. Both teachers and students need to know and understand how to incorporate the plethora of available materials in a responsible fashion. Whether digital materials form the primary or adjunct learning space, it is critical that content, if not created by the primary institution, be curated carefully, to ensure that what students study is of high quality, accurate, up-to-date, and aligned with local laws, regulations, ethical requirements, and the eventual working environment for which the student is being prepared. This is becoming even more important in the era of artificial intelligence (AI), where the use of AI will not only become an option or available tool for ad hoc use but also embedded in software that is widely used, such as search engines and word processors. Creating an environment that can adapt to these new and transformative developments will be essential to ensure that the learning environment remains in touch with the times and sustainable [2, 12]. Understanding the way in which the digital learner learns and thinks is very important here. Digital learners grow up hyperconnected, with the Internet, gaming platforms and social media, a virtual extension of their identities, their selves, and their way of being in this world. Teaching methods need to consider and meet their needs of collaboration in groups, augmented reality, gamification of learning, and the widespread use of AI in the future [13, 14].

In the generation of AI, it is important not only to equip students to use AI to enhance their learning, but teachers must ensure that the students' soft skills (or uniquely human skills) are developed. The World Economic Forum (WEF) has stated that in 2023, the following are the top ten job skills:

 1. analytical thinking,
 2. creative thinking,
 3. resilience, flexibility, and agility,
 4. motivation and self-awareness,
 5. curiosity and lifelong learning,
 6. technological literacy,
 7. dependability and attention to detail,
 8. empathy and active listening,
 9. leadership and social influence, and
10. quality control.

Many of these are uniquely human skills that cannot be replaced by AI [5], transfusion education programs may build these skills into their "hidden curriculum," to ensure that students are equipped with these skills. Education must keep abreast with change. The WEF states that up to 44% of workers' core skills will change in the next 5 years, and while many transfusion tasks may not change, current day reality includes electronic cross-match, drones delivering blood, and big data analytics in blood transfusion that may have not been considered a decade ago. Students must be future-ready, and that is a moving target [5].

The efficacy of these components lies in the regular assessment and feedback of students' knowledge and abilities [15]. Scheduled assessments and evaluations provide students with a measure of their progress and identify areas that require further attention. Feedback to learners should be timely, clear, and specific; feedback that is delayed and vague feedback is not helpful and does not guide improvement. Feedback should be based on direct observations and offer examples illustrating the point and avoid assumptions. Additionally, feedback must be balanced, offering both positive feedback and addressing areas that need improvement, this can be done by means of a two-way discussion where the learner is given an opportunity to reflect on both the performance as well as the feedback. Considering the aforementioned, feedback should include giving the learner goals to strive for, with measurable and actionable suggestions (e.g., referring the learner to a specific learning resource or activity, highlighting that learning is a continuous process and that improvements are incremental over time. Lastly, feedback should be professional, supportive, encouraging, and respectful.

It is crucial to recognize that the social learning environment consists of interactions between students, instructors, other members of the interdisciplinary healthcare team, and the institutional culture [16]. An optimal learning environment for clinical transfusion medicine, therefore, fosters patient-centeredness, continuous improvement, encourages professional development, and champions innovation, but also considers that one deals with students who are human beings with their own backgrounds, frailties, challenges, and dreams.

In the following sections, some of the broad issues above will be discussed in more detail.

1.4 The Psychosocial Aspects of the Learning Environment (The Climate)

The psychosocial culture aspect in a learning environment can be thought of as the prevailing climate in our metaphorical garden. Although these may be less tangible and measurable, they are no less important, as they are often ignored, or perhaps in one's blind spot, but have a major impact on the overall atmosphere that is experienced within the learning environment [17]. As long as we deal with humans rather than with "intelligent," but unemotional machines, these factors will play a major role in the success of any training program. The foundation of a high-quality psychosocial learning environment is effective communication and interpersonal skills. This starts with proper orientation of the student to their new environment and summarized nicely in the article by Gifford et al., providing practical examples of orienting students by answering questions like, *Why am I here?, Who is the team?, What do I do?, Where are things?, When do things happen?*, and *How do I navigate patient care and learning?* [18] This includes things like Instructor Talk, recognized as the ways in which language, tone, attitude, perceptions, and positive or negative phrasing affect and alter the students' learning experience and outcomes [19]. These need to be practiced, modelled, and taught. The ability to convey information clearly and empathetically, not just among peers and mentors but also with patients and their families, lays the foundation for trust and mutual understanding, which are critical in the field of clinical transfusion medicine. Building on this foundation, a learning environment should encourage collaboration and teamwork. Working in clinical transfusion medicine is seldom a solitary endeavor; it relies heavily on the coordinated efforts of various professionals, each bringing their own expertise to the table. By fostering a culture of collaboration, the learning environment ensures that trainees are prepared to work in diverse teams.

While fostering communication and teamwork, the environment should also cultivate empathy and respect. These qualities are essential in a field like clinical transfusion medicine, where sensitive decisions and interactions are commonplace. By nurturing these values, we can ensure that our future healthcare professionals are not just technically competent but also compassionate in their practice. The importance of emotional well-being and resilience cannot be understated in such a high-stakes field. Medical training is known to be rigorous and can often take a toll on one's mental health. Therefore, a supportive learning environment that emphasizes self-care, work-life balance, and provides resources for mental health is crucial in building resilience among trainees. The immediacy and availability of staff to support students when needed is very important here [2, 6]. Practically, an environment characterized by appropriate use of humor and mindfulness training and similar modalities can improve mental health and decrease anxiety [6]. In tandem with emotional support, creating a culture of safety and trust is paramount. Important here is understanding the concept of "power distance," and the degree to which differences in "power distance" beliefs and fear of authority affects communication is very important in clinical transfusion medicine, where mistakes can have significant consequences [20]. Learners need to feel secure in acknowledging their errors, asking questions, and seeking guidance. This atmosphere of openness is key to continuous learning and improvement, and ultimately, to patient safety. Woven into all these aspects is the thread of ethical practice. Transfusion medicine brings with it a unique set of ethical challenges and considerations that all practitioners need to navigate. A learning environment that instils a deep understanding of these issues and promotes the accepted values and ethical underpinnings of approaches to these are essential in preparing trainees to uphold the highest ethical standards in their practice [21].

As we shape this environment, we must also ensure that it is inclusive and respectful of diversity. This diversity refers not only to the trainees but also to the patients they will eventually serve. Recognizing and respecting diversity—cultural, racial, and others—enriches the learning experience and equips trainees to provide culturally competent care. In addition to these elements, the environment should also cultivate leadership skills. This also speaks to the importance of having a sense of belonging, which, together with a sense of security and healthy self-concept, has been shown to affect student experience, progress, and achievement [8, 22, 23]. As they progress in their careers, medical professionals often find themselves in situations where they must make critical decisions, advocate for their patients, or guide a team. Here one should recognize the importance of mentorship, not just the organizational and management forms of leadership. As humans are imitating beings in their nature, we tend to become more and more like those we spend time with, which can be both to our benefit or detriment. Finally, the learning environment should promote a culture of feedback and reflective practice. Constructive feedback helps learners understand their strengths and areas for improvement, while reflective practice allows them to learn from their experiences and continually refine their professional identity.

In combining these elements—culture, communication, collaboration, empathy, caring, emotional support, safety, ethical practice, inclusivity, leadership, and reflective practice—we can create a robust and enriching psychosocial learning environment [2]. This environment not only prepares learners for the technical aspects of transfusion medicine but also nurtures the softer, yet equally important, skills that define a compassionate and effective healthcare professional.

1.5 The Stakeholders (All Parties with a Vested Interest in the Success of the Garden)

Various stakeholders intricately involved in high-quality clinical transfusion medicine education shape its success. In terms of the garden one can think of them as those who have some interest in seeing the garden function optimally and becoming a successful and fruitful venture. Each entity brings unique perspectives, needs, and interests, but they are united by a common goal: to ensure students are adequately prepared to deliver safe and effective patient care in transfusion medicine.

Students, being the direct recipients of the education, hold an essential position in this ecosystem. They are the primary stakeholders whose proficiency in the field hinges on the quality of the program. Educators, comprising teachers, professors, and clinical instructors, are responsible for imparting instruction. Their educational skill and dedication directly influence the success of the program and the efficacy of the students. Institutions such as universities, colleges, hospitals, or training centers constitute another significant stakeholder group. By offering the necessary infrastructure and resources, these institutions enable the educational program to operate effectively. Patients, as the ultimate beneficiaries of high-quality clinical transfusion medicine education, stand as vital stakeholders. The goal is to offer them safe and effective care, delivered by well-trained transfusion medicine practitioners and medical specialists.

The public plays a dual role in this context. On the one hand, they contribute to transfusion services through donations of blood and other resources. On the other hand, they often fund blood services and educational institutions through taxes. Importantly, the public (as patients), is essentially the greatest beneficiary of adequate transfusion medicine training. Recognizing the importance of public engagement is essential for anyone working in transfusion medicine.

Professional associations like the Association for the Advancement of Blood and Biotherapies (AABB), the International Society for Blood Transfusion (ISBT), Africa Society for Blood Transfusion (AfSBT), Asian Association of Transfusion Medicine (AATM), and other medical associations and professional societies also significantly influence the education landscape. They set standards, promote continuing education and research, and represent the profession to the public and other stakeholders.

Healthcare institutions such as hospitals and clinics are invested in high-quality clinical transfusion medicine education as they depend on competently skilled transfusion medicine practitioners and medical specialists to ensure their patients receive safe and effective care. Blood services are integral stakeholders as the education provided directly impacts the functioning of these services, the provision of safe blood and blood products, and their appropriate clinical usage. Government agencies including health departments, and regulatory boards and blood establishments are important as they ensure the safety and quality of blood products, the qualifications and accreditation of transfusion medicine practitioners, and compliance with regulations. For these institutions to function optimally, practitioners need to be competently skilled, but their training must also be ongoing and current, to ensure patient safety and component quality.

While each stakeholder brings their own perspective and interest, they all share the commitment to fostering high-quality education towards an excellent "product" delivered to the public. This collective goal ensures the preparedness of future professionals to provide the best patient care in the field of clinical transfusion medicine.

1.6 The Regulatory and Legislative Framework Within Which a Learning Environment Operates (The Fence)

A legislative and regulatory framework is vital in an educational setting, underpinning the creation of secure, equitable, and efficient learning environments. It shapes and guides the educational standards, such as curriculum specifications, learning outcomes, qualifications for educators, and accreditation requirements, thereby maintaining the quality of education. It safeguards students' rights, ensuring nondiscrimination, equal access to education, and student safety and welfare. The legislative framework also promotes accountability. By requiring responsibility from educational institutions through oversight and reporting, it helps ensure that learning environments are conducive to intellectual growth. The framework also delineates a clear scope of practice for each discipline, supporting recognition of qualifications by professional societies and academic institutions.

Another key role of the legislative framework is establishing funding mechanisms, thereby increasing access to resources for all students. In transfusion medicine, it sets rigorous requirements for healthcare professionals, ensuring competence and capacity to provide high-quality patient care. The framework facilitates the creation of professional healthcare board-accredited career opportunities, such as transfusion safety officers, blood banking laboratory professionals, and transfusion physicians [24]. It also regulates blood donation and transfusion, stipulating safety standards and patient rights while guiding curriculum development and assessment.

1.7 Entry Criteria and Its Role in the Educational Environment (The Entry Gate)

If we think of the legislative and regulatory environment as the protective wall of the garden, entry criteria can be represented by the entrance gate where the prospective students (plants) that enter are evaluated for their suitability for the environment and where the student can consider the suitability of the environment to them.

Entry criteria serve as a vital cornerstone in the educational landscape, defining the prerequisites for students to undertake a specific course or join a particular academic institution. They play a pivotal role in ensuring that students possess the requisite knowledge, skills, and aptitudes to flourish in their chosen field of study. Moreover, the completion of the study program should pave the way for career advancement, enrichment, and expansion, with an overarching aim to provide advisory capacity and support in the field of transfusion medicine.

Some ways in which entry requirements can shape the educational milieu in clinical transfusion medicine may include the following:

First, they bolster the quality of education. Entry criteria that are aligned with the program's

standards and intended outcomes ensure that students have an appropriate foundation and are adequately equipped to navigate the level of coursework necessitated by the program. This strategic alignment serves to enhance the quality and uphold the standards of the education program. Secondly, they facilitate student success. By admitting students who meet predefined entry criteria, educators can increase the probability of student success, higher graduation rates, and improved student outcomes in their chosen fields of study. The third aspect is the preservation of academic rigor. Through well-defined entry criteria, educators can maintain a consistent, challenging, and demanding academic rigor within the program. This can foster deeper learning, enhance critical thinking skills, and improve students' future employability prospects.

Entry criteria also promote fairness and accessibility. Clear and consistent entry standards can ensure a fair, equitable, and accessible admission process for all students, regardless of their backgrounds or prior experiences. In the healthcare sector, particularly in transfusion medicine, safety is a primary concern. By admitting students who meet these specific predetermined criteria, the likelihood that future practitioners are competent and have the necessary skills to practice safely and ethically can be increased, thereby ensuring patient and public safety. It must be acknowledged that students in the same program may all have fulfilled similar entry requirements, however, their training backgrounds are likely diverse. The learning environment must acknowledge this and assist students who may have knowledge gaps to bridge these gaps by offering additional tutorials or referring the student to appropriate resources and/or opportunities for the student to acquire the necessary knowledge and skills. In the context of a garden, such plants may require a little extra fertilizer to help them to catch-up with their growth. Setting realistic expectations is another essential role played by entry criteria. They can guide students in choosing programs that align best with their preparation level and commitment, helping them avoid investing time and resources in courses that may not suit them.

Finally, entry criteria can create opportunities for career development. The education system must acknowledge clinical transfusion medicine qualifications and offer career prospects for individuals with such professional qualifications to practice as specialist practitioners, such as Transfusion Practitioners, Blood Banking professionals, Transfusion Safety Officers and others. Alignment of the training program and its entry criteria with available, local career options and needs can enhance the employability of graduates [25]. These career development opportunities can incentivize enrolment into clinical transfusion education programs, and the learning gained can bolster the transfusion medicine knowledge and practices among the qualified individuals and provide valuable advisory capacity and strengthen their respective healthcare settings.

1.8 The Role and Competence of Teaching Staff (The Gardeners)

The proficiency of the teaching staff, our metaphorical gardeners, is an integral part of the equation towards success for any clinical transfusion medicine education program. Their importance cannot be overstated and is manifested in various ways. Enhancing the quality of education hinges heavily on the teachers' knowledge and expertise in clinical transfusion medicine. Teachers should be able to deliver accurate and current information and make complex concepts understandable. This capacity to translate intricate subject matter into digestible content undeniably elevates the overall educational experience. Moreover, the competence of teachers, including peer instructors and mentors, directly influences student success [26]. Skilled educators can discern the individual learning needs of students and provide tailored instruction accordingly [27]. This personalized approach often leads to better educational and eventually better patient outcomes, given that the students are better equipped to excel in their chosen field.

Patient safety is another crucial facet of healthcare education. Knowledgeable and experienced teaching staff can assure this by providing the right blend of learning methods, education, and guidance on the correct procedures and protocols in transfusion medicine [28]. By doing so, they minimize the risk of errors and instil in students the confidence to deliver safe and effective care to patients. Furthermore, the role of educators extends beyond the classroom and into modelling professionalism. Teachers possessing the necessary experience in clinical transfusion medicine and teaching can serve as mature exemplars of professional conduct for students, thereby fostering and encouraging the growth of attitudes and behaviors conducive to effective patient care, interprofessional teamwork and collaboration with colleagues from diverse backgrounds.

The clinical experience of teachers also comes to bear in shaping the students' learning experience. Teachers, armed with their own rich repertoire of real-world experiences, can share practical insights, enriching the understanding of students and aiding in the development of their clinical reasoning skills. Teachers and instructors should be able to make use of blended teaching modalities, as this has been shown to improve student engagement and success [8]. Also of importance is the commitment to continuous learning and professional development (CPD) on the part of the teaching staff. Their dedication to stay current with the latest guidelines, research, and best practices in clinical transfusion medicine and educational methods can keep students at the forefront of knowledge, will reinforce a culture and commitment to lifelong learning. This includes teachers modelling a humble approach with regards to their own limitations, needs for learning and continuous professional development.

Last, but certainly not least, is the psychological well-being of the teachers, which has been linked to student outcomes. The psychological adaptability of teachers, defined as "a process of change manifested by individuals in the face of changes in the environment" has been shown to be essential to the well-being (e.g., stress, burnout), work engagement, and sense of autonomy of an individual [29–31]. Psychological adaptability has been shown to be an important issue for training institutions, teachers, and students as it has been linked to teacher attrition, productivity, engagement with work, career adaptability, adoption of new technologies and embracing changes in the learning environment. A key factor to recognize is that authorities and leaders that provide teachers with a sense that they have autonomy have a positive effect on their commitment to their jobs and to their well-being [1, 32, 33].

Globalization of education may reduce pressure on teachers in under-resourced areas. The not-for-profit organizations, such as Project ECHO, provide a platform for medical education, continuous collaboration, and professional growth, linking professionals across the world. ECHO aims to reduce disparities in healthcare, by sharing educational resources [34]. They follow the principles of amplification (the use of technology to leverage scarce resources), best practices (to reduce disparities), case-based learning (to master complexity), and data (monitoring of outcomes to increase impact). This platform may be useful to improve teaching burden and access to transfusion education, globally and has already been used in Patient Blood Management (PBM) education in Sub-Saharan Africa.

1.9 The Role of Auditing and Accreditation (Guarding the Garden)

Accreditation serves as an integral process in which an independent accrediting body evaluates an educational or training program, verifying that it meets defined quality standards. Having internal and external procedures to audit the training program according to acceptable criteria, has many benefits, both to the training institution, the students and all other stakeholders. As a start, it ensures quality assurance, verifying that a training program complies with specific quality criteria, thus providing education on par with other programs within the same field. In case of deficiencies in the program, interventions can be

planned in a focused and appropriate manner [35]. It has the potential to bolster a program's reputation, making it more enticing to both students and employers. In the healthcare industry, accreditation can positively influence patient outcomes by ensuring that a training program imparts the necessary knowledge and skills for safe and effective patient care and treatment. It further promotes student mobility, especially in a world where there is great mobility of the healthcare workforce globally, making it easier for them to transfer credits or diplomas to other schools or continue their studies [36]. It also facilitates the transition of graduates into a competent workforce by demonstrating that they are well-prepared for their roles. Keeping quality high instead of limiting mobility to retain graduates in a specific country can yield better graduates and enhance the institution's reputation.

In many instances, accreditation is necessary for compliance with laws and regulations governing a profession. For example, in many countries' healthcare professions, certain accreditation is mandatory for practice. The requirement for accreditation encourages training organizations to engage in continuous self-evaluation and quality improvement. Regular assessments, both internal and by the accrediting body, can help identify areas of improvement and ensure continued compliance with the accrediting body's quality standards, fostering a culture of continuous improvement. It also provides a measure of accountability for a training program to the institution, students, stakeholders, and society at large and ensures that the program adheres to established ethical standards, providing education that is inclusive and fair for all students. Accreditation may also increase cultural responsiveness, making certain that the program provides education that is sensitive to the cultural diversity of the patient population it serves. Both internal and external auditing processes should also actively seek feedback from students and their experience of the learning environment and teaching program [8].

Beyond these aspects, accreditation offers an invaluable external perspective on an education (teaching and training) program. The accrediting bodies, usually composed of experts in the field, can provide insights and suggestions for improvement that may not be easily seen from within the program. This helps keep the program updated and relevant. It is perhaps important to note that the accreditation process itself is a wonderful learning opportunity not only for the institution and the instructors but also for the trainees who may very likely be involved in accreditation processes during their careers as well.

It should also be remembered that the sustainability of a learning program and environment is affected by a broad range of factors that need to be proactively considered and managed. Some of these factors include financial sustainability, attrition of good teachers, recognition and accreditation of program, and resource requirements [37].

1.10 Outcomes and Assessment as Key Elements of the Learning Environment (The Exit Gate)

The outcomes set and the assessment methods used can significantly influence the learning environment, shaping how learners engage with the material, interact with instructors and peers, and ultimately, how they comprehend and apply their knowledge and skills. We can think of these as the exit gate of our garden.

Outcomes provide a roadmap for learning, guiding the content, activities, and methods used in instruction and, as stated by Henry and West, facilitate the creation of a "shared mental model of what is to be learned between learners and supervisors" [38]. They articulate the expected knowledge, skills, and abilities learners should demonstrate upon completion of a course or education program [39].

Clear, specific outcomes can give learners a sense of purpose and direction, helping them to understand what they are working towards, why it is important, and how they will use it in their future practice. In clinical transfusion medicine, for example, outcomes may include understanding the principles of blood transfusion, demonstrating technical skills in blood administration, or making informed decisions about transfusion needs. These goals can influence the combination of teaching strategies used, such as case studies, practical demonstrations, or simulations, and encourage active engagement and real-world application.

Assessment methods, on the other hand, provide a mechanism for learners and instructors to gauge progress towards these outcomes. The way assessment is designed and implemented can shape learners' attitudes towards their studies, their motivation, and their approach to learning. For example, assessments that only focus on rote memorization may lead to superficial learning and anxiety, while assessments that encourage critical thinking, problem-solving, and real-world application can promote deeper learning and engagement. One of the key characteristics of a good learning environment is one where outcomes and assessment are aligned properly, as "assessment drives learning" [40]. It can be incredibly demotivating to students if they are provided a set of outcomes, but are evaluated and assessed on something else. Applying proven methods of standard setting to assessment practice and communicating these clearly to learners is essential to maintain fairness and comparability across different assessments over time and among different groups.

Formative assessments, which provide ongoing feedback during the learning process, can support continuous learning and improvement. They can help identify areas of strength and areas needing improvement, allowing for timely intervention and support. Summative assessments, conducted at the end of a course or program, help determine whether the learner has achieved the desired outcomes. Assessments that are learner-centered and competency-based can promote a more personalized and meaningful learning experience. These assessments consider individual progress and needs, focusing not just on knowledge acquisition, but also on practical skills, decision-making abilities, and professional behaviors. This can provide a point of departure to have fruitful feedback sessions with students that can help and encourage them to remain motivated, focused, improve on areas of weakness, but also gain confidence when achieving success on predetermined outcomes.

The outcomes set and the assessment methods used in a learning environment significantly influence the learners' experiences, their engagement with the content, their approach to learning, and ultimately, their competency and readiness to practice. By thoughtfully designing these elements, we can create a learning environment that promotes effective, meaningful, and lifelong learning. These critical aspects of clinical transfusion medicine education are discussed in more detail in other chapters.

1.11 Continuous Professional Development (Beyond the Garden)

It is crucial to understand that the learning environment expands beyond the confines of the institution, extending further in both time and place. In the realm of clinical transfusion medicine, it is essential to promote and sometimes even require continuous medical and professional education, both on- and offline [41]. This ensures that practitioners stay up-to-date with the latest breakthroughs and best practices in the field. Such ongoing education helps practitioners keep pace with new research, maintain professional competence, and improve patient outcomes [42]. Moreover, it aids in adapting to evolving regulations, provides networking opportunities, and equips students for certification examinations. Encouraging successful students, now independent practitioners, to remain part of a community of practice not only maintains the sense of belonging and community but also provides a platform that may function as a sounding board, place to ask questions, and share information as described above.

An example of a successful long-term community of practice in clinical transfusion medicine is the Sub-Saharan Africa Patient Blood Management (PBM) group. This group has a flat structure and is interdisciplinary (including doctors, nurses, laboratory professionals, transfusion educators and policy makers), international, and inclusive (members vary from heads of departments and professors to new graduates or students). The purpose of the group is only to engage regarding matters related to PBM. This includes sharing information regarding educational opportunities, congresses, policies, blood shortages, invitations to participate in or contribute to research, recent PBM publications, and at times just asking PBM-relevant questions. While no specific rules exist in the group, members are respectful of each other and maintain professionalism.

Continuous professional development (CPD) significantly enhances the prospects of long-term career success. Importantly, the pursuit of continuous professional development is propelled by both internal and external forces in the environment [43]. Internally, it could be self-directed learning or curiosity, and externally, it could be enforced by legislation or regulations [2, 44].

1.12 Conclusion

This chapter aimed to demonstrate that the learning environment is not a "nice-to-have," but an essential element of effective clinical transfusion medicine education. It is therefore very important to understand that the individual elements thereof cannot be assumed, but need to be carefully planned for and designed into any envisaged training program. In existing programs where this was not previously formerly considered, it would be very useful to direct focus on the learning environment as an important element of program review and renewal.

Acknowledgments We would like to thank Prof. Cees Smit Sibinga for his encouragement, support, and editorial guidance during the writing of this chapter.

References

1. Friedman CP, Donaldson KM, Vantsevich AV. Educating medical students in the era of ubiquitous information. Med Teach. 2016;38(5):504–9.
2. Johnston SC. Anticipating and training the physician of the future: the importance of caring in an age of artificial intelligence. Acad Med. 2018;293(8):1105–6.

3. Ryan E, Poole C. Impact of virtual learning environment on students' satisfaction, engagement, recall, and retention. J Med Imaging Radiat Sci. 2019;50(3):408–15.

4. Dai Z, Xiong J, Zhao L, Zhu X. Smart classroom learning environment preferences of higher education teachers and students in China: an ecological perspective. Heliyon. 2023;9(6):e16769.

5. World Economic Forum. The Future of Jobs Report. 2023. https://www.weforum.org/publications/the-future-of-jobs-report-2023/infographics-2128e451e0/#report-nav.

6. Smit Sibinga CT, Louw VJ, Nedelcu E, et al. Modeling global transfusion medicine education. Transfusion. 2021;61(10):3040–9.

7. Smit Sibinga CT. Chapter 8. Transfusion medicine: from AB0 to AI (artificial intelligence). In: Digital health. Brisbane, AU: Exon Publications; 2022. https://www.ncbi.nlm.nih.gov/pubmed/35605070.

8. Al-Riyami AZ, Peterson D, Vanden Broeck J, et al. E-learning/online education in transfusion medicine: a cross-sectional international survey. Transfus Med. 2022;32(6):499–504.

9. Al-Riyami AZ, Louw VJ, Indrikovs AJ, et al. Global survey of transfusion medicine curricula in medical schools: challenges and opportunities. Transfusion. 2021;61(2):617–26.

10. Hauser RG, Kwon RJ, Ryder A, et al. Transfusion medicine equations made internet accessible. Transfus Med Rev. 2020;34:15–9.

11. Eichbaum Q, Shan H, Goncalez TT, et al. Global health and transfusion medicine: education and training in developing countries. Transfusion. 2014;254(7):1893–8.

12. Pershing S, Fuchs VR. Restructuring medical education to meet current and f. uture health care needs. Acad Med. 2013;88(12):1798–801.

13. Han ER, Yeo S, Kim MJ, et al. Medical education trends for future physicians in the era of advanced technology and artificial intelligence: an integrative review. BMC Med Educ. 2019;19(1):460.

14. The Blood Project. What is an electronic crossmatch? 2022. https://www.thebloodproject.com/ufaq/what-is-an-electronic-crossmatch/.

15. Al-Riyami AZ, Al-Nomani I, Panchatcharam SM, et al. Transfusion knowledge of medical and surgical specialty board residents: a cohort study. Transfus Med. 2018;28(6):440–50.

16. Flott EA, Linden L. The clinical learning environment in nursing education: a concept analysis. J Adv Nurs. 2016;72(3):501–13.

17. Buhari M, Nwannadi I, Oghagbon E, Bello J. Students' perceptions of their learning environment at the College of Medicine, University of Ilorin, southwest, Nigeria. West African J Med. 2014;33(2):141–5.

18. Gifford KA, Choi E, Kieffer KA. Resources for clinical learning environment orientation. Med Educ Online. 2022;27(1):2013404.

19. Ovid D, Rice MM, Luna JV, et al. Investigating student perceptions of instructor talk: alignment with researchers' categorizations and analysis of remembered language. CBE Life Sci Educ. 2021;20(4):ar61.

20. Dai Y, Li H, Xie W, Deng T. Power distance belief and workplace communication: the mediating role of fear of authority. Int J Environ Res Public Health. 2022;19(5):2932.

21. Hoff TJ, Pohl H, Bartfield J. Creating a learning environment to produce competent residents: the roles of culture and context. Acad Med. 2004;79(6):532–9.

22. Pienaar M, Orton AM, Botma Y. A supportive clinical learning environment for undergraduate students in health sciences: an integrative review. Nurse Educ Today. 2022;119:105572.

23. Levett-Jones T, Lathlean J. The ascent to competence conceptual framework: an outcome of a study of belongingness. J Clin Nurs. 2009;18(20):2870–9.

24. Rambiritch V, Vermeulen M, Bell H, et al. Transfusion medicine and blood banking education and training for blood establishment laboratory staff: a review of selected countries in Africa. Transfusion. 2021;61(6):1955–65.

25. Louw VJ. The difference in scope of practice between a specialist in transfusion medicine and the clinician who deals with transfusion on an ad hoc basis. Transfus Apher Sci. 2014;51(3):33–7.

26. Moscaritolo LM. Interventional strategies to decrease nursing student anxiety in the clinical learning environment. J Nurs Educ. 2009;48(1):17–23.

27. Rivard SJ, Kemp MT, Evans J, Sandhu G. Resident perceptions of faculty behaviors promoting learner operative skills and autonomy. J Surg Educ. 2022;79(2):431–40.

28. Jumpp S. Evidence-based competency training program for blood product administration. Worldviews Evid-Based Nurs. 2021;18(4):308–10.

29. Fan SY, Yu ZY, Zheng X, Gao CH. Relationship between psychological adaptability and work engagement of college teachers within smart teaching environments: the mediating role of digital information literacy self-efficacy. Front Psychol. 2023;14:1057158.

30. Li J. Analysis of professional psychological adaptability of students majoring in hotel management and digital operation for higher vocational education under deep learning. Wirel Commun Mob Com. 2022;2022:e7114630.

31. Collie RJ, Granziera H, Martin AJ. Teachers' perceived autonomy support and adaptability: an investigation employing the job demands-resources model as relevant to workplace exhaustion, disengagement, and commitment. Teach Teach Educ. 2018;74:125–36.

32. Holliman AJ, Revill-Keen A, Waldeck D. University lecturers' adaptability: examining links with perceived autonomy support, organisational commitment, and psychological wellbeing. Teach Educ. 2022;33(1):42–55.

33. Martin AJ, Strnadova I, Nemec Z, Hajkova V, Kvetonova L. Teacher assistants working with students with disability: the role of adaptability in enhancing their workplace wellbeing. Int J Inclusive Educ. 2021;25(5):565–87.

34. Project Echo. Moving knowledge, not people. 2023. https://hsc.unm.edu/echo/.
35. Joubert J, Joubert S, Raubenheimer J, Louw V. The long-term effects of training interventions on transfusion practice: a follow-up audit of red cell concentrate utilisation at Kimberley Hospital, South Africa. Transfus Apher Sci. 2014;51(3):25–32.
36. Gushulak B, Weekers J, Macpherson D. Migrants and emerging public health issues in a globalized world: threats, risks and challenges, an evidence-based framework. Emerg Health Threats J. 2009;2:e10.
37. Louw VJ, Nel MM, Hay JF. Postgraduate education in transfusion medicine in the absence of formal residency training: assessment of factors needed to develop and sustain a postgraduate diploma program. Transfus Apher Sci. 2013;49(3):681–6.
38. Henry D, West DC. The clinical learning environment and workplace-based assessment: frameworks, strategies, and implementation. Pediatr Clin N Am. 2019;66(4):839–54.
39. Louw VJ. Determining the outcomes for clinicians completing a postgraduate diploma in transfusion medicine. Transfus Apher Sci. 2014;51(3):38–43.
40. Wormald BW, Schoeman S, Somasunderam A, Penn M. Assessment drives learning: an unavoidable truth? Anat Sci Educ. 2009;2(5):199–204.
41. Yeung KCY, Kapitany C, Charge S, et al. Transfusion camp: a retrospective study of self-reported impact on postgraduate trainee transfusion practice. Transfusion. 2023;63(4):839–48.
42. Sargeant J, Wong BM, Campbell CM. CPD of the future: a partnership between quality improvement and competency-based education. Med Educ. 2018;52(1):125–35.
43. Kathuria I, Mandal S, Negi S, et al. An audit to estimate the quality of practices followed during bedside blood transfusion in a tertiary care hospital and role of continuous medical education in it. Transfus Clin Biol. 2022;29(3):209–12.
44. Robinson JD, Persky AM. Developing self-directed learners. Am J Pharm Educ. 2020;84(3):847512.

Outcomes-Based Clinical Transfusion Medicine Education

Vernon J. Louw, Claire L. Barrett, and Vanitha Rambiritch

Brief

Outcome defined education in clinical transfusion medicine:

The importance of predefined teaching outcomes is determining the quality of education—professionalism. What needs to be in the curriculum and what competence does the teaching cadre need to offer to assure that these predefined outcomes are achieved.

2.1 Introduction

Medical education has undergone major changes, driven by rapid advancements in healthcare, technology, globalization, and changing societal expectations. The language of learning outcomes has emerged as a catalyst for change, shifting the focus from the traditional approach emphasizing course *duration* and *content* to a more defined, *outcomes*-based education (OBE).

2.1.1 Background

OBE is a learner-centered, performance-based approach that structures the educational system around prespecified goals that students are expected to achieve during their course of study, answering the essential question: What kind of healthcare professional do we want to produce? The emphasis in OBE, therefore, is on the *product* of education rather than the educational *process*. In the traditional model, medical courses lacked clear statements of learning objectives, sometimes leading students on a vague learning path without clear expectations. However, OBE has forced educators to reconsider the validity of what and how they teach. Unlike traditional education, where the focus was primarily on the teacher's actions, OBE centers on what the student can do at the end of the teaching and learning process. The outcomes may include specific skills, knowledge, and attitudes tailored to the specific field of study. This shift from a process-focused to a product-focused model emphasizes the learning *outcomes* of the educational experience over the *methods* used. It's a move from a situation "WHERE, WHEN and HOW students learn took precedence over WHAT is learned

V. J. Louw (✉)
Division of Clinical Haematology, Department of Medicine, Groote Schuur Hospital, University of Cape Town, Cape Town, South Africa
e-mail: vernon.louw@uct.ac.za

C. L. Barrett
School of Medicine, University of the Free State, Bloemfontein, South Africa

V. Rambiritch
South Africa National Blood service (SANBS), Roodepoort, South Africa
e-mail: vanitha.rambiritch@sanbs.org.za

and WHETHER it's learned well" [1, 2]. Attributes such as decision-making and self-assessment, previously neglected, are now considered essential competences for a healthcare professional.

An outcome represents the projected realization of an intention, distinguishing it from a mere intention or objective [2]. In the field of medicine, OBE has brought about a significant transformation, aligning education with the broader needs of the healthcare environment and society. It ensures that what is expected to be learned is explicitly stated, and that the course of study is arranged to achieve the intended goals. By focusing on the end-product and clearly defining learning outcomes, the teaching and learning approach becomes more adaptable, effective, and aligned with the continuously evolving landscape of medicine and healthcare, with the ultimate aim of improved patient safety, resource utilization, and overall healthcare delivery.

2.1.2 What OBE Is Versus What It Is Not

Outcome-Based Education (OBE) represents a shift in educational emphasis towards what can be achieved by the learner at the end of an educational experience. It is a learner-centered approach that focuses on clearly defined and measurable outcomes, whether they are knowledge, skills, or attitudes. While traditional models may focus on the process, content, time spent, and teacher's control, the emphasis in OBE is on the learner, the achievements, the end-goals, and the flexibility in reaching them. By aligning education with defined outcomes, OBE ensures that learning is purposeful, measurable, and aligned with real-world requirements and competencies. It is about ensuring that students do not only receive an education but also achieve mastery in defined areas, preparing them effectively for their future roles and responsibilities (Table 2.1).

Table 2.1 Outcome-based education (OBE)

What OBE is:
1. **Learner-centered**: OBE puts the learner at the center, focusing on what students should know and be able to do at the end of a learning process.
2. **Performance-based**: Success is measured by actual accomplishments and performances rather than simply course completion or time spent on tasks.
3. **Goal-oriented**: It emphasizes predefined goals and competencies that students must achieve, clearly stating the expected outcomes from the outset.
4. **Flexible in approach**: OBE allows for various teaching and learning methods, as long as they align with achieving the defined outcomes.
5. **Assessment-aligned**: In OBE, assessment strategies are carefully designed to evaluate whether the intended learning outcomes have been achieved, leading to a close alignment between learning and assessment.

What OBE is not:
1. **Not teacher-centered**: Unlike traditional education where the teacher's role is primary, OBE shifts the focus from what the teacher does to what the student learns.
2. **Not time-bound**: Traditional education often measures success by time spent in classes or on tasks. In contrast, OBE focuses on achievement, regardless of the time it takes for different students.
3. **Not content-driven**: While content is essential, OBE does not prescribe a rigid curriculum. It prioritizes the outcomes, not merely covering a fixed set of topics.
4. **Not process-oriented only**: While traditional education emphasizes the learning process, OBE places the emphasis on the product or outcome of that process.
5. **Not one-size-fits-all**: OBE acknowledges that learners are different and may need various paths and time frames to achieve the same outcomes. It is not limited to a uniform way of teaching and learning

2.2 Principles of Outcomes-Based Education

When designing a curriculum, certain principles need to be kept in mind if an outcomes-based approach is used.

The Principles of OBE in General, Include the Following:

1. **Clarity of focus**: The skills, knowledge, and attitudes envisaged should be clearly defined before the instruction begins.
2. **Design down, deliver up**: Start with the end in mind and design the curriculum backward, starting with a clear vision of what successful learning at graduation will mean.
3. **High expectations**: Set high, challenging, and clearly defined standards of performance that are applied to all students.
4. **Expanded opportunities**: Understanding that different students learn in different ways and times, and providing numerous opportunities to learn and demonstrate learning.
5. **Alignment**: Outcomes should be aligned with the student's career goals and needs of the healthcare system, the workplace, and society. It also needs to be carefully aligned with assessment.

2.2.1 Clarity of Focus

Clarity of focus when designing outcomes is important for creating a useful curriculum. When outcomes are articulated in a thoughtful, clear, and unambiguous manner, they provide a strong foundation for the systematic organization of curricular content, envisaged teaching methods, and assessment strategies. A clear focus on outcomes ensures that the curriculum is not only aligned with the essential competencies required but also remains responsive to the evolving needs of the health services and society. By precisely defining the outcomes, educators can create a roadmap that outlines the specific skills, knowledge, and attitudes students must develop. Such a roadmap will guide the selection of content and organization, ensuring that every aspect of the curriculum serves the ultimate goal of the educational program. It also enables a seamless alignment of teaching and assessment methodologies, fostering an environment where learning objectives and evaluation are interconnected and mutually reinforcing.

A well-defined set of outcomes functions as a guide for students and educators, ensuring that the educational pathway is purpose-driven and relevant. It also paves the way for continuous curriculum review and improvement. By periodically evaluating the alignment of the outcomes with the broader needs of the health sector and society, educators can make informed decisions about any revisions or enhancements that may be required. This ensures that the teaching and learning approach taken remains adaptive and responsive to internal (e.g., student) and external (e.g., healthcare system, societal) needs, meeting both the current demands of the profession and the future needs of patients and the community. A clear and unambiguous focus on outcomes is the cornerstone of a robust, responsive, and relevant curriculum. It serves as the starting point, the guiding principle, and the continuous point of reference for all aspects of education, from content and teaching methodologies to assessment strategies and ongoing improvement processes, connecting academic learning with real-world application and societal needs.

2.2.2 Design Down, Deliver Up

Outcomes-based education in clinical transfusion medicine adheres to the principle of "Design Down, Deliver Up," a method that ensures both the cohesiveness of the curriculum and the practical relevance of the teaching. By starting with the end in mind, educators first identify the specific skills, knowledge, and abilities that students must attain to become successful professionals in transfusion medicine. This end goal then guides the design of the entire curriculum, working backward from the desired outcomes. The "Design Down" phase encompasses a thorough analysis of professional competencies and standards required in the field of transfusion medicine. From understanding the complex procedures of blood typing and cross-matching to promoting the ethical considerations and patient safety in clinical transfusion practice, the curriculum is constructed to align with real-world demands. "Deliver Up" focuses on the sequential and systematic delivery of this content, ensuring that each stage of learning builds on the previous one. This progression reinforces both theoretical understanding and hands-on skills needed in clinical settings. It's not just about learning in a vacuum; it's about preparing students for the multifaceted realities of clinical transfusion medicine practice.

This principle acknowledges that education in transfusion medicine is not a linear process but a dynamic and integrative one. The curriculum is flexible yet targeted, adapting to emerging trends and technologies while maintaining alignment with essential competencies. It offers a structured pathway to bridge the gap between academia and practice. It creates a learning environment where theoretical knowledge is coupled with real-world application, fostering a more competent and confident workforce that is well prepared to meet the continually evolving demands of clinical transfusion medicine.

2.2.3 High Expectations

Setting high expectations in terms of outcomes in clinical transfusion medicine education involves establishing clear and challenging goals, which encourage students to aim to reach their full academic and career potential. High standards also reflect the real-world demands of the profession, mirroring the high stakes of safe and ethical transfusion practice. This may involve outcomes as diverse as mastering complex laboratory techniques to dealing with ethically difficult situations in day-to-day patient care. High expectations must be balanced with the necessary support, resources, guidance, and mentorship. Expectations must be reasonable and reflect the real needs of the workplace and healthcare environment. By setting and maintaining high expectations, educators foster and encourage continuous improvement and lifelong learning, which are essential in an evolving field.

The hope is that the principle of "High Expectations" will act as a catalyst for excellence, fostering a culture of ambition and growth. In clinical transfusion medicine, where precision, knowledge, and ethics are vital components of good clinical practice, this principle is more than just a guideline; it reflects the profession's core values while providing the means and guidance to reach them.

2.2.4 Expanded Opportunities

The principle of expanded opportunities in outcomes-based clinical transfusion medicine education recognizes the diverse learning paces, preferences, and abilities of students. It emphasizes the importance of an inclusive and flexible educational environment, offering a range of ways in which to learn and demonstrate that outcomes have been achieved. This may mean using a variety and combination of teaching methods, such as, lectures, workshops, simulations, and self-paced learning, to cater to different learning styles. Personalized learning paths allow students to progress at their own pace, focusing on areas where they need development without being held back. Multiple assessment strategies, including written exams and practical demonstrations, ensure various opportunities to show competence. Opportunities for real-world application through internships or placements in environments where blood is transfused regularly or in blood establishments can provide context and practical experience. Utilizing technology and virtual labs can further enrich the learning experience, offering flexibility, as it is not limited to place and teaching can be delivered asynchronously, i.e., on the student's own time. The flipped classroom model and massive open online courses have been exciting developments in the area of asynchronous learning "at your own pace". Continuous feedback, support, and the inclusion of different approaches to learning ensure that no student is left behind.

Importantly, this principle is not about diluting the rigorous standards that clinical transfusion medicine demands. Instead, it is about aligning varied learning opportunities with the desired outcomes, ensuring that all students, regardless of their learning style, can achieve the necessary competencies. By creating a curriculum that offers various pathways to success, without compromising essential skills, the principle of "expanded opportunities" connect directly to outcomes, ensuring that education is both robust and adaptable. In essence, expanded opportunities in clinical transfusion medicine education foster an environment where each student's uniqueness is recognized and honored. This approach enriches the educational experience and prepares students to be adaptable, well-rounded professionals, reflecting the multifaceted challenges and core outcomes of the clinical transfusion medicine. It is a forward-thinking principle that aligns the processes of learning with the desired outcomes, maximizing the potential of every student.

As David Leach, executive director of the Accreditation Council for Graduate Medical Education (ACGME), puts it, "The 'substance' of medicine is enduring," but it is the forms through which that substance is conveyed which necessitate modification throughout time. OBE is one of those forms that bring together competencies and "substance" [3].

2.2.5 Alignment

Alignment is a cornerstone in OBE, ensuring that the educational process resonates with the student's career goals, the healthcare system's needs, and broader societal demands. In clinical transfusion medicine, a field integral to patient care and public health, this alignment is particularly vital.

Alignment with the student's career goals and the needs of the workplace guarantees that the education is not just theoretical but practical and directly applicable to the real-world context. It ensures that students are prepared to perform the key functions required in their future workplace, meet the healthcare system's standards, and contribute positively to the healthcare environment.

Aligning outcomes with stakeholders' needs, including patients, society, students, and the learning environment, creates a more holistic educational approach. In clinical transfusion medicine, this can mean creating outcomes that reflect ethical considerations, patient safety, efficiency in practice, and collaboration with other healthcare professionals.

One of the most important elements of OBE is the alignment of assessment with outcomes as a key that unlocks success. Since it has been recognized that "assessment drives learning" and that students tend to study what they will be tested on, it is essential that assessments and evaluations are designed to reflect precisely what has been taught and what the students are expected to learn [4]. In clinical transfusion medicine, this might involve assessments that test both theoretical knowledge, such as understanding blood compatibility, and practical skills, like doing a cross-match, performing a transfusion, or taking informed consent. In other words, if students know they will be tested on specific outcomes, they will focus their efforts on those areas. The assessments, therefore, must be clearly defined, thoughtfully designed, and perfectly aligned with the outcomes shared with the students in advance [4]. This principle of alignment serves as a blueprint to construct a curriculum that doesn't just teach but prepares students for their future roles in the healthcare system. It recognizes that education is not an isolated process but interconnected with various facets of life and work. In clinical transfusion medicine in particular, where the stakes are high, and precision is paramount, alignment helps in bridging the gap between the classroom and the clinic, between learning and practice, and between theory and the critical real-world application.

2.3 Role of Professional Organizations in OBE in Medical and Transfusion Medicine Education

Outcomes-based education has been supported and/or incorporated by the activities of many international societies involved in medical education. A few examples of OBE in general medical and specialist education are the following:

1. The Accreditation Council for Graduate Medical Education (ACGME): ACGME is a professional organization responsible for the accreditation of post-MD medical training programs in the United States. ACGME has defined a set of core competencies that residents must demonstrate during their training, which is an example of an outcomes-based approach [5].
2. The Royal College of Physicians and Surgeons of Canada: This organization launched the Competence by Design (CBD) initiative, which embraces the outcomes-based education model. The CBD framework describes different stages of postgraduate medical education, each associated with specific expected outcomes [6].
3. Association for Medical Education in Europe (AMEE): The AMEE is an organization that incorporates members from more than 90 countries and five continents. It has supported outcomes-based education in its conferences and literature, and has produced very useful guidelines and documents on the topic. It has played a role in advancing the Outcome-Based Education (OBE) approach in medical education [2].
4. The General Medical Council (GMC) in the UK: The GMC has established outcomes for graduates which they call the "Outcomes for Graduates 2018." It describes the knowledge, skills, and behaviors that the new UK medical graduates must be able to show [7].
5. The Medical Council of India (MCI): The MCI has adopted a competency-based medical education approach, which is an application of the outcomes-based education model [8].

Examples of learning objectives and curricula published for undergraduate and graduate education include:

1. US Medical Licensing Examinations (USMLE): contains a relatively short list of transfusion medicine topics for medical stu-

dents [9]. Significant gaps in clinical application of transfusion have been noted [10].
2. Association for Pathology Chairs: Provides learning objectives with strong emphasis on blood banking side of transfusion medicine [11].
3. Academy of Clinical Laboratory Physicians and Scientists (2010): Learning objectives with stronger focus on clinical transfusion medicine [12].

These are only a few examples of large organizations that have adopted various forms of an outcomes-based educational approach. Many other specialties have published transfusion medicine-related outcomes within their respective curricula.

2.4 Importance of and Need for Implementation of Outcomes-Based Education in Clinical Transfusion Medicine

Outcomes-based education (OBE) in clinical transfusion medicine is fraught with unique challenges, reflecting the complexity and multifaceted nature of this essential medical field. Transfusion medicine is a broad discipline that involves a diverse range of role players, including blood services, hospitals, medical professionals, laboratory technologists, regulators, and funders, each contributing their expertise. Moreover, transfusion medicine finds application across various medical specialties, incorporating a wide array of products, each possessing distinct indications, risks, and costs. This diversity adds layers of complexity to teaching and learning in this field. Among the most pressing challenges is the significant shortage of teaching time dedicated to transfusion medicine within medical curricula [13]. Most studies echo this concern of inadequate training time, revealing substantial gaps in knowledge among both junior and senior healthcare workers [14, 15]. This issue is particularly alarming considering that nearly all healthcare workers, across specialties, engage in the active practice of clinical transfusion medicine regularly, if not on a daily or weekly basis. Compounding these challenges is the rapid evolution of the field itself. With dramatic advancements in immunology, molecular biology, technology, artificial intelligence, transfusion alternatives, and patient blood management, transfusion medicine is continually reshaping itself, further complicating the educational landscape.

Despite these obstacles, the targeted implementation of OBE in transfusion medicine is not merely advisable but essential. By methodically determining the specific knowledge, skills, and attitudes a healthcare worker must possess, educators can ensure that vital elements are incorporated into time-limited curricula. This strategic approach provides a robust framework to advocate for dedicated teaching time for this crucial subject. The benefits of this focus on outcomes are profound. By aligning educational goals with the realities of practice, we pave the way for healthcare workers who are proficient in clinical transfusion medicine. Standardized learning objectives lead to enhanced patient safety and outcomes, responsible resource utilization, especially concerning the precious commodity of freely donated blood, and tangible cost savings.

The importance of OBE in clinical transfusion medicine can therefore not be overstated. It represents a critical tool in bridging the gap between the demands of a dynamic and vital field and the limitations of current educational structures. It not only addresses the existing shortcomings in training but also sets a clear and defendable path towards a more competent, ethical, and efficient practice of clinical transfusion medicine. The future of patient care in this area depends on embracing this thoughtful and systematic approach.

2.5 The Importance of Outcomes Applied to Clinical Transfusion Medicine

2.5.1 Education Outcomes

Education outcomes are important for clinical transfusion medicine education as they can provide assurance that students learn and develop the appropriate mix of skills and knowledge needed to promote and preserve health in a safe and efficient manner. It must be emphasized that "health is about people" [16]. It is about people who need services and people who are entrusted to deliver the needed services. This trust is earned through a special blend of technical competence and service orientation, and developing such a blend requires a lengthy period of education, training, and service orientation [17]. Education and learning in health services is necessary to ensure that the required knowledge, skills, and behaviors are developed through adequate training programs; the overall intent is to assure excellence in healthcare delivery [18].

The National Heart Lung and Blood institute's State of the Science in Transfusion Medicine symposium held in 2015 was aimed at identifying important research questions that could be answered in the next 5–10 years and which have the potential to transform the clinical practice of transfusion medicine. One of the overarching themes identified in the symposium was that there is a need for enhanced training and education in transfusion medicine to facilitate and promote research in transfusion medicine, train transfusion medicine physicians, and educate physicians and nurses who prescribe and use blood [19]. Enhanced education for all health professionals involved in the "vein-to-vein transfusion chain" is in fact necessary to minimize or prevent harm to patients [20].

Well-structured, fit for purpose, curriculum-driven transfusion medicine education and training programs with clearly defined, measurable outcomes are essential. Education outcomes must be aligned to present day health needs, and the quality of education and training provided is key to assuring best practices and patient safety. By creating precise and quantifiable learning goals, educators can ensure that curricula are in line with global and country-specific health needs, demands, and challenges [21]. This will enable students to acquire the knowledge and skills required for safe and efficient patient care by applying best practice standards appropriate for their respective roles in delivery of healthcare. The bottom line is that healthcare education curricula and learning outcomes must focus on the patient. Transfusion medicine education outcomes must be tailored to ensure that knowledge gained is translated into daily clinical practices and results in quality patient care.

A set of outcomes for a graduate course in clinical transfusion medicine has previously been published by one of the authors [22].

2.5.2 Quality Patient Care

Patient safety and quality health outcomes are of the highest priority. In terms of clinical transfusion practices, efforts must be directed at minimizing harm to patients by preventing transfusions that are inappropriate, meaning that they are not clinically indicated. Education that drives sound clinical reasoning skills, and practices that focus on early detection and correction of underlying conditions, considering transfusion alternatives and collaborating with clinical colleagues to achieve best patient outcomes are paramount.

To manage blood, and to appropriately care for patients, requires that clinicians have a sound knowledge of good clinical transfusion practices [23]. Literature on transfusion practices globally indicate that the majority of transfusion decisions are made by clinicians with little or no formal training in transfusion medicine [24, 25]. Audits of clinical transfusion practice consistently demonstrate knowledge deficiencies amongst clinicians, contributing to variations in transfusion practices, inappropriate, overuse, and even wastage of blood and blood components, all associated with potential harm to patients [26–28].

As far back as 2002, the WHO strategy for global blood safety [29] advocated the need for training in the clinical use of blood for all clinicians involved in the transfusion process and for Blood Transfusion Service staff commitment to the prevention, early diagnosis, and treatment of conditions that could result in the need for transfusion (obstetrical complications, trauma, gastrointestinal or perioperative blood loss, etc.). Moving ahead, in 2010, the WHO endorsed patient blood management as a standard of care, [30] and in 2021, the WHO released a policy brief with a call to action for all member states to urgently adopt patient blood management (PBM) to improve the population health status and individual patient outcomes while reducing overall health care expenditures [31].

PBM is a patient-centered, systematic, evidence-based approach to improve patient outcomes by managing and preserving a patient's own blood, while promoting patient safety and empowerment (see also Chap. 7) [32]. It involves the timely, multidisciplinary application of evidence-based medical and surgical concepts aimed at:

1. screening for diagnosing and appropriately treating anemia;
2. minimizing surgical, procedural, and laboratory sampling blood losses and managing coagulopathic bleeding throughout the care episode;
3. supporting the patient while appropriate treatment is initiated [32].

The WHO 2021 policy brief explains that one barrier to adoption of PBM as a standard of care is the lack of awareness and education among healthcare professionals and patients; emphasizing that PBM and its multiple benefits should be promoted amongst all members of multidisciplinary healthcare teams, health authorities, and patients [31].

Undergraduate and postgraduate medical education curricula for the various healthcare professionals involved need to include educational outcomes that target knowledge and application of the principles of PBM, as appropriate in their various domains of practice. Knowledge, understanding, and routine application of these principles will foster an evidence-based culture of patient care aligned to best medical practice standards and enhanced health outcomes. Having at least one broad PBM-centered educational outcome in the various health professions training curricula will target a host of healthcare needs and priorities. These include responding to the global disease burden of anemia, team-based patient care, application of multidisciplinary blood conservation modalities, awareness in weighing transfusion risks and benefits with consideration of appropriate alternatives in clinical transfusion decision-making; all underpinned by the overarching outcome of quality healthcare.

2.5.3 Ethical Considerations

The safety of blood and blood products is a promise made, overtly or tacitly, by all who collect, store, and distribute these unique entities. Included in this promise is to do what is right because it is right; to fulfil the professional obligation to help those in need. Such obligations are ancient, rooted in the Hippocratic and other ethical traditions [33]. The medical ethical principle of "first do no harm" must underpin the education and practices of all health practitioners. Although not directly involved in the bedside care of patients, health professionals responsible for collecting, processing and testing of blood and blood products must understand the impact of poor laboratory practices and laboratory errors.

Competence, quality, and hygiene during the entire blood donation process, preparation, storage, delivery, and transfusion have always been and will continue to be of paramount importance for transfusion safety [34]. Education outcomes can help ensure that students learn the proper procedures and apply the protocols for safe transfusion medicine practices. This would lead to a reduction in errors and adverse events.

There are several causes of transfusion related adverse events and the best prevention is to avoid transfusions, except when there are no suitable alternatives. Often, patients are not adequately informed about the wide range of risks associated with blood and blood components transfusions; nor are they involved in the transfusion decision-making process. Clinicians owe a duty of honest care to patients and in doing so, they need to involve, advise and empower patients in their care plan by discussing with them the diagnosis, available treatment options, the risks, benefits and available alternatives. This must be done in a manner that allow individual patients to understand their health condition, enable them to ask the right questions and ultimately give proper informed consent to the treatment. Such principles of care must be deliberately taught to students at an early onset of clinical practice and remain entrenched as they progress in their careers ahead.

Doing what is best for individual patients, and not what has been historically done nor what is convenient, must be a continuous underlying educational paradigm that is carried through from undergraduate into postgraduate and specialist phases of education and training. Convenient and/or poor decisions, not aligned with good clinical practices, come with potential harm and can have significant legal ramifications, particularly in an era of more empowered patients and a more empowered society.

2.5.4 Developing Competence

Educational outcomes and assessment of learning should focus not only on knowledge generation but should also ensure that students are competent to perform critical tasks as required in the relevant employment sector. Entrustable Professional Activities (EPAs) should be developed to ensure that students acquire not only knowledge and competence but also trustworthiness, which is tested robustly to ensure safe transfusion practice. Whilst competencies describe personal qualities involving knowledge, skills, attitudes, and values, EPAs are units of professional practice, which can be described as responsibilities or discrete tasks that supervisors entrust trainees with once they achieve adequate competencies [35]. EPAs are not meant to replace competencies but are a mode of translation of competencies into clinical practice; their aim being to ground competencies in multiple day-to-day skills [18, 19]. EPAs should be observable, measurable, executed within a designated time frame, and suitable for entrustment decisions by qualified personnel [35].

Frenk et al. [16] describe three groups of competencies that graduates should develop as outcomes of the teaching and learning process:

1. Foundational competencies involve establishing a comprehensive knowledge of theories, concepts, and facts that are widely accepted

by the scientific community and that form the basis for professional practice.

2. Specialized competencies refer to the knowledge and skills required for the practice of different professions or specializations.

3. Integrative competencies refer to complex capabilities, such as critical thinking, numeracy, creativity, innovation, communication proficiency (including intercultural communication), teamwork, emotional intelligence, ethical deliberation, and social responsibility.

Such competencies cannot be developed all at once, rather they should be developed as outcomes of a teaching and learning framework directed at developing "complete competence" in graduates. Simply put, developing this "complete competence," which encompasses knowledge, skills, clinical reasoning, and professional and behavioral development should be a phased approach, where one phase serves as a foundation and scaffold upon which more complex competencies are developed. Central to this is the reflection of learning and learning experiences, which is a key aspect of the learning process and is needed to entrench deep, lifelong learning.

2.5.5 Developing Professionalism

Professional competence is the habitual and judicious use of communication, knowledge, technical skills, clinical reasoning, emotions, values, and reflection in daily practice for the benefit of the individual and community being served [36]. Knowledge and skills (knowing and doing) aspects are key to protecting and preserving health. Behavioral aspects ("how to be" attributes) are key in shaping professionalism, creating self-awareness, enabling and sustaining a team-based work culture, and fostering social responsibility and service orientation. Professionalism is an important component of medicine's contract with society [37, 38]; the "how to be" aspects must therefore be deliberatively taught and assessed with ongoing feedback given to students. This will provide student readiness for the world of work in the healthcare environment and improve interactions with clinical

colleagues, patients, communities, and society at large.

Grooming graduates with adequate workplace readiness, competence and resilience is nonnegotiable. Rather than being linear and philosophical, education programs must be action and practice orientated, having a sound connect between what is learnt in the classroom and the reality of the actual healthcare environment. Values such as empathy, care, and ethical and professional behaviors must accompany the knowledge and skills aspects of clinical practice. Assessment methods must be tailored to ensure that they are all-encompassing and reliable in terms of measuring complete competence. This will allow translation of learning gained into daily practice. By ensuring that students are meeting the necessary education outcomes, educators can ensure that students are developing the required competence, professional practice, and that they are adequately prepared to meet the ethical, professional and legal requirements of the profession.

2.6 Student Success

Student success, which is ultimately associated with improved patient care, is a product of sound education outcomes that serve as a roadmap for student learning and grooming them towards their chosen field of study. The healthcare profession is one of care and service orientation and those who enrol to serve must be willing to serve. When students choose to join the healthcare profession, it is essential that they develop a clear concept of their professional identity, their roles and responsibilities, and bring with them certain nonnegotiable "must-have" qualities such as empathy, commitment, and dedication. They must understand that health practitioners have an altruistic obligation to patients [33], and as such, healthcare roles require the right type of person for the job. Key to student success is the understanding of their role and purpose in health and patient care. The rewards and the demands associated with their chosen profession must be clear at an early phase of study.

There is no doubt that the demands and challenges faced by healthcare professionals are many. Health systems worldwide are struggling to keep up with the demands, as healthcare needs become more complex and costly, thus placing added demands on health workers [17]. These challenges are magnified in low- and middle-income countries (LMICs), which have high disease burdens, larger patient populations, health resource limitations, and inadequate funds. Despite the changing health paradigms, health professions education has not kept pace with these challenges and demands, largely due to fragmented, outdated, and static curricula that produce ill-equipped graduates [17].

Ill-equipped graduates are likely to become overwhelmed and/or challenged in executing their roles and responsibilities, creating frustration, anxiety, and poor performance outcomes, all leading to the potential detriment of health practitioners and patients. Dissatisfaction and disinterest in their chosen careers may set in. Student health and well-being is key and it is likely that some students and novice health practitioners may become overwhelmed by the demands of their chosen profession. Training of health professionals is an economic and healthcare investment, and countries across the globe seek a return on this investment as it impacts population health. Sklar [39] explains that we lose potential physicians all along the expensive and stressful medical education continuum, for example:

1. those who are eliminated during large science lecture courses in premedical, programs because they lack adequate preparation, or
2. the students who survive the admissions process but leave medical school because of the mental and physical distress they experience, which leads to burnout, or
3. those students who survive medical school but fail to match in their desired specialties and lose their enthusiasm for a medical career.

These factors apply also to student nurses, laboratory professionals, and all other health profession groups. It is therefore essential that education and training programs provide students with the readiness to embrace the demands of their chosen profession, whilst staying rooted to their purpose, managing work–life balance and enabling them to cope with periods of stress and adversity. Measures to ease the burden of tasks and responsibilities through approaches such as collaborative team-based care should be embedded at an early stage of study and entrenched throughout teaching and learning. The much-advocated multidisciplinary team-based healthcare approach addresses the silo approach to patient care and brings on board shared expertise with direct benefits to patients. This approach harmonizes patient care and can help in building collaborative partnerships, respect, and value amongst clinical partners within multidisciplinary teams.

Education curricula directing teaching and learning and the outcomes for training programs should have a dual purpose with focus on both patient care and self-care. Mechanisms for self-care are essential for the mental well-being of health professionals to cope with stress and adversity and avoiding burnout. Early exposure to the clinical environment and a clear understanding of the expectations of the profession can help students in shaping their careers and allow best execution of their purpose.

2.7 Continuous Medical and Professional Education

A key outcome of any educational program is to ensure that students and trainees become lifelong learners. This past century has presented the world with more medical advances than previously thought possible, making it a challenge to keep pace with new and improved best practices without continuous active learning [40]. Like other fields of medicine, transfusion medicine is a rapidly evolving field that now interfaces with virtually every clinical discipline and with many of the basic medical and social sciences and has had a major impact on public health, political, legal and regulatory systems around the globe [41, 42].

Mueller and Seifried [41] explain that there are numerous positive reasons for the increasing complexity of transfusion medicine; modern medical therapies like stem cell transplantation, cellular therapy, transplantation of solid organs, regenerative medicine, and surgery cannot exist without a safe supply of blood products and high quality standard as well as special blood products and laboratory services provided by blood banks and transfusion medicine specialists. The added aspects of good laboratory practice (GLP), good manufacturing practice (GMP), quality management systems, and quality control on the pharmaceutical manufacturer's level are only a few examples of the high standards required in today's blood banking environment [34, 43]. Continuous medical education on these aspects is critical to apply and maintain best practice standards across the vein-to-vein chain.

In the past, maintaining one's competence was not as problematic because relevant knowledge accumulated slowly; today, however, without a program of active learning one will not remain competent for more than a few years after graduation [26]. Continuous medical and professional education therefore plays a vital role in supplementing clinical transfusion medicine education programs. It is needed to help students stay up-to-date with the latest developments, guidelines, protocols, and best practices in the field and to apply the new knowledge to their practices. By staying current with new developments and best practices, students who participate in continuing education can be better equipped to provide safe and effective care, leading to improved patient outcomes.

Continuing education also plays a vital role in preparing students for certification examinations. Many transfusion medicine practitioners seek certifications to demonstrate their knowledge and competency in the field. Not only does it help students prepare for these examinations, continuous education also serves in maintaining their certifications. Furthermore, the field of transfusion medicine is highly regulated and it is important for practitioners to stay current with any changes to the regulations and guidelines that govern their practice. Continuous medical and professional education can help practitioners remain compliant and avoid penalties and even litigation.

Education outcomes can provide a basis for ongoing and lifelong learning. Students who are well-versed in the knowledge and skills outlined in the education outcomes will have a better understanding of the importance of continuous learning and be more equipped to adapt to new developments, guidelines, and best practices in the field of transfusion medicine. As a result, they will be able to deliver safe and better care for the duration of their careers. Additionally, educators can use the educational results as a foundation for ongoing program evaluation and development, which can result in more effective and efficient training that ultimately benefit the patients, the healthcare facility, and society at large. Continuous education activities must be tailored to solidify existing knowledge and serve as a window for new knowledge and practices.

Continuing medical education is now accessible through a variety of online platforms, bringing along opportunities for building professional networks. Continuing education can create avenues for students to network and learn from other health professionals and experts from across the globe in their field of interest. This can provide valuable insights and opportunities for teaching, knowledge expansion, collaboration, research, innovation, process, and practice improvements; all aimed at improving population health.

2.8 Conclusion

From the above, it should be clear that OBE applied to clinical transfusion medicine can achieve the end-goals of ensuring student success, safe clinical transfusion practice, and good quality patient care. Ensuring that both the teacher and the student understand exactly what is expected will allow for robust curriculum development, goal-oriented teaching strategies, and appropriate assessment that is aligned with what is expected.

Acknowledgments We would like to thank Prof Cees Smit Sibinga for his encouragement, technical support, and editorial guidance during the writing of this chapter.

References

1. Spady WG. Outcome-based education: critical issues and answers. Arlington, VA: The American Association of School Administrators; 1994.
2. Harden RM. Outcome-based education: the future is today. Med Teach. 2007;29(7):625–9. https://doi.org/10.1080/01421590701729930.
3. Leach DC. Changing education to improve patient care. Qual Health Care. 2001;10(II suppl):54–8.
4. Wormald BW, Schoeman S, Somasunderam A, Penn M. Assessment drives learning: an unavoidable truth? Anat Sci Educ. 2009;2(5):199–204. https://doi.org/10.1002/ase.102.
5. ACGME. ACGME common program requirements. 2021. https://www.acgme.org/What-We-Do/Accreditation/Common-Program-Requirements. Accessed 4 Aug 2023.
6. Royal College of Physicians and Surgeons of Canada—Competence by Design (CBD). https://www.royalcollege.ca/ca/en/cbd.html. Accessed 4 Aug 2023.
7. General Medical Council. Outcomes for graduates 2018. 2018. https://www.gmc-uk.org/education/standards-guidance-and-curricula/standards-and-outcomes/outcomes-for-graduates. Accessed 4 Aug 2023.
8. Medical Council of India. Competency-based undergraduate curriculum for the Indian medical graduate. 2018. https://www.nmc.org.in/information-desk/for-colleges/ug-curriculum. Accessed 4 Aug 2023.
9. Examination USML: USMLE content outline. https://www.usmle.org/step-1/#content-outlines. Accessed 11 Aug 2023.
10. Peedin AR. Update in transfusion medicine education. Clin Lab Med. 2021;41(4):697–711. https://doi.org/10.1016/j.cll.2021.07.010. Epub 2021 Sep 29.
11. Knollmann-Ritschel BEC, Regula DP, Borowitz MJ, et. al. Pathology competencies for medical education and educational cases. Acad Pathol 2017;4:2374289517715040.
12. Smith BR, Aguero-Rosenfeld M, Anastasi J, et. al. Educating medical students in laboratory medicine: a proposed curriculum. Am J Clin Pathol 2010;133:533–42.
13. Karp JK, Weston CM, King KE. Transfusion medicine in American undergraduate medical education. Transfusion. 2011;51(11):2470–9. https://doi.org/10.1111/j.1537-2995.2011.03154.x. Epub 2011 May 4.
14. Al-Riyami AZ, Louw VJ, Indrikovs AJ, et al. Education Sub. Committee of the AABB Global Transfusion Forum. Global survey of transfusion medicine curricula in medical schools: challenges and opportunities. Transfusion. 2021;61(2):617–26. https://doi.org/10.1111/trf.16147. Epub 2020 Oct 22.
15. Halford B, Pinheiro A, Haspel RL. Hospital medicine providers' transfusion knowledge: a survey study. Transfus Med Rev. 2021;35(2):140–5. https://doi.org/10.1016/j.tmrv.2021.04.003. Epub 2021 Apr 20.
16. Frenk J, Chen LC, Chandran L, et al. Challenges and opportunities for educating health professionals after the COVID-19 pandemic. Lancet (London, England). 2022;400:1539–56.
17. Frenk J, Chen L, Bhutta ZA, et al. Health professionals for a new century: transforming education to strengthen health systems in an interdependent world. Lancet (London, England). 2010;376:1923–58.
18. Graham JE. Transfusion e-learning for junior doctors: the educational role of 'LearnBloodTransfusion'. Transfus Med. 2015;25:144–50.
19. Spitalnik SL, Triulzi D, Devine DV, et al. Proceedings of the National Heart, Lung, and Blood Institute's state of the science in transfusion medicine symposium. Transfusion 2015;55:2282–90.
20. Smit Sibinga CT, Louw VJ, Nedelcu E, et al. Subcommittee on education of the AABB global transfusion forum. Modelling global transfusion medicine education. Transfusion. 2021;61(10):3040–9. https://doi.org/10.1111/trf.16641. Epub 2021 Sep 1.
21. Louw VJ. Determining the outcomes for clinicians completing a postgraduate diploma in transfusion medicine. Transfus Apher Sci. 2014;51(3):38–43. https://doi.org/10.1016/j.transci.2014.10.009. Epub 2014 Oct 16.
22. Karafin MS, Bryant BJ. Transfusion medicine education: an integral foundation of effective blood management. Transfusion. 2014;54:1208–11.
23. O'Brien KL, Champeaux AL, Sundell ZE, Short MW, Roth BJ. Transfusion medicine knowledge in postgraduate year 1 residents. Transfusion. 2010;50:1649–53.
24. Panzer S, Engelbrecht S, Cole-Sinclair MF, et al. Education in transfusion medicine for medical students and doctors. Vox Sang. 2014;104:250–72.
25. Strauss RG. Transfusion medicine education in medical school: only the first of successive steps to improving patient care. Transfusion. 2010;50:1632–5.
26. Morgan S, Rioux-Masse B, Oancea C, Cohn C, Harmon J Jr, Konia M. Simulation-based education for transfusion medicine. Transfusion. 2015;55:919–25.
27. Yudelowitz B, Scribante J, Perrie H, Oosthuizen E. Knowledge of appropriate blood product use in perioperative patients among clinicians at a tertiary hospital. Health SA Gesondheid. 2016;21:309–14.
28. WHO. Blood safety. Aide-memoire for national health programmes. 2022.
29. WHO. Sixty-third World Health Assembly. Resolutions, decisions and annexes. WHA63. Geneva: World Health Organization; 2010.
30. World Health Organization. The urgent need to implement patient blood management: policy brief. Geneva: World Health Organization; 2021.
31. Shander A, Hardy JF, Ozawa S, et al. A global definition of patient blood management. Anesth Analg. 2022;135(3):476–88. https://doi.org/10.1213/ANE.0000000000005873. Epub 2022 Feb 10.

32. Macpherson CR, Domen RE, Perlin TM. Ethical issues in transfusion medicine. Bethesda, MD: AABB Press; 2001.
33. Seifried E, Mueller MM. The present and future of transfusion medicine. Blood Transfus. 2011;9:371–6.
34. Shorey S, Lau TC, Lau ST, Ang E. Entrustable professional activities in health care education: a scoping review. Med Educ. 2019;53:766–77.
35. Kirk LM. Professionalism in medicine: definitions and considerations for teaching. Proc (Bayl Univ Med Cent). 2017;20:13–6.
36. Ten Cate O. Nuts and bolts of entrustable professional activities. J Grad Med Educ. 2013;5:157–8.
37. Sklar DP. Creating a medical education continuum with competencies and entrustable professional activities. Acad Med. 2019;94:1257–60.
38. Hathaway EO. Changing educational paradigms in transfusion medicine and cellular therapies: development of a profession. Transfusion. 2005;45:172S–88S.
39. Storch EK, Custer BS, Jacobs MR, Menitove JE, Mintz PD. Review of current transfusion therapy and blood banking practices. Blood Rev. 2019;38:100593.
40. Busch MP. Transfusion-transmitted viral infections: building bridges to transfusion medicine to reduce risks and understand epidemiology and pathogenesis. Transfusion. 2006;46:1624–40.
41. Mueller MM, Seifried E. Blood transfusion in Europe: basic principles for initial and continuous training in transfusion medicine: an approach to an European harmonisation. Transfus Clin et Biolog. 2006;13(5):282; quiz 6–9.
42. Norman GR, Shannon SI, Marrin ML. The need for needs assessment in continuing medical education. BMJ. 2004;328:999–1001.
43. Supe AN. Networking in medical education: creating and connecting. Indian KJ Med Sci. 2006;62:118–23.

The Role of Knowledge Economy in Clinical Transfusion Practice

Cees Th. Smit Sibinga and Yetmgeta E. Abdella

3.1 Introduction

Knowledge economy is focused on essential importance of human capital in the society of the twenty-first-century [1]. The rapid expansion of knowledge and the increasing reliance on computerization, big data analytics, robotics, and automation are changing the advanced world to one that is more dependent on intellectual capital and managerial skills, and less dependent on the technical production process, adding on to the existing knowledge gaps in the less-developed world. The emphasis is on specific knowledge and skills, data analysis and measurable performance, and strategic management by objectives.

Knowledge economy is characterized by the presence of a higher percentage of highly educated and skilled employees whose jobs require advanced and special knowledge and skills. Unlike in the past, when the economy depended heavily on low- and unskilled labor jobs and consisted primarily of producing physical goods, the modern economy is comprised more of services and jobs that require thinking and analysis of data produced by robotics and computerized processes and procedures. The modern economy is also known as the post-industrial economy or the information economy—a reference to the importance of information and communication technology (ICT) and artificial intelligence (artificial neural networks, deep learning and machine learning) in the economies of advanced nations, and an important platform for applied research and science to build on evidence [2]. Specialized knowledge and skills may serve as either productive asset to deploy or as products to offer and market on a cost-recovery principle, e.g., pathogen reduction and inactivation technologies, cellular engineering, and cellular therapies, and personalized medicine including the application of nanotechnology in clinical diagnostics and therapeutic approaches.

3.2 Comparing Transfusion Practices

Blood collected in an anticoagulant can be stored and transfused to a patient in an unmodified state. This is known as whole blood transfusion. However, blood may be used more effectively if it is separated into components (red cell concentrates, fresh plasma, cryoprecipitate, and platelet concentrates), so that it can meet the specific needs of more than one patient.

C. T. Smit Sibinga (✉)
International Development of Transfusion Medicine, University of Groningen and IQM Consulting, Zuidhorn, Netherlands

Y. E. Abdella
Self-employed, Freelance Consultant in Blood and other Products of Human Origin, Addis Ababa, Ethiopia

Many factors influence the requirements for blood to meet the health care needs of a population, as with all other treatment modalities. These include health care policies, income levels, current status and rate of development of the health care system, and accessibility of health care facilities to the public, all intimately related to the Universal Health Coverage (UHC) program and the Sustainable Development Goals (SDG) [3, 4]. The need for, demand for, and use of blood in a country could be affected by geography, population migration, and epidemiology of diseases for which blood is needed but also competency of governance and stewardship, levels of knowledge acquirement, and transfusion medicine education and its environment. Therefore, it is important to agree on definitions of need for, demand for, and use of blood [5] (Fig. 3.1).

Need:
An estimation of the amount of blood needed (supplied) to meet the transfusion requirements of the patient population according to current policies, clinical guidelines, and best practices.
Demand:
The amount of blood that would be transfused if all prescriptions for blood were met. Demand may reflect appropriate or inappropriate indications and practices.
Use:
The actual amount of blood currently transfused; use may be appropriate or inappropriate.

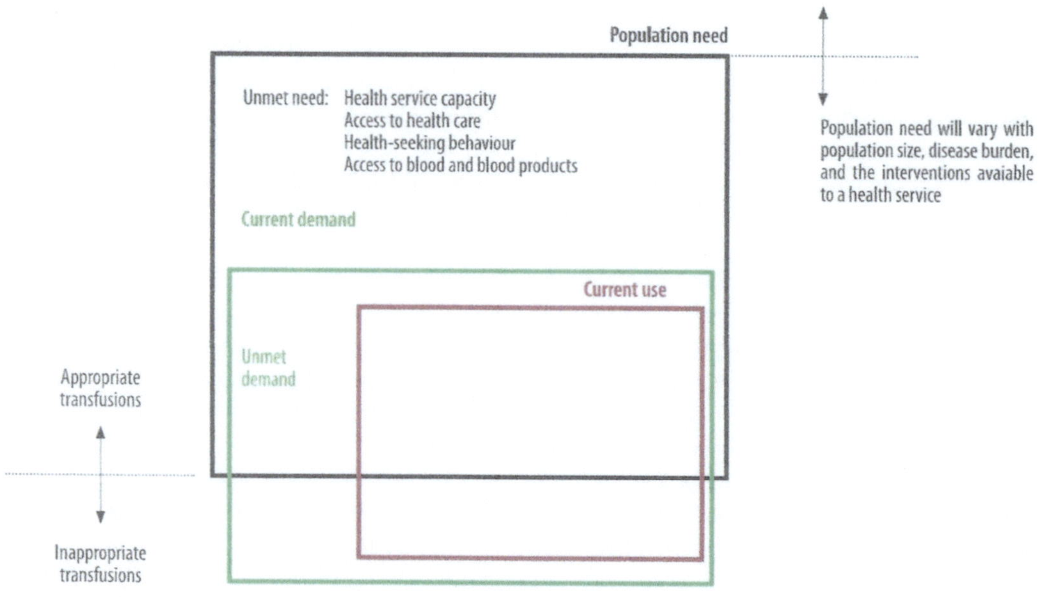

Fig. 3.1 Paradigm or model of need for, demand for, and use of blood [6]

Ideally there should be a balance between the demand and the need, translated into a demand–supply equilibrium based on appropriate and evidence-based use and demand-based manufacturing of collected units of blood; hence the two important interfaces to which the blood establishments are connected—clinical and societal.

3.2.1 Need

Based on data reported to the GDBS by 157 countries [5], 89% of whole blood donations collected globally were processed into components to meet the need: 96% in high-income countries, 96% in upper-middle-income countries, but 75% in lower-middle-income countries, and only 38% in low-income countries. Across the six WHO regions, the percentages for processing blood into transfusable components were 42% in the African Region (AFR, 18/43 countries), 50% in the South-East Asia Region (SEAR, 5/10 countries), 57% in the Eastern Mediterranean Region (EMR, 8/14 countries), 60% in the Western Pacific Region (WPR, 12/20 countries), 71% in the Region of the Americas (AMR, 22/31 countries), and 95% in the European Region EUR, 37/39 countries). These data provide a global picture of clinical blood component need and demand in the six WHO regions in the world.

3.2.2 Demand

Shortages of blood, whether real or potential, have impacted all countries at different times and periods, including more recently during the COVID-19 pandemic and ongoing humanitarian emergencies. In the early stages of the pandemic, there were major concerns about lack of availability of blood for transfusion. Strategies and recommendations for responding to potential blood shortages must be incorporated into resilience planning for blood supply by countries and blood system and service operators [7–9] to mitigate the risk of harm.

3.2.3 Use

Data reported indicate significant differences in the age distribution of patients transfused. In high-income countries, the most frequently transfused patient group is aged over 60 years, which accounts for up to 76% of all transfusions. In low-income countries, up to 54% of all transfusions are for children aged under 5 years (mostly for anemia due to malaria), usually followed by females aged between 15 and 45 years (obstetrics). The WHO 2018 data [5] on distribution of units of blood transfused in different clinical departments in hospitals or other transfusion prescribing and performing health facilities from 19 countries in the AFR revealed that among 2,248,721 units of blood, 466,625 (21%) were transfused to patients in pediatrics departments, and 427,289 (19%) were transfused to patients in obstetrics and gynecology departments. In 5 of the 19 countries, more than 30% of blood was transfused to pediatric patients: Democratic Republic of the Congo 60%, Benin 58%, Burkina Faso 39%, Congo 33%, and Comoros 31%. Five countries reported that more than 30% of blood was transfused to gynecological and obstetric patients: Burkina Faso 61%, Cameroon 55%, Comoros 40%, Eswatini 32%, and Burundi 32%. Blood use for trauma and major bleeding varied considerably, although generally at lower rates than for patients in pediatrics, and obstetrics and gynecology departments. The same data from the WHO AFR suggest that rates of usage in emergency and resuscitation departments in some countries approaches 23% to 34% (Madagascar 23%, Gabon 26%, Sao Tome and Principe 28%, and Cabo Verde 34%). Although these data indicate that children and women are the recipients who are most frequently transfused in low-income countries, it should be noted that these results are dependent on the accuracy of coding and documentation—e.g., it is possible that blood use in emergency departments is covered by surgery departments in some countries [5].

Globally in 2018, the proportion of whole blood transfusions among all red cells transfused was 7.7%. By WHO region, this proportion was 28.3% in Africa, 27.9% in the Eastern Mediterranean, 27.3% in South-East Asia, 2.1% in the Western Pacific, 0.4% in Europe and 0.3% in the Americas.

- South-East Asia reported a reduction in the proportion of whole blood transfusion from 32.2% in 2013 to 27.3% in 2018.
- The Americas, Europe, and the Western Pacific reported low percentages of whole blood transfusion in both years, and a slight to mild reduction between 2013 and 2018 (respectively 0.3, 0.2, and 4.9%).
- In the Eastern Mediterranean, the proportion of whole blood transfusion increased from 22.3% in 2013 to 27.9% in 2018. However, this was based on data from only seven countries and might not reflect the actual regional trend.
- Africa reported a minimal increase in the proportion during the period (0.3%).

Another, often disrespected, fact is the almost daily occurring under-transfusion and late transfusion due to poor logistics, organization of the blood system, and poor to failing communication between prescribing and treating clinicians and blood suppliers. A number of studies have highlighted the burden of severe anemia in under 5 years of age children, often due to malaria. Mortality rates are significant, and deaths may occur within a few hours of arrival in hospital, indicating the importance of access to timely blood transfusion support, which is often not available [10–12]. Failure to recognize the presence of severe anemia resulted in lack of transfusion in some cases [13]. Currently, there are very limited data or studies available on unmet needs for blood transfusion in low- and middle-income countries.

The prevention and treatment of postpartum hemorrhage requires a multiplicity of interventions, including timely blood transfusion [14]. The WOMAN trial report published by Picetti et al. [15] assessed the clinical and contextual factors surrounding the deaths of 483 women (of the 20,060 patients assessed in the trial) following postpartum hemorrhage in developing coun-

tries. It found that lack of timely transfusion and insufficient transfusion are still factors that lead to maternal deaths [15]. An earlier review by Bates et al. [16]. estimated that overall 26% (ranging from 16 to 71%) of maternal hemorrhage deaths were due to lack of blood for transfusion (need}.

The paucity of publications on the clinical impact of lack of available blood for transfusion in low- and middle-income countries, hence lack of effective knowledge economy, urges for evidence-based action. It is also important to establish data collection mechanisms based on a sound documentation system to systematically monitor and eventually evaluate and correct the situation. The expansion of the scope of hemovigilance and patient blood management (PBM) should be considered to include monitoring and evaluating unmet needs and demands through a structured reporting system [17].

The questions, however, are the following:

- How appropriate and evidence-based the prescriptions (demands) have been?
- To what extent these reflect accurate and appropriate clinical knowledge and effective knowledge economy of transfusion medicine (use)?
- How well is transfusion medicine, as a vein-to-vein science practiced with proper functioning interfaces (demand and need), perceived and governed?

3.3 Knowledge Economy: A Fact or a Fiction?

Knowledge economy is an economy in which growth is dependent on the quantity, quality, and accessibility of the information or knowledge available, rather than the means of production. This means that available information or knowledge through education (teaching knowledge and training skills) is of paramount importance. In 2018, UNDP published a Statistical Update on the Human Development Indices and Indicators in which the state of the art of all indicators and indices are provided [18].

This Update has shown a snapshot of conditions today as well as key trends in human development indices and indicators. Five key findings emerge from the analysis of which two are relevant to this chapter:

- Quantitatively, most people today live longer, are more educated, and have more access to goods and services than ever before. Even in countries with low human development index, human development has improved significantly.
- But the quality of human development reveals large deficits. Living longer does not automatically mean more years spent enjoying life. Being in school longer does not automatically translate into equivalent capabilities and skills. So shifting the focus towards the quality and essential conditions of human development will be important in monitoring future progress.
- Progress in human development cannot be sustained without addressing environmental degradation and climate change, which the recent progress on the HDI has exacerbated.
- For human development to become truly sustainable, the world needs to break with "business-as-usual" approaches and adopt innovative sustainable production and consumption patterns, the health care included.

The universalism *"Every human being counts, and every human life is equally valuable"* is at the core of the human development concept. With the 2030 Agenda for Sustainable Development, the Sustainable Development Goals and the promises "to leave no one behind," this universal perspective is more critical than ever, particularly in a world that is increasingly unequal, unstable, and unsustainable [4].

One of the tools to achieve the goals set in knowledge economy is the sharing of acquired knowledge and skills, the human capacity and its intellectual capacity. The question raised is one of quality and no longer just quantity. This means that education should be a national investment to develop and sustain the outcomes for which a structure is needed, governed by the ministry of education and an oversight body to protect the quality of education and educators at all levels—primary, secondary, and tertiary (Table 3.1). With the outcomes achieved, knowledge economy could play a paramount role in sustaining—intellectual assets and higher skills to improve on the quality in all aspects of life, including the health care and clinical transfusion medicine in line with the old adagio *"first do no harm."*

However, the 2018 Update still shows dramatic differences in quality and quantity of education.

The lower the HDI the greater the decrement in secondary and particularly tertiary (higher education, medical school, university) education enrolment. Tertiary education in the very high-HDI countries shows 72% enrolment, where enrolment in the medium and low HDI parts of the world, respectively is only 24% and 8%, and enrolment in the high HDI countries is 50% (Table 3.2). This illustrates the impressive paucity in education, hence knowledge and a weak economy of available and accessible knowledge.

The root cause analysis discloses a major area of attention to bridge and narrow the existing knowledge gaps. Education in these countries has been focused almost exclusively on vocational education of laboratory skills (testing and processing) with limited theoretical attention (knowledge), and rudimentary attention to topics such as governance, stewardship, human capacity investment, and appropriate clinical use of blood [5].

Table 3.1 Analysis of the vocational and professional backgrounds of staff to be employed in clinical transfusion medicine

Steering processes:
- Top management
  - Medically qualified competent leader
  - Secretariat (qualified secretary, secondary education)
- Quality management
  - Qualified quality management officer (vocational/academic)
  - Quality management trained personnel (document management and control)
  - Ancillary (secretariat, secondary education)
- Costing and financing of the vein-to-vein activities in blood establishments and hospital blood banks
- Clinical consultation service
  - Medical (preferably clinical specialist—internist, hematologist, clinical transfusion medicine specialist)

Supportive/secondary processes:
- Human resource management and education
  - Qualified HRM (vocational HE)
- Maintenance and engineering (building, equipment, vehicles)
  - Qualified mechanic or engineer (vocational)
  - Mechanics
- Domestic services (cleaning and hygiene, waste disposal, laundry, canteen, wellness)
  - Qualified domestic economy
  - Primary or secondary education personnel
- ICT (equipment, network, barcoding, printing, programming, logistics, inventory management, management information systems, artificial intelligence)
  - Qualified ICT officers (vocational)

Primary processes:
Clinical use
- Ordering (diagnosis, indication, alternatives, decision, informed consent)
  - Medical
  - Nursing/midwifery
  - Ancillary (administration, cleaning, runners)
- Component selection and immunohematology testing (blood group serology, antibody screening and identification, quality testing, crossmatching)
  - Medical technical (medical or pathology responsibility)
  - Ancillary (administration, cleaning/waste, runners)
- Transfusion (bedside)
  - Medical
  - Nursing/midwifery
  - Ancillary (administration, cleaning, waste)

Table 3.2 UNDP (2018) education enrolment rates of school-age populations (%) in the four HDI groups for primary, secondary, and tertiary education

Human development groups	Education enrolment ratio		
	Primary school-age population (%)	Secondary school-age population (%)	Tertiary school-age population (%)
Low HDI	98	*43*	*8*
Medium HDI	*110*	*73*	*24*
High HDI	103	96	**50**
Very-high HDI	102	106	72

3.4 Impact of Knowledge Economy on Clinical Transfusion Practice

Knowledge economy is a system of consumption and production that is based on intellectual capital. It is an economy where knowledge is acquired, created, disseminated, shared, and used effectively to enhance economic development whether for profit or not for profit, private or public [1].

It has been found that successful transition to knowledge economy typically involves elements such as long-term investments in education, developing innovation capability, modernizing the information infrastructure, and having an environment that is conducive to market transactions [2]. These elements have been termed by the World Bank as the pillars of the knowledge economy and together they constitute the knowledge economy framework defined according to these four pillars:

1. An *institutional and educational incentive regime* that provides good economic policies, and institutions that permit efficient mobilization and allocation of resources, and stimulate creativity and incentives for efficient creation, dissemination, sharing intellectual assets and skills, and use of existing knowledge.
2. *Educated (knowledge) and skilled (trained) workers* who can continuously upgrade and adapt their skills to efficiently create and apply knowledge.
3. An *effective innovation system* of institutions, research centers, universities, consultants, and other organizations that can keep up with the knowledge revolution and tap into the growing stock of global knowledge, assimilate and adapt it to local needs, e.g., health care and transfusion medicine.
4. A *modern and adequate information infrastructure* that can facilitate the effective communication, dissemination, sharing, and processing of information and knowledge, e.g., the development and implementation of artificial intelligence (AI) and digital foot printing (see Chap. 5 and 6).

This knowledge economy framework thus suggests that investments in the four knowledge economy pillars are necessary for sustained creation, adoption, adaptation, and use of knowledge in domestic economic processes, which will consequently result in higher value-added goods and services as exemplary for the blood supply and consumption in the health care.

Clinical transfusion practice differs substantially over the globe as illustrated earlier based on the latest Global Status Report of 2021 [5]. When analyzing the details of the indications and decisions to transfuse it becomes clear that these differences are not limited to less advanced countries. Several surveys among clinicians demonstrate the weaknesses in knowledge of transfusion medicine. Not only because of shortcomings in medical education but also the poor and inappropriate use of knowledge economy. Knowledge economy of transfusion medicine could contribute to a better understanding, patient blood management (PBM) and a more focused prescription of blood components. Looking in detail at the four knowledge economy pillars designed by World Bank, the impact on and values of clinical transfusion practice recognizable are the following:

1. **Institutional and educational incentive regime:**
   Creating in the institutional and educational environment a climate of attractivity of, appetite for, and interest in the values and risks of clinical transfusion medicine in educational institutions and hospitals (continuous professional development or CPD) will lead to more and better attention to be given to the risks and supportive values of prescribing and transfusing blood and blood components in health care. Whatever the clinical condition of a patient, physiology remains active albeit sometimes weak, and needing supportive interventions to bridge the time period of insufficient and inadequate self-support in hematopoiesis and protein synthesis. This happens both in acute situations as well as in protracted and chronic pathology.

2. **Educated (knowledge) and skilled (trained) workers:**

When the employees of all levels, from those enhanced in steering, policy making and governance to those in the supportive functions and the professionals in the primary process functions are well educated and skilled, team spirit and curiosity will grow, quality of service and care will improve and most likely adverse events (hemovigilance) will diminish and prevented. This will have a major impact on the costs related to clinical blood transfusion (e.g., outcomes, admission times).

3. **Effective innovation system:**

Educated and competent employees are needed for the development and implementation of an innovative system of progress. The team will strive for the best and have the results peer reviewed. Documentation plays a paramount role, accurate and quality to build innovation on and step by step develop and show superiority in knowledge and practice, becoming the "primus inter pares" in the field. To sustain and upgrade knowledge and an innovative system the team needs to be susceptible to knowledge economy and explore actively the sources e.g., literature, scientific exchanges, and discussions on how to achieve and what has been achieved (applied research). Networking through recognition and visibility is essential to develop an effective and innovative system—mitigating and eliminating avoidable harm through appropriate and well-documented patient blood management [19].

4. **Modern and adequate information infrastructure:**

An effective and competent team knows how to communicate and share information and knowledge. Therefore, documentation, both written and digital, is of paramount importance. Knowledge economy functions better when knowledge is disseminated electronically and digitally, which includes the availability of social media, artificial intelligence using deep learning algorithms and machine learning, radiofrequency identification (RFID), and implementing a digital footprint in clinical transfusion medicine. Again, networking and sharing are of essential importance to contact the sources and senders or disseminators of the knowledge stream, securing access to and implementing sustained communication—internal and external.

The impact of knowledge economy depends highly on keeping up with the knowledge revolution and taping into the growing library of global knowledge to be assimilated and adapted to local needs e.g., health care and transfusion medicine.

3.5 The Facts and the Fictions

Although many factors operate to explain the considerable variations in transfusion practice among and within countries, one key factor is variable uptake and implementation of evidence-based best practice, the knowledge of clinical transfusion medicine informed by high-quality research. There is an expanding body of literature, informed by high-quality randomized trials, to provide clearer recommendations on which patients benefit from transfusions. A 2016 update of earlier Cochrane systematic reviews on the use of red blood cell transfusions was further revised in a 2021 update [20]. This 2021 review identified and reported on a total of 48 randomized clinical trials of red cell transfusion, involving data from 21,433 participants, across a range of clinical contexts (e.g., orthopedic, cardiac, or vascular surgery; critical care; acute blood loss, including gastrointestinal bleeding; acute coronary syndrome; and cancer). Other randomized trials have evaluated both the timing of transfusion administration and transfusion volume in African children with severe anemia [21, 22].

Knowledge economy is an economy in which growth is dependent on the quantity, quality, and accessibility of the information available, rather than the means of production and provision. It is a system of consumption and production that is based on intellectual capital. In particular, it refers to the ability to capitalize on scientific discoveries, innovation, and applied research. De facto knowledge economy represents a large share of the activity in most highly developed countries. In a knowledge economy, a significant component of value may consist of intangible assets such as the value of health care and transfusion medicine workers' knowledge or intellectual property. A well-developed outcomes-driven education structure at national level is a key requirement.

However, it is a fiction to think that knowledge economy is commercial and owned by the national and international commercial structure and companies; however, knowledge economy may contribute to development in which the financial economy or welfare plays a role.

It is a fiction to classify knowledge economy as describing the contemporary commercialization of science and academic scholarship, education, and professionalism.

It is a fiction to state that in knowledge economy, innovation based on research is commodified via patents and other forms of intellectual property.

Knowledge economy deals with an intangible asset or knowledge that can be classified as either indefinite or definite. An institution's "brand name" is considered an indefinite intangible asset because it stays with the institution for as long as it continues operations and services. An example of a definite intangible asset would be a legal agreement to operate under another institution's name, with no plans of extending the agreement, e.g., universities or tertiary hospitals. An agreement has a limited life and is classified as a definite asset.

3.6 Conclusion and Recommendations

A knowledge economy depends on skilled and competent labor and education, strong communications networks, and institutional structures that incentivize innovation and progress.

Clinical transfusion practice differs widely over the globe, largely dependent on poor to mediocre education of transfusion indicating, prescribing and practicing clinicians. As a consequence, patient care including supportive blood transfusion lacks behind in its development and the prevention of avoidable transfusion adverse events.

Quality and outcomes-based education remains the essence to overcome this situation. Knowledge economy could play a paramount role in updating the meagre and fragmented knowledge of those already practicing.

3.6.1 Recommendations

1. There is strong evidence for avoiding unnecessary transfusions with allogeneic red cells in most patients at hemoglobin thresholds between 7.0 and 8.0 g per deciliter, and implementation of restricted transfusion policies. Research is ongoing.

2. Strategies to implement this research would minimize risk of exposure to unnecessary blood for transfusion, which is particularly important given variability in practices of laboratory screening for potential TTIAs in many countries.

3. Evidence-based guidelines are important tools in the education of those indicating and prescribing blood and/or blood components. They are prerequisites for establishing systems for appropriate clinical use of blood, such as clinical audits. In 2018, 128 countries reported the existence of national guidelines on the clinical use of blood. Across WHO regions, 9 (90%) in the South-East Asia Region, 33 (79%) in the European Region, 19 (76%) in the Western Pacific Region, 32 (74%) countries in the African Region, 23 (70%) in the Region of the Americas, and 12 (67%) in the Eastern Mediterranean Region reported the existence of national guidelines on the clinical use of blood. However, there is little known about the implementation of these guidelines.

4. GDBS data reported by 92 countries (33 high-income countries, 29 upper-middle-income countries, 21 lower-middle-income countries, and 9 low-income countries) indicated that hospital transfusion committees (HTC) were present in 48% of hospitals prescribing and performing transfusion. Across World Bank

economic groups, the percentage was 25% in low-income countries, 31% in lower-middle-income countries, 35% in upper-middle-income countries, and 62% in high-income countries. However, there is limited information on the active performances of these HTCs.

5. A well-structured system for quality in higher and tertiary education for those deployed in hospitals and involved in clinical transfusion practice is fundamental.

6. The education sequence should conclude with knowledge economy to secure dissemination and sharing of advanced knowledge to improve clinical transfusion practices and allow progress in that part of the national health care.

References

1. Hayes H. The role of libraries in the knowledge economy. Serials. 2004;17:231–8.
2. Chen DHC, Dahlman CJ. The knowledge economy, the KAM methodology and World Bank operations. Stock No. 37258. Washington, DC: World Bank Institute; 2006.
3. WHO. Universal health coverage program. 2012. http://www.who.int/universal_health_coverage/en/. Accessed 30 Dec 2022.
4. UN. Sustainable development goals 2016–2030. 2015. https://sustainabledevelopment.un.org/?menu=1300. Accessed 30 Dec 2022.
5. Global status report on blood safety and availability. Licence: BY NC-SA 3.0 IGO. Geneva: World Health Organization; 2022.
6. WHO experts' consultation on estimation of blood requirements. Geneva: meeting report. Geneva: World Health Organization; 2010. http://www.who.int/bloodsafety/transfusion_services/estimation_meeting-report.pdf?ua=1. Accessed 30 Dec 2022.
7. Stanworth SJ, New HV, Apelseth TO, et al. Effects of the COVID-19 pandemic on supply and use of blood for transfusion. Lancet Haematol. 2020;7(10):e756–e64.
8. Action framework to advance universal access to safe, effective and quality-assured blood products, 2020–2023. Licence: CC BY-NC-SA 3.0 IGO. Geneva: World Health Organization; 2020.
9. Guidance on ensuring a sufficient supply of safe blood and blood components during emergencies. Licence: CC BY-NC-SA 3.0 IGO. Geneva: World Health Organization; 2023.
10. Kiguli S, Maitland K, George EC, et al. Anaemia and blood transfusion in African children presenting to hospital with severe febrile illness. BMC Med. 2015;13:21–31.
11. Thomas J, Ayieko P, Ogero M, et al. Blood transfusion delay and outcome in county hospitals in Kenya. Am J Trop Med Hyg. 2017;96(2):511–7. https://doi.org/10.4269/ajtmh.16-0735.32.
12. Cheema B, Molyneux EM, Emmanuel JC, et al. Development and evaluation of a new paediatric protocol for Africa. Transfus Med. 2010;20:140–51.
13. Educational modules on clinical use of blood. Licence: CC Y-NC-SA 3.0 IGO. Geneva: World Health Organization; 2021.
14. WHO recommendations for the prevention of postpartum haemorrhage. Geneva: World Health Organization; 2012. http://apps.who.int/iris/bitstream/handle/10665/75411/9789241548502_eng.pdf. Accessed 30 Dec 2022.
15. Picetti R, Miller L, Shakur-Still H, et al. The WOMAN trial: clinical and contextual factors surrounding the deaths of 483 women following post-partum haemorrhage in developing countries. BMC Pregnancy Childbirth. 2020;20:409. https://doi.org/10.1186/s12884-020-03091-8.
16. Bates I, Chapotera GK, McKew S, van den Broek N. Maternal mortality in sub-Saharan Africa: the contribution of ineffective blood transfusion services. BJOG. 2008;115(11):1331–9. https://doi.org/10.1111/j.1471-0528.2008.01866.x.
17. User guide for navigating resources on stepwise implementation of haemovigilance systems. Geneva: World Health Organization; 2021.
18. UNDP. Human development indices and indicators. 2018 Statistical update. New York; 2018. http://hdr.undp.org/en/content/human-development-indices-indicators-2018-statistical-update. Accessed 30 Dec 2021.
19. Global patient safety action plan 2021–2030. Towards eliminating avoidable harm in health care. 2021. https://www.who.int/docs/default-source/patient-safety/global-patient-safety-action-plan-2021-2030_third-draft_january-2021_web.pdf?sfvrsn=948f15d5_17. Accessed 30 Dec 2022.
20. Carson JL, Stanworth SJ, Dennis JA, et al. Transfusion thresholds for guiding red blood cell transfusion. Cochrane Database of Systematic Reviews 2021, Issue 12. Art. No.: CD002042. https://doi.org/10.1002/14651858.CD002042.pub5. Accessed 15 Apr 2023.
21. Maitland K, Kiguli S, Olupot-Olupot P, et al. Immediate transfusion in African children with uncomplicated severe anemia. N Engl J Med. 2019;381(5):407–19.
22. Maitland K, Olupot-Olupot P, Kiguli S, et al. Transfusion volume for children with severe anemia in Africa. N Engl J Med. 2019;381(5):420–31.

Part II

Artificial Intelligence and a Digital Footprint in Clinical Transfusion Medicine

Cees Th. Smit Sibinga

Cees Th. Smit Sibinga and Yetmgeta E. Abdella

4.1 Introduction

Before the industrial revolution, craft workers made their products one by one and only those products that fulfilled their requirements and satisfied the customers were sold (100% quality control). With the introduction of bulk production, 100% quality control became too expensive and no longer feasible. Statistical quality control was introduced.

With the increase of product reliability, the system of quality assurance (QA) or Good Manufacturing Practice (GMP) was introduced for the pharmaceutical and military industry [1]. Later a generic quality system (ISO 9001:2000) has been developed [2], including the involvement of external parties or stakeholders like customers and general public, suppliers and regulators.

In many countries pharmaceutical industries by law must comply to the requirements of cGMP and are regularly inspected by the Competent Authority like FDAs.

Blood products consist of living cells and proteins in a matrix called plasma. As they are used for supportive therapeutic purposes, they must be produced in accordance with the pharmaceutical production rules. This includes the introduction of the quality system Good Manufacturing Practice (GMP), originally developed by FDA for the pharmaceutical and military industry [1]. Not all requirements of the International GMP apply to the blood system. Therefore, the Dutch blood establishment organization developed a guideline "GMP for blood banks" [3]. In 2005 the European Union (EU) accepted the Directive 2005/62/EU containing the quality requirements for blood establishments [4]. However, this quality system is product oriented and not all departments of a Blood Establishment nor the hospital blood transfusion service are involved in this quality system. Therefore, it is advisable to look at other quality systems as well, like ISO 9001 and the European Foundation of Quality Management (EFQM) [5]. With the version of ISO 9001 issued in 2002 most of the specific elements of EFQM became part of ISO 9001:2000. However, EFQM contains a specific method of self-auditing by analyzing the various phases of the departments or processes of an organization (see below).

The strong points of ISO 9001:2000 and later versions are the management involvement (annual management review is required) and the supplier chain [supplier—producer—customer (internal or external)] and customer satisfaction.

C. T. Smit Sibinga (✉)
International Development of Transfusion Medicine, University of Groningen and IQM Consulting, Zuidhorn, Netherlands

Y. E. Abdella
Self-employed, Freelance Consultant in Blood and other Products of Human Origin, Addis Ababa, Ethiopia

Until the development of quality assurance (QA) principles there was no real management of the system. Operational documents such as SOPs (Standard Operating Procedures) and other documents were written when necessary, wanted or for any other reason. This resulted in two major questions:

1. Is documentation complete?
2. How to write a quality manual?

The EFQM or European Forum for Quality Management is de facto not a quality system but a management system. It recognizes five different development stages of quality management development [6]:

1. **Activity or product oriented**: The system is restricted to SOPs and EOPs, and related records and forms. The focus is on quality control (QC), just the collection of data.
2. **Process oriented**: SOPs and EOPs are more cohesive as the focus is on quality assurance (QA). Collected data are interpreted intellectually.
3. **System oriented**: Processes are cohesive and the focus is on GMP. Supplier-customer principles introduced.
4. **Chain oriented**: External stakeholders like suppliers and customers are involved in the quality system, which has now become ISO based. Market principles apply.

5. **Recognized for Excellence**: Results and employees are involved in the quality system and the focus is on holistic management of all aspects and integrated in the society.

The Pyramid documentation model includes all these phases.

4.2 The Pyramid Concept

The Pyramid documentation model consists of four layers or levels (Fig. 4.1).

4.2.1 The Managerial Levels 1 and 2

Level 1 contains first of all the **Mission and Vision Statements** describing the ultimate goals and objectives, and the future expectations of the institution. These statements must be approved and authorized by top management of the institution and where appropriate by the ministry of health. However, it can be developed by a broad group of coworkers of the institution. This is very helpful in getting a high level of commitment and stewardship within the organization and good relationships with the customers if they are involved in the writing-up of the statement. The Mission and Vision Statements must be brief and comprehensive (maximum 1 or 2 sentences); they should be valid for at least 5–10 years. As a

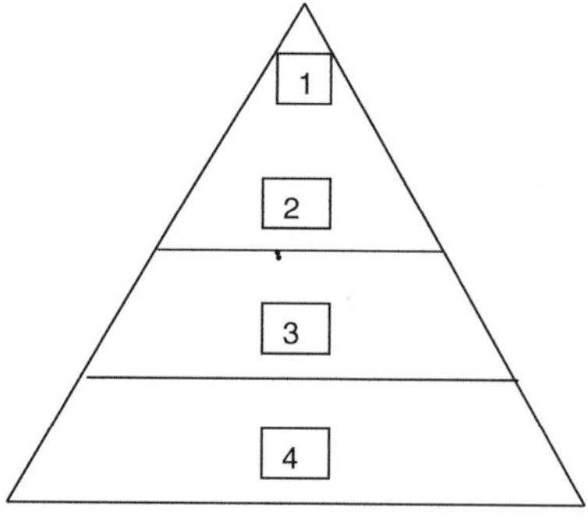

Fig. 4.1 Pyramid documentation model

consequence these goals must appear in the organogram as the core business.

The second element of the first level is the **Quality Policy and Strategy**. This is the translation of the Mission Statement into the "way how" the goals and objectives are to be achieved. The director (CEO) and the management team should write this document. The type of the organization must be described transparently and an organogram showing the lines of command included. All plans and processes used must be described— blood ordering or request (bedside, demand); blood selection and compatibility testing/immunohematology (blood transfusion laboratory, need); and patient transfusion (bedside, use). But also the supportive plans like the education plan including continuous education, the human resource plan, the finance and budget plan, the contingency and emergency preparedness and response plan, the hygiene and cleanliness plan, the hemovigilance plan, the patient blood management (PBM) plan, and the waste management plan. It is important that all processes are analyzed and described in this document. Processes not mentioned cannot be described in the next layers, the levels 2 and 3 documents.

Finally, this level contains the **Annual Quality Plan**. The Quality Manager supported by the Director/CEO should write this document. It must contain the plans for the coming or current year in terms of the development and improvement of the quality system(s). The document must contain measurable objectives in terms of quality and a time schedule (SMART principle). At the end of each period, the Quality Manager should write an evaluation report and there has to be transparent and good arguments and explanations for not achieving one or more of the objectives (root cause analysis); the **Management Review.**

Level 2 contains the **Process Descriptions (PD),** including the basic performance requirements of personnel (managerial part of job description/JD). The processes and outcomes mentioned in the Quality Policy and Strategy must be described in detail. The principle and scope of the process, used abbreviations and definitions of words with a special meaning of usually unknown words, tasks, authorization, responsibilities and accountability of all type of employees involved in the process, list of related processes and the final description of the process including mentioning all Standard Operating Procedures (SOPs) and Equipment Operating Procedures (EOPs) needed to perform the process, and list of forms or records needed to document outcomes of activities performed (Fig. 4.2).

These process descriptions should be written by the heads of departments, e.g., the clinician in charge of the blood transfusion practice in the healthcare facility with, where necessary, the help of operational staff (nurses and Blood Transfusion Laboratory professionals).

Job descriptions (JD) like operating procedures consist of two parts: the managerial part name and description of the function, required education level and accountability, and the list of specific tasks, which is part of level 3.

Level 1 and 2 together contain all elements that must be in the Quality Manual. So, time can be saved because the Quality Manual does not need to be written separately as it already exists in its elements.

4.2.2 The Operational Levels 3 and 4

Level 3 contains the **SOPs, EOPs, and JDs** (operational or functional part). Once the processes have been in detail described, the work-instruction "how to perform" a procedure or "how to operate" equipment can now easily be written by the operators who perform the procedures or operate the equipment, e.g., therapeutic apheresis machine and blood warmer. As a consequence the language in which the work-instructions are to be written should be transparent and clear to those who need to understand and operate the procedure or run the equipment.

SOPs and EOPs contain as a minimum an introduction and the work instructions. Where necessary and/or appropriate some tasks, responsibilities, and authorization can be repeated from the process description(s).

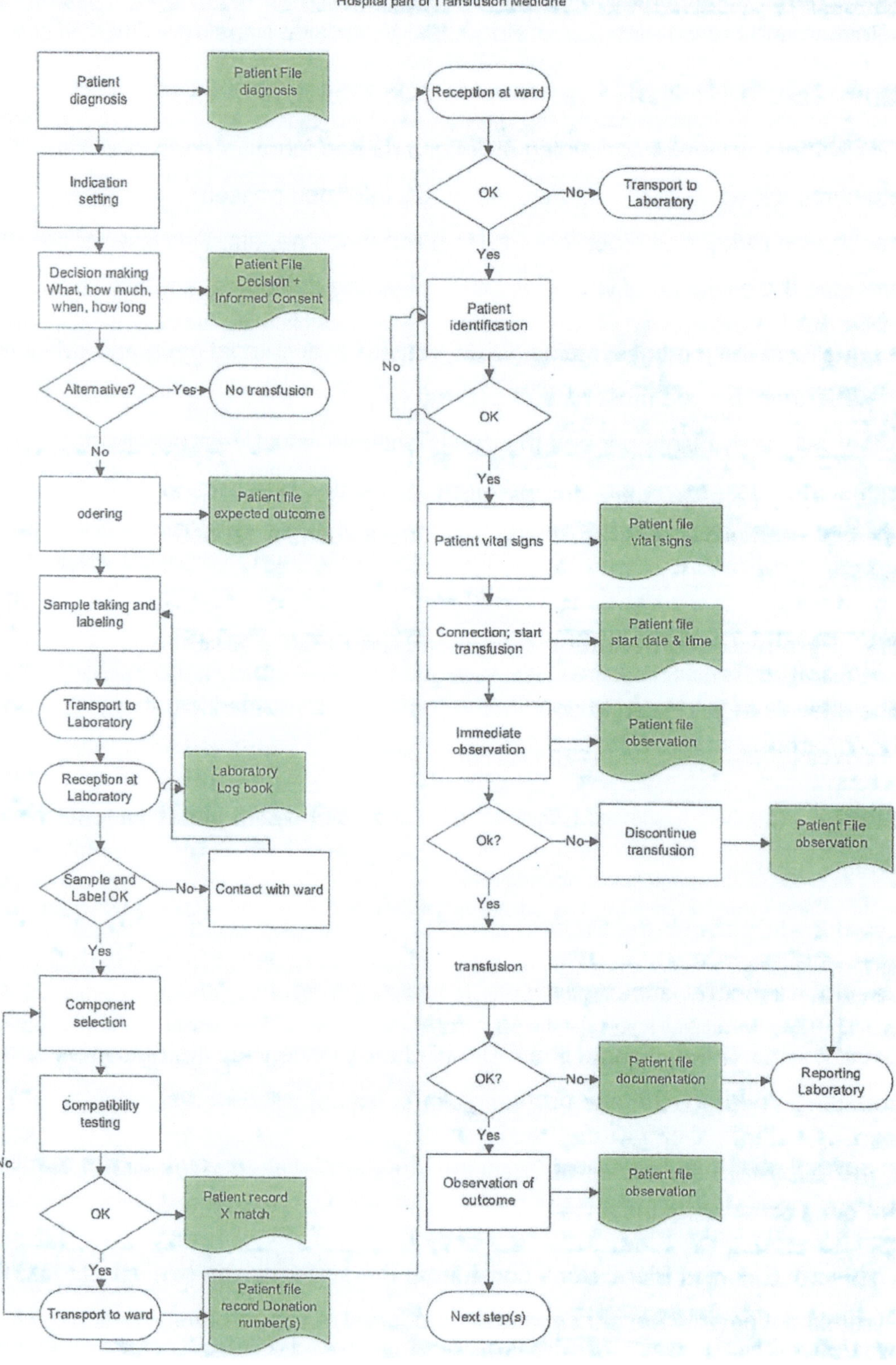

Fig. 4.2 Clinical process of blood transfusion. The 12 green symbols represent documentation. The seven diamond symbols are decisions or critical control points (CCP). (Author owned)

The job descriptions (JD) should have as a minimum the following subjects:

Name of the organization, name of the department, title of the function, educational/vocational requirements or level, salary scale, short description of the organization, department and function, and tasks, authorities, responsibilities and accountability (TARA). For each and every function such description must be available. It can be used for making up an advertisement to attract employees and can be used during the interview with candidates for a defined function as well as for operational evaluation.

First 3 green documentation symbols: ordering (bedside/expectation); Second 3: selection and crossmatch (Laboratory); last 6: bedside transfusion (bedside/reality).

Finally there is **level 4** containing all level 3 related forms, reports, records, attachments, equipment operating manuals, informed consent information, transfusion request or order form, transfusion outcome, etc. This level of documents provides the evidence of what has been done, the outcomes, and allows traceability.

As quality management systems (QMS) require to document each and every activity or performance, there must be a structured way to do so. Small pieces of random paper will easily disappear and the documentation is lost. Appropriate and identifiable forms, records, reports, etc., are therefore necessary. Handwriting is often poorly readable and easily allows mistakes and errors such as transcription errors and poor readability.

4.3 Pyramid Documentation Model and the EFQM Phases

The four levels of the Pyramid documentation model translated into the EFQM phases of development could be presented as follows:

Level 1—This is the level of Excellence and transformation phase into the System an Chain phases.

Level 2—This level is the Process phase.

Level 3—This level is the Activity or Procedure phase.

Level 4—This is the ultimate first Product phase, evidencing the outcomes or results, both tangible (products) and non-tangible (services), allowing traceability.

This model has been discussed and introduced in several countries. The reactions are quite different. Some instances are the following:

The North Estonian Blood Bank considered the system as an eye-opener and the Pyramid documentation principle was introduced to support their existing quality system.

In some countries in sub-Saharan Africa, Eastern Europe, the Middle East, and Asia it seems to be more difficult to transfer the theory into practice. People reported to have fully understood the system, though kept writing their SOPs in the old and traditional way omitting or ignoring the levels 2 (PDs) and 1 (governance). More broad-based intensive education to achieve the right perception of the principle and process analysis will be needed in these countries. That means a more holistic view and approach.

The Pyramid documentation model was also introduced in a Hospital Blood Bank in Nicosia, Cyprus. The system was very well understood and implemented after full explanation. Two more short educational sessions followed and process analysis revealed that some SOPs were missing because they were not mentioned in the related process description (PD).

Practice has demonstrated that this documentation model works well. The system proved that documentation is bottom up complete to the level of process description (level 2); however, collection of the data is not always of quality and complete.

> The Pyramid documentation model is a clear and well-functioning system to manage the required quality documentation at all levels—managerial and operational. It is simple, practical, enables to prove that the documentation is complete, and provides and maintains the quality manual.

4.4 Copying and Reproducing

Quality system management (QSM) consists of five elements:

1. organization, (infra-)structure, and governance;
2. standards (quality and technical, guidelines);
3. documentation (traceability);
4. education (competence); and
5. assessment (monitoring and evaluation/M&E, hemovigilance);

Documentation is the core of quality management. It documents policies and strategies, processes and procedures, and the evidence of performances and activities. When a necessity arrives to copy one of the many documents (managerial, instructive or outcome) it must be done such that the copy clearly shows to be a copy e.g., color paper or watermark. The quality manager should be informed and explained why and when reproducing an official document is needed.

4.5 Document Control and Archiving

Because of the crucial role of documents in the quality system and the legal importance (customer or patient rights protection) documents need to be controlled and securely archived for any future retrieval (consultation, evidence).

Quality of data is a prime requirement for Artificial Intelligence (AI) whether machine or deep learning application. As a serious consequence also document control, archiving and retrieval need to be documented. These procedures need an SOP and where digital an additional EOP under the responsibility of the quality manager and director/head of the department in the health care institution.

4.6 Who Is Responsible?

Documentation is the nucleus of a quality system and its management. Anecdotally, documentation is characterized by the phrases "write up what you do" so that "you can do what has been written" but "not written is not done." WHO in its Quality Management Training [7] course states: A job is not done until the paperwork is complete" and added "Do what is documented" and "document what you do.

> **Principles of documentation:**
> - Write up what you do.
> - Do what has been written.
> - Not written is not done.
> - A job is not done until the paperwork is complete.

The overall responsibility is with the Director/CEO, delegated to the Quality Manager and hierarchical down to the heads of departments. However, every employee is responsible for his/her authorized task, which includes the elements of the quality system and management, and should therefore account to both head of the department and quality manager.

4.7 Standardizing Documents

In clinical transfusion practice there are a number of documents, largely of the level 4 message and outcome type that need standardization and transparency, besides the level 3 and 2 documents dealing with the instructions (SOPs, EOPs, and JD), and strategies (PDs) based on a step wise analysis of the transfusion medicine in-hospital flow (Fig. 4.2). Following the flow they are:

1. **Blood Request Form** is a message form accompanied by a labelled test tube with patient blood for immunohematology and compatibility testing. The message is addressed to the Blood Transfusion Laboratory. This message form should have three parts and a response, and should be self-copying in threefold—one for the patient file as a proof of having ordered blood and why, two are sent to the Laboratory to be completed with the immunohematology and compatibility test outcomes of which one copy is

archived at the Laboratory (evidence), and the last one accompanies the blood units (cold chain) to the ward, OR, or ICU, wherever the 'patient in need' might be. The three information parts are:

(a) Patient demographic information including ABO and Rhesus type if known (who);

(b) History and indication (why);

(c) Request of blood (components and number of units), where and when to be delivered (what and where).

(d) The response section with the laboratory immunohematology tests and compatibility outcomes of the unit(s) requested (donation numbers and collection dates) (Fig. 4.3).

This completed part of the form and the crossmatched selected units are received by the nurse (ward, OR. ICU) and compared to the first one (patient file) and the blood or blood components it accompanies, to be sure that the right units have been delivered for the right patient at the right place and time.

Amazingly (*first do no harm*), all over the globe this does not prevent the human errors in writing, completing and the phenomenon of "wrong blood in tube" or "wrong name on tube" [8, 9].

2. **Transfusion (or hemovigilance) Report Form** is separate from the patient file and provides in writing the course of the transfusion and clinical outcome, whether adverse or as expected. This form fuels the hospital hemovigilance documentation system. Usually it is sent to the Blood Transfusion Laboratory where all these forms are compiled and anonymously sent to the supplying blood establishment. They collect these forms from all hospitals supplied, compile them into a report, and send the report to the responsible division of the Ministry of Health.

3. **Patient file** is the overall and personal document of a patient which follows exactly the day-to-day course of the admission and the outpatient visits, either hand written or electronical/digital. Treating doctors and caring nurses have to document all information during the lifetime of the patient (customer). The patient file stays in the healthcare facility and has to be archived in compliance with the law and rules in the country (privacy protection).

These documents preferably need a standardization or at least a uniformity on a national level, identifying the respective hospital or healthcare institution, and be transparently, properly, and identifiably used and archived. That is a matter of good education, comprehension, and professional discipline and respect.

HOSPITAL: _______________________   Date of request: _______________

PATIENT DETAILS

Family name: _______________   Date of birth: _________   Gender: _________

Given name: _______________   Ward: _______________

Hospital reference no.: _______________   Blood group (if known):   ABO [   ]

Address: _______________   Rh D [   ]

HISTORY

Diagnosis: _______________   Antibodies: Yes/No _______________

Reason for transfusion: _______________   Previous transfusions: Yes/No _______________

Haemoglobin: _______________   Any reactions: Yes/No _______________

Relevant medical history: _______________   Previous pregnancies: Yes/No _______________

REQUEST

[   ] Group, screen and hold patient's serum   Whole blood [   ] units

[   ] Provide product   Red cells [   ] units

Date required: _______________   Plasma [   ] units

Time required: _______________   Platelet concentrate [   ] units

Deliver to: _______________

NAME OF DOCTOR (print): _______________   **SIGNATURE:** _______________

IMPORTANT: *This blood request form will not be accepted if it is not signed or any section is left blank* .

LABORATORY USE ONLY

Patient   ABO [   ]
       Rh D [   ]

Donation pack no.	Donor typing		Compatibility testing					Date of issue	Time of issue
	ABO	Rh	Antibody screen	AHG XM	RT Saline XM	Date of match	Time of match		

Signature of tester: _______________

Fig. 4.3 Example of a blood request form with its four sections: (a) Patient demographics; (b) History and indication; (c) Request, and (d) the Laboratory response. (Author owned)

4.8 Document Identification and Retrievability

The Pyramid documentation system is well structured from level 1 to level 4 with a number coding system that allows easy traceability, retrievability, and transparency. For each level, the numbering is horizontal where a code for the institution and the department or process links the documents vertically from level to level. Each document belongs to a vertical family of documents, which makes it easy to position and retrieve. An example from Montenegro is the process description of the clinical transfusion chain "PD BO-BT 2.01 – Clinical Transfusion Chain" where PD indicates the level 2 with its process descriptions (PD), BO the blood ordering or requesting and BT the actual bedside blood transfusion. Every document has a code that links it to its process or procedure horizontally and vertically. No document is stand-alone and therefore should be recognizable.

4.9 Importance of Quality Data

4.9.1 Handwriting vs. Machine Writing and Printing

Documentation of outcomes of performances, interventions, and procedures provide the evidence of what has been done. Standards provide the minimum level of quality and quantity of the outcomes achieved. In general, outcome data have to be transferred from the source to a document. Transcription is a well-known source for human errors due to the fact that generated data have to be transcribed on to a form or record for further interpretation and archiving [10, 11]. Patient files are an example of handwritten documentation. Reliability and quality of these data are therefore questionable. Today more and more these files are replaced by electronic or digital files. Data from laboratory processes are electronically transferred or uploaded into a patient electronic file protected by a unique bar code, block code or radiofrequency identifier (RFID) to guarantee that the right individual has been targeted [12] (see Chap. 6). However, there are interventions and performances which need to be manually documented. Usually they have a high subjective content (interpretation) which forces the performer e.g., an anesthetist in the OR, or an intensivist in the intensive care unit (ICU) to write a report either manual or using a computer. Printing of data provides good readability easing proper interpretation and decision-making, improving patient care.

4.9.2 Interpretation

Data are not stand-alone evidences of a process, intervention, or performance, they contain a message or a story to be received and interpreted. When data are illegible, of poor quality and incomplete, the story they tell and the message they bring will not be interpreted or received correctly as intended. However, there is also a fair chance of misreading and misinterpretation and taking the wrong decision. The introduction of artificial intelligence (AI) with artificial neural networks (ANN) in deep learning and the use of algorithms might bring the human interpretation error rate down to an acceptable minimum (see Chaps. 5 and 6).

4.9.3 Legal Aspects

Documents are written evidences of what has been done and therefore have a legal aspect. The legal aspect requires transparency and optimal readability, harmonizing the interpretation and judgment. Remember the quote "not written, not done."

Error typology according to H.F. Taswell [10]
- Identification.
- Performance.
- Transcription.
- Interpretation.
- Storage retrieval.

4.10 Conclusion and Recommendations

Documentation is the core of quality system management (QSM), and it needs to be transparent, legible, and retrievable. The Pyramid documentation system provides a framework for a well-ordered documentation with two managerial levels and two operational levels.

The managerial levels cover the policies and strategies which include the analysis-based process descriptions (PD, Quality and Technical standards or Guidelines, and the various plans e.g., education, contingency/emergency preparedness and response plan, human resource plan and waste management plan).

The two operational levels cover the primary functions with the SOPs, EOPs, and JDs, and the evidence-based outcome documents (standardized forms, records, reports, etc.). Preferably today these should be digital or electronic to minimize handwritten errors and misinterpretations, improving the quality of and confidence in the institution and the system.

4.10.1 Recommendations

- Every healthcare institution performing clinical blood transfusion should have a qualify system (QS) developed and implemented, with a transparent and reliable documentation system such as the Pyramid documentation system.
- Documents used shall be standardized and number coded to allow easy traceability and retrievability (managerial, operational, and for legal reasons).
- The use of a digital or electronic documentation system based on AI and RFID prevents human transcription errors, allowing more accurate interpretation of data and improve on decision making (see Chaps. 5 and 6).
- Good and reliable documentation supports patient safety and prevents even minimum avoidable patient harm in clinical transfusion practice.

Key Points

- Documentation is the core and gatekeeper of quality management.
- Documentation needs to be systematic and orderly organized.
- Documentation shall be transparent and unambiguously interpretable.
- Digitalization of documentation prevents human errors.
- The Pyramid system is a well-organized and structured recommendable system.
- Human errors are avoidable using a transparent documentation system.

References

1. The Rules Governing Medicinal Products in the European Union. Volume 4: Good manufacturing practices. Brussels: European Commission; 1989.
2. ISO standard 9001: quality management systems—requirements. International Standardisation Organization, Geneva 2000.
3. Guideline GMP for blood banks. Sanquin blood supply foundation. Sanquin Blood Supply Foundation, Amsterdam; 2001.
4. EU Commission Directive 2005/62/EC of 30 September 2005; Implementing directive 2002/98/EC of the European Parliament and of the council as regards community standards and specifications relating to the quality system of a blood establishment. Brussels: European Commission; 2005.
5. European Foundation of Quality Management (EFQM). EFQM, Brussels; 2001.
6. ISO/TR 10013. Guidelines for quality management system documentation. International Standardization Organization. Geneva; 2001.
7. Quality management training for blood transfusion services. Facilitator's Toolkit. WHO/EHT/04.13. 2004.
8. Dzik WH, Murphy MF, BEST working party, International Society of Blood Transfusion. An international study on the performance of patient sample collection. Transfusion. 2002;42:26S.
9. Bolton-Maggs PH, Wood EM, Wiersum-Osselton JC. Wrong blood in tube—potential for serious outcomes: can it be prevented? Br J Haematol. 2015;168(1):3–13. https://doi.org/10.1111/bjh.13137. Epub 2014 Oct 4.
10. Taswell HT, Sonnenberg CL. Blood bank errors: a new functional classification. Transfusion. 1979;19:652–3.

11. Sonnenberg CL, Taswell HF. Error analysis: methods of detection, analysis and control. In: Smit Sibinga CT, Das PC, Taswell HF, editors. Quality assurance in blood banking and its clinical impact. Breda NL: Martinus Nijhoff; 2010. p. 239–46.

12. Guidelines for the use of RFID Technology in Transfusion Medicine. Vox Sang. 2010; 98(Suppl 2):1.

Clinical Blood Transfusion and Artificial Intelligence

José A. Cancelas, Effimia Gkoumassi, and Cees Th. Smit Sibinga

5.1 Introduction

An effective planning process will continuously combine top-down plans and milestones with detailed bottom-up plans that are developed as the main processes evolve. This "big-picture/out of the box thinking" is needed to look for the best structures, identify, and manage the implications of key interactions during the clinical blood transfusion chain. Artificial intelligence based on big data, deep and machine learning, and algorithms might be a valued asset starting off in a well-designed project setting and selection [1].

Project selection has an enormous impact on operational performance in a health care setting since this ensures that the organization puts its resources in the optimum portfolio of investments (short-term as well as long-term elements).

This plays a role, not only when projects are initially selected for investment (e.g., hemovigilance, patient blood management (PBM), development, and introduction of artificial intelligence) but also in enabling rapid algorithmic decision-making (machine learning) once the project is up and running, including closing down a project that is no longer delivering what is wanted by the organization to properly manage the related processes. In this way, successful project-based health care institutions promote a robust portfolio management discipline that continuously addresses the question of which processes best satisfy the strategic objectives and what processes need to be in place to achieve excellence in the clinical transfusion of human blood and blood components, particularly in emergency situations (e.g., humanitarian emergencies, pandemics).

5.2 Data, Artificial Intelligence, Deep Learning

In the vein-to-vein clinical field of transfusion medicine, documentation is of paramount importance. Yet, in many poor economic countries and cultures, documentation is one of the least developed systems for data collection and management; numerous handwritten cahiers and files, loose paper sheets, and incompletely documented request forms and records (Fig. 5.1).

J. A. Cancelas
Hoxworth Blood Center Research Division, College of Medicine, University of Cincinnati, Cincinnati, OH, USA
e-mail: cancelje@ucmail.uc.edu

E. Gkoumassi
Digital Competence Centre, University Medical Centre Groningen, Groningen, The Netherlands
e-mail: e.gkoumasi@umcg.nl

C. T. Smit Sibinga (✉)
International Development of Transfusion Medicine, University of Groningen and IQM Consulting, Zuidhorn, Netherlands

In quality system management, documentation is the core, interconnecting all elements and steps, whether manufacture or clinical consumption and allowing managerial and operational guidance (process descriptions, standard operating procedures) and standardization (standards), interpretation of outcomes (assessment) and initiatives to improve quality [2]. Today data and documents are mostly stored in hardware and operate through hardware networks with appropriate entrance restrictions, e.g., test results from unauthorized access, safeguarding the privacy of both donor and recipient. Problems faced

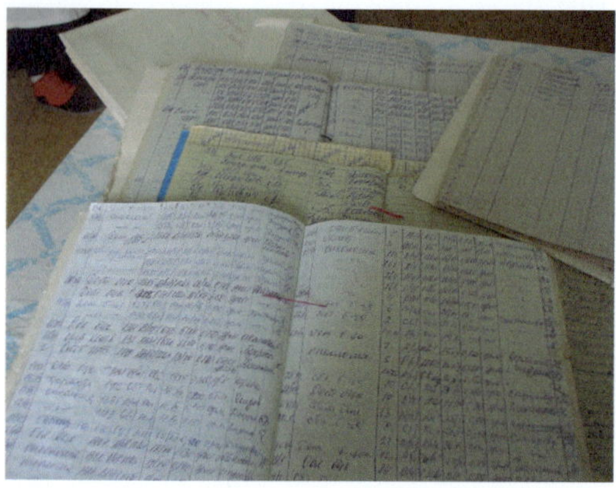

Fig. 5.1 Manual documentation, still existing in many LMICs. (Image credit Cees Smit Sibinga)

are the limited capacity and speed of computers and the unreliable power supply in a considerable part of the world. However, over the last decade, computer capacity has gone through a tremendous development, which still continues to grow. That paved the way for a machine-based handling of the daily mass of clinical data (diagnostic and therapeutic) applying artificial intelligence (AI) by building artificial neural networks (ANN) and allowing complex layered grouping of artificial neurons process wise—input layers → hidden layers → output layer [3]. Input layer receives and supplies the "raw data"; hidden layers process or compute these data mathematically into outcomes, which appear in the output layer (Fig. 5.2). One of the challenges in creating neural networks is deciding the number of hidden layers, as well as the number of neurons for each layer. Deep Learning refers to having more than one hidden layer. The output layer returns the output data. In our case, it gives us, e.g., prediction of the need to transfuse a patient in a given medical situation.

5.2.1 Deep Neural Networks

To build and condition such DNN, a meticulous and detailed analysis of all three categories of

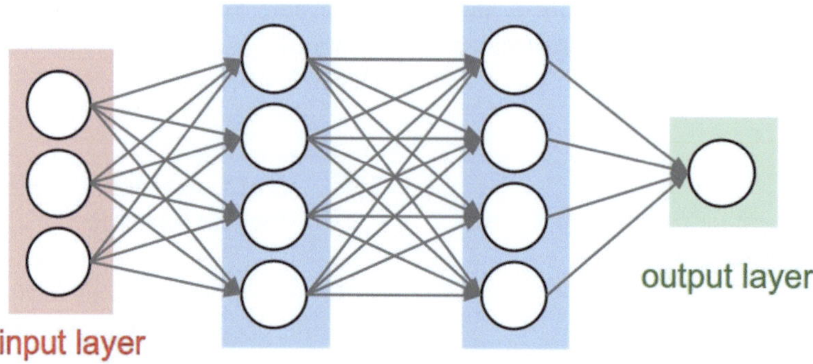

Fig. 5.2 Deep learning model with two hidden layers, an input and an output layer. The more the hidden layers the deeper the computerized learning; the ANN becomes a DNN or deep neural network. The magnitude of input, mathematical computations, speed of analyzing, and quality of outputs depend on the capacity of the hardware available, the architecture and training or conditioning of the ANN, and the infrastructural environment allowing an

undisturbed computation or deep learning process. Deep learning is a class of machine learning algorithms that uses multiple layers to progressively extract higher-level features from the raw input. The magnitude of raw data depends on the operational size or economy of scale of the vein-to-vein process in all its complexity of primary, supportive, and steering processes. (Image credit Radu Racea) processes, steering, supportive, and primary, and their interrelations and interconnections is paramount. Conditioning AI and the needed DNN is actually the hardest part because one needs

1. a large and quality data set (big data);
2. a large amount of computational capacity and power; and
3. to condition the DNN to provide 100% correct quality outcomes.

To condition AI and its DNN one needs to give the inputs from the existing data set and compare the output or outcome with the known historic outcome of the used data set. Since at onset AI and DNN are not yet conditioned, the outcome will be wrong. Going through the whole data set you may create a function that shows how the outputs differ from the real outputs, the so-called Cost Function. Ideally, the Cost Function should be zero. This can be achieved by adjusting the so-called weights of the neurons, which could efficiently be done using a technique called Gradient Descent (Fig. 5.3). This works by changing the weights in small increments after each data set iteration by computing the derivative or gradient of the Cost Function to see in which direction the minimum will be. This is a time-consuming process, which needs a large computational power, where fortunately the changing of the weights is done through Gradient Descent in an automatic way [4].

To minimize the cost function, you need to iterate through your data set many times. This is why you need a large amount of computational power.

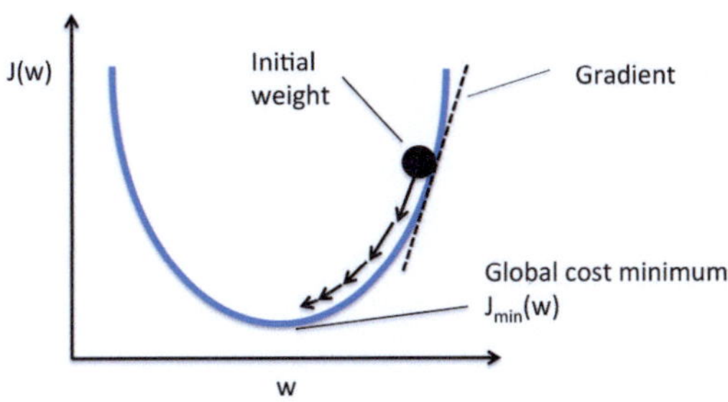

Fig. 5.3 Gradient descent scheme to set the ideal weight [3]. (Image credit Sebastian Raschka)

5.2.2 Statistical Basis of Big Data-Based Predictions

Over the past few years, the amount of data generated is increasing exponentially, increasing the need for good data management practices. The data produced needs to adhere to certain standards to ensure that reliable conclusions are being drawn. As Good Clinical Practice set ground rules for clinical research, Good Manufacturing Practice for medicinal product manufacturing and Good Laboratory Practice for laboratory procedures, so do the FAIR data guidelines offer the baseline for data management.

The importance of good data management is paramount when big data is concerned. As described in the rest of this chapter, AI and big data can provide a valuable source for research and predictions on transfusion practices. Big data requires good data management from the start: big data is created by combining existing datasets, for which data needs to adhere to basic quality standards, the FAIR principles.

5.2.3 Where Are We Now?

Over the past decades the most significant change has been the acceptance of transfusion medicine (TM) as a medical subdiscipline focusing on the patient to determine appropriate therapy. In the early years of the twenty-first century greater emphasis was placed on patient blood management (PBM) [5, 6], hemovigilance [7, 8], cost [9], blood usage, especially red cell transfusion, has decreased over the last two decades, further affected by the SARS-COV-19 pandemic.

As integrated healthcare delivery evolves, efficient suppliers, including blood establishments, have to become LEAN [10] and practice continuous improvement. The prime goal is efficiency embraces stewardship. A blood availability and safety digital footprint driving efficiency, safety, patient satisfaction, and lower cost might be the road to the new Rome and contribute to achieving a number of the 2016–2030 UN

Fig. 5.4 Artificial (AI) structure with Machine Learning (ML) and Deep Learning (DL) elements. AI = mimicking the intelligence or behavioral patterns of humans or any other living entity; ML = a technique by which a computer can "learn" from data without using a complex set of different rules. The approach is mainly based on training a model from data sets; DL = a technique to perform machine learning inspired by our brain's own natural network of neurons. (Image credit Cees Smit Sibinga)

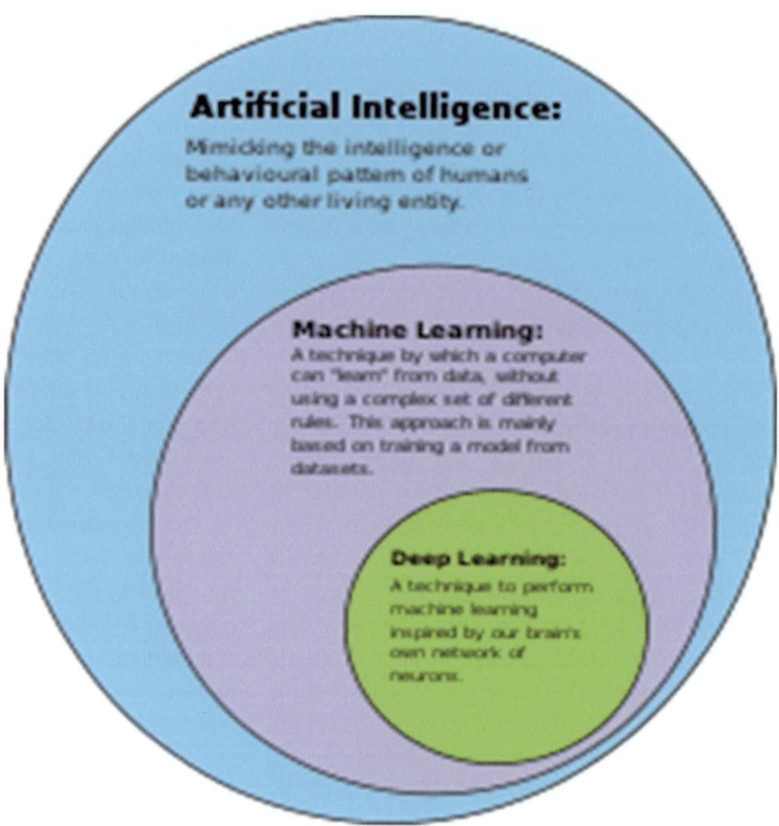

Sustainable Development Goals (SDG) [11] as well as the 2030 UN Universal Health Coverage (UHC) goal [12].

With the rapid development and extension of the use of AI with its Machine Learning and Deep Learning capacities (Fig. 5.4), the approach might help accelerate the bridging of the global gaps existing in the blood supply and clinical use between the more advanced world and the developing world [13].

5.3 FAIR Data Principles: The Statistical Basis of Big Data-Based Predictions

The FAIR data principles were established to set the ground rules for research data management and data quality [14]:

Findable—The creation of big data requires the combination of a large number of smaller datasets, which have been generated under slightly different conditions (e.g., different research groups, countries, hospitals, transfusion services in the context of the current book). Datasets need to be findable in the first place to be combined.

The ultimate goal for findable data is machine-readable data: allowing them to be searchable by machines (and eventually to be combined by using AI tools).

Data can be made findable by uploading the metadata (descriptive information about the dataset) to a data catalogue. National data catalogues are increasingly being used, however, are still not universal practice.

Accessible—After datasets are made findable, they need to be accessible to be able to be combined. That would often mean data being uploaded to a data repository (e.g., xenodo) or being otherwise available to access through institutional procedures, if restrictions apply.

However, when sensitive and/or personal data is concerned, as often clinical transfusion data is, uploading in a repository is not possible unless the dataset is sufficiently anonymized/pseudonymized.

In these cases, the possibility of access to the data can be achieved by federated analysis, such as the Data shield system [15].

Interoperable—Data needs to be interoperable. Interoperability is relevant (and required) on difference levels for the datasets.

When collecting data, the ontologies used to describe the data are of importance. E.g., how is the blood group annotated? If the data is in a spreadsheet, is the column annotation according to standards?

Interoperability also refers to file formats and proprietary software/hardware. Can the data file be accessed using open source software and hardware? Will the data be readable after the software/hardware developer has ceased to exist or the specific laboratory equipment model is discontinued?

The data needs to adhere to a minimum amount of requirements, to be able to be interoperable and reusable. The MIABIS convention sets the minimum amount of required data for biobanks and sample collections [16–19].

Reusable—The ultimate goal of FAIR data is reusability, allowing the data to be used for new research or reanalyzed to confirm the results of the initial study.

In principle, the FAIR data principles are not very different from the GxP quality standards [20]. As in every GxP quality system, FAIR data is assuring quality by ensuring traceability: "not described is not done." Consequently, describing what has happened with the data, how it was collected (for example, experimental conditions and data cleaning procedures) as well as how it was analyzed (including any software/scripts specifically developed for analysis or data cleaning).

The creation of big data is only possible when the datasets to be combined are compatible and used. The data needs to be findable through catalogues, eventually available through repositories and need to be interoperable.

Metadata schemas, clear and unambiguous descriptions of the data, are indispensable for creating large combined data sets [21].

5.4 Machine Learning and Robotics

Machine learning refers to the ability of a machine, usually a computer, to learn using large data sets (big data) instead of using hard coded rules. This type of learning takes great advantage of the processing power and speed of the modern computer generation, able to process easily and fast large data sets (big data). The learning can be done in a supervised (using labelled data sets) or unsupervised way (using data sets with no specified structure). In the blood supply and clinical consumption generally we use specified data sets, so should apply supervised machine learning.

In the advanced world, machine learning has been introduced in the clinical decision-making for transfusion, using data sets and stochastic dynamic programming [22] to predict the need [23–27]. ANNs have been shown to provide an acceptably reliable mechanism to evaluate preoperatively the potential for perioperative transfusion across a wide range of surgical interventions, reducing unnecessary crossmatching and out of stock of blood components for a considerable amount of time during the day [26]. Pretransfusion compatibility testing is also entering AI through machine learning, with the introduction in the late twentieth century of computerized or electronic crossmatching; saving time, reagents, and labor [28, 29]. This is considered as safe as the classic immediate spin crossmatch, provided there are no clinically significant alloantibodies present and there is no ABO discrepancy. Increasingly, robotics has been introduced in almost all manufacturing processes of blood, e.g., automated mixing/weighing machines in blood collection, blood grouping and infectious disease marker testing robots using algorithms, advanced blood cell separators and centrifuges, computerized labelling machines, and machine learning-based cold chain management. There are certainly similar applications in the clinical transfusion setting securing error prevention in decision-making, selection of blood components, wrong blood in tube events and prediction of the need and demand. The use of robots in surgery, both macro and the innovative needle steering, continuum robotics, and medical microrobotics is growing, allowing more focused and precise surgery, minimizing the invasive aspect, and less blood loss and tissue damage.

5.5 Applications in Blood Banking and Transfusion Medicine

AI algorithm approaches are expected to help the blood bank operations throughout the cycle of demand prediction, just-in-time inventory management, and resource allocation. Some major applications of AI/ML are as follows:

5.5.1 Blood Inventory Management

Blood inventory management is one of the areas where AI/ML can make a significant impact. By leveraging historical data, seasonal trends, and other relevant factors, AI/ML algorithms can predict the demand for different blood types more accurately. This enables blood banks and healthcare facilities to maintain optimal inventory levels, reducing wastage and ensuring that they have the required blood types readily available when needed for transfusions and emergencies. AI/ML can be used to predict the demand for different blood types based on historical data, seasonal trends, and other local relevant factors (i.e., incidence and/or prevalence of specific pathologies in a hospital or a region). In theory, these algorithms would enable blood banks to maintain optimal inventory levels, reducing wastage and ensuring that the required blood types are always available when needed. The AI-powered blood inventory management system could continuously analyze data and make real-time predictions, allowing blood banks to respond quickly to fluctuations in demand and supply. AI/ML would also help optimize storage and distribution processes, ultimately ensuring that patients receive the appropriate blood in a timely manner.

In addition to demand prediction, AI/ML can assist in tracking expiration dates and managing the shelf life of blood products, further reducing wastage, and improving the overall efficiency of blood bank operations. This combination of data-driven decision-making and automation enhances the effectiveness of blood inventory management and contributes to better healthcare outcomes.

5.5.2 Donor Matching and Mobilization

AI/ML algorithms can analyze donor data and identify suitable donors based on compatibility with recipients. This helps in efficient donor mobilizing and matching mobilizing efforts. AI/ML can play a crucial role in donor mobilization and matching for various medical procedures, including blood transfusions, organ transplants, and bone marrow donations. Specific examples on how AI/ML can assist in these processes include, but not limited to, donor compatibility analysis and optimal donor mobilization.

Donor compatibility analysis and matching could benefit of AI/ML algorithms by analyzing extensive vein-to-vein clinical transfusion data which include donor and recipient relevant information, including phenotypically and genotypically identified blood type, laboratory data relevant to the past medical history (i.e., hemoglobinopathies, presence of allo- or auto-antibodies in the recipient's plasma, clinical context, diagnosis and therapeutic indications). Traditional methods of donor matching can be time-consuming and may not consider all relevant factors simultaneously. Provided a large pool of blood units is available, AI/ML algorithms can identify potential matches between donors and recipients, ensuring that the most suitable donors are selected for the medical procedure, a process that may be especially relevant in situations of medical emergency.

AI/ML can assist in donor mobilization efforts by identifying individuals who are likely to be compatible donors based on their medical history, genetics, and other clinically relevant factors. This targeted approach ensures that the mobilization process is more effective, saving time and resources for both healthcare providers and potential donors. Applications in this context may be especially relevant in the context of hematopoietic stem cell transplantation in which worldwide databases of histocompatibility typed unrelated donors are available, resulting in improved accuracy of donor matching, and potential improved outcomes.

5.5.3 Blood Quality Monitoring

AI/ML can be used to analyze data from various blood tests to assess the biochemical, biophysical, and morphological characteristics of blood cell products. Blood cell degradation during storage is an objective fact that has been extensively studied during the last 40 years. Unfortunately, classical approaches to determine blood product degradation and define thresholds of acceptability are subjective and labor-intensive. Machine learning algorithms can overcome the limitations of conventional RBC assessment methods. ML algorithms can specifically target specific tasks directly associated with blood product quality outcomes, including infectious disease testing data collection and analysis, analysis of cell contaminants (e.g., leukocyte content) or through the use of trained neural networks to extract chronological progressions of morphological or biochemical changes in stored blood cells during storage (the so-called storage lesion), without human input [30] and using continuous improvement protocols to improve accuracy and performance.

5.5.4 Predictive Maintenance in Blood and Blood Product Collection and Storage

Refrigerators and storage systems are critical for maintaining the integrity and quality of blood products, and any equipment failure or malfunction can lead to clinically relevant consequences on safety. AI can help predict equipment failures or maintenance needs in blood bank refrigerators and storage systems. By identifying potential issues in advance, blood establishments can prevent equipment breakdowns and ensure the integ-

rity of blood storage. Specific areas in which AI can help is accurate and timely collection of data related with sensors, and monitoring systems can be installed in blood bank refrigerators and storage units to collect various data points, such as temperature, humidity, door openings, and compressor performance. This data can be continuously recorded and stored for analysis and individualized to specific blood products by using radio-frequency identification (RFID) systems [31, 32].

AI/ML algorithms then can analyze stored data to identify patterns and anomalies that may indicate potential issues with the equipment. By processing historical data, the algorithms can learn the normal behavior of the refrigerators, detect any deviations from the expected performance, and establish models to predict when specific equipment components may fail or when maintenance is needed based on early warning signs and performance trends. Predictive maintenance enables blood banks and transfusion services to optimize their maintenance schedules, and instead of following a fixed calendar-based approach, the AI-driven system can prioritize maintenance tasks based on actual equipment condition, which can lead to prolonged equipment longevity, cost savings, reduced downtime, and improvements of overall cost-effectiveness.

5.5.5 Routing and Transportation Optimization

In connection with the use of RFID technologies of tracking mentioned above, AI can optimize the routing and transportation of blood units from collection centers to the manufacturing facility, distribution depots, and then to hospitals. This ensures timely delivery while minimizing transportation costs.

AI can significantly improve the efficiency of blood transportation by optimizing routing and logistics. Blood units need to be transported quickly, safely, and with maintaining special temperatures from collection centers to the central blood establishment and then to hospitals where they are required. AI can identify ways to generate real-time traffic analysis including weather conditions and road closures to identify the most efficient and fastest routes for blood transportation, allowing geospatial optimization (optimizing the number of trips, minimizing the distance traveled, and balancing the workload among different transportation vehicles), adaptation to changing conditions, prediction of potential congestion or delays, and selection of the optimal plan for delivery including most appropriate routes and types of vehicle needed for transportation by including dynamic approaches to dispatching vehicles based on real-time information on demand and adjusting routes to accommodate and optimize routes in a short notice. This may be especially important in situations of natural or man-made disasters, where blood supply is critical. AI can quickly adjust routing and prioritize deliveries to ensure that blood units reach affected areas promptly. Shipment optimization also includes approaches to demand forecasting potentially reducing stat orders and reduce costs by proactively allocating blood units based on anticipated needs, reducing the probability of shortages or overstocking in hospital-based transfusion services. Altogether, the expectation is that the use of AI could reduce transportation costs, including fuel expenses and maintenance, reducing carbon footprint and traffic jamming.

By leveraging AI for routing and transportation optimization, blood establishments can enhance their ability to meet the urgent needs of hospitals and patients while efficiently managing resources. This results in better distribution of blood units, reduced transportation costs, and improved patient care during emergencies and routine operations.

5.5.6 Data Analytics and Decision Support

Blood establishments generate vast amounts of data, including information on blood inventory levels, donor demographics, donation frequency, donor deferral, donor medical history, patient transfusion records, and medical history. AI algorithms can efficiently process and analyze this data, providing a comprehensive view of blood establishment operations. These algorithms are expected to boost areas in which our blood centers remain distant from generating satisfactory outcomes. These areas include the following:

(a) Donor engagement in which AI can segment donors based on various characteristics, such as donation frequency, age, or location. These insights are expected to help blood establishments tailor their donor engagement strategies, improving donor retention and mobilization efforts;

(b) Usage patterns and demand prediction in which AI is expected to identify usage patterns previously unidentified, by analyzing historical data and seasonal trends, enabling them to maintain optimal inventory levels and avoid shortages or wastage;

(c) Quality control in which AI can monitor and analyze data related to blood quality, storage conditions, and testing results, aimed to meet the required safety and regulatory/accreditation standards.

To achieve these goals, AI/ML can specifically provide a major service to blood establishments: resource allocation, operational efficiency, identification of trends and insight generation, and real-time decision support from analysis and interpretation of critical metrics.

5.5.7 Automated Documentation and Record-Keeping

AI can streamline the process of maintaining accurate records of blood donations, inventory, and donor information, potentially resulting in a reduction in the administrative burden on staff and maintaining a comprehensive and up-to-date, accurate database.

Specific processes that can benefit from the use of AI are the following:

(a) Data entry and validation: Done by extracting relevant information from multiple databases, such as donor forms, laboratory reports, and other records, and validate the accuracy and completeness of the data, reducing the likelihood of errors and inconsistencies;

(b) Application of natural language processing (NLP): Here NLP technologies enable AI systems to understand and process unstructured text data, such as donor notes or medical histories, potentially allowing a better categorization and analysis of donor information;

(c) Data integration: AI can integrate data from donor and laboratory databases, creating a comprehensive and unified database and making it easier for staff to access relevant information in real time;

(d) Data cleaning and deduplication: AI can identify and resolve duplicate or redundant records, ensuring a clean and accurate database, helping blood center electronic systems to maintain accurate databases, eliminating confusion sources, and reducing the risk of errors in decision-making;

(e) Record maintenance and updates: AI can automatically update donor records, inventory levels, and other information in real time by interconnecting existing databases in blood banks among themselves, and potentially with other public health services databases;

(f) Personalized donor communications: AI can analyze donor preferences and engagement history to automate personalized communication, such as appointment reminders, thank-you messages, and updates on blood drives;

(g) Analytics and reporting: AI-driven analytics tools can generate comprehensive reports and dashboards, offering insights into operational key performance indicators (KPIs), supporting informed decision-making and strategic planning; and

(h) Compliance and privacy: AI logical language may be built to ensure compliance with data privacy regulations through the implementation of secure access controls and anonymization of sensitive information as needed.

5.5.8 Blood Group Prediction and Electronic Crossmatch

AI/ML algorithms can predict a donor's blood group based on genetic data, and this can be especially useful in identifying donors with rare blood types. These algorithms will also be useful for tissue/organ typing. The process would include first genetic/genomic data collection, an area in which modern blood banking has already advanced significantly and has been used extensively in the potential matching of blood donors and chronically transfused recipients. Genetic/genomic data is then to be curated through a preprocessing algorithm in charge of extracting relevant features and preparing it for training the machine learning model. An ML model is to be trained in pattern recognition in the genetic/genomic data, and once the model is trained, the AI/ML algorithm would be designed to predict the blood donor's or patient's group. These iterative processes may be extremely helpful to identify rare blood types for which current reagents may not be sensitive and/or specific enough to detect. Based on the use of large, national or international databases, ML-based blood group prediction could, at least in theory, help identify individuals with rare blood types more efficiently and indirectly increase the effective donor pool and enhance blood transfusion matching effectiveness, potentially reducing the risk of alloimmunization and transfusion-related adverse events.

It is important to highlight that while ML can be a powerful tool for predicting blood groups, it is not a replacement for traditional blood group testing methods. Confirmatory tests and verification in a laboratory setting are and will still be necessary to ensure accuracy and safety.

5.5.9 Personalized Medicine

Personalized medicine is a rapidly emerging field that leverages AI to analyze individual patient data and tailor treatment plans for better outcomes. In the context of blood typing and other relevant factors, AI can be instrumental in optimizing personalized transfusion treatment plans. AI algorithms can assist data integration by analyzing a wide range of patient datasets, including blood type, genetic information, medical history, lifestyle factors, and treatment responses, and integrating and processing this data into comprehensive patient profiles, enabling a more holistic understanding of each patient's unique health needs. In addition, AI can identify correlations and patterns in patient data, helping healthcare professionals make more informed treatment decisions and predict how patients may respond to specific treatments based on their unique characteristics, including blood type, potentially improving therapeutic outcomes and minimizing trial-and-error approaches.

AI algorithms can also identify personalized dosage approaches in which blood component\ transfusion volumes can be estimated based not only on hematological parameters and body weight/height/gender but also on other patient medical characteristics (for instance, cardiac or renal function parameters, metabolism parameters, drug interactions, pediatrics, and neonatology). AI-driven risk assessment models can identify potential risks and alert towards the use of proactive, targeted interventions and preventive measures. As new patient data becomes available and treatment outcomes are recorded, AI systems can continually learn and improve their predictive capabilities, leading to better personalized treatment recommendations over time. Finally, AI can facilitate personalized patient education by tailoring health information and treatment plans to individual patients, increasing patient engagement into the blood transfusion process.

5.6 Technical and Human Resources

5.6.1 Metrics and Key Performance Indicators (KPIs) in Blood Banking and Transfusion Medicine: Prediction and Interpretation Algorithms

Metrics and KPIs play a crucial role in ensuring the efficient and safe management of the blood supply chain. These concepts help blood establishments and healthcare organizations assess their performance, identify areas for improvement, and make data-driven decisions to enhance patient care. Understanding and defining the right metrics and KPIs are crucial steps to the successful application of AI/ML and implement decision-making approaches based on analytics and predictions generated by such algorithms.

Metrics are quantitative measurements used to track and assess the performance, effectiveness, and/or productivity of a particular aspect of blood banking management. These are usually specific, measurable, achievable, relevant, and time-bound (SMART) indicators that provide insights into the organization's performance [33]. Metrics can range from simple counts, percentages, and averages to more complex calculations based on the context and goals of the business. These metrics include but are not limited to the following:

- **Blood inventory levels**: Tracking the quantity of blood units available in inventory to ensure an adequate and safe supply for patient needs.
- **Blood utilization rate**: Measuring the rate at which blood units are utilized or issued to patients, indicating the demand for blood products.
- **Turnaround time**: Measuring the time it takes to process and distribute blood units from the time of donation to the time of issue, to assess efficiency.
- **Wastage rate**: Calculating the percentage of blood units that are discarded or wasted due to expiration or other reasons, to optimize inventory management.
- **Inventory days on hand:** Inventory days on hand is a critical metric in blood banking that indicates the number of days' worth of blood and blood product units available in inventory.
- **Out of stock incidents:** Measuring and monitoring the frequency of out-of-stock incidents is a critical aspect of blood banking to assess the availability and accessibility of specific blood types and products.
- **Adverse events**: Monitoring and recording adverse events related to blood transfusions to ensure patient safety and quality assurance.

KPIs are a subset of metrics that are deemed critical for evaluating the success of a blood establishment in achieving its objectives. Metrics parameters intend to measure effectiveness in:

1. **Blood component and blood type inventory levels**: Tracking blood inventory levels is a critical aspect of blood banking and hospital transfusion services to ensure a sufficient and safe supply of blood components for patients in need. A well-maintained blood inventory ensures that blood products/components are readily available when needed, reducing the risk of delays or shortages during critical medical procedures. Blood establishments must manage a diverse range of blood types and products, including red blood cells, platelets, plasma, and other specialized components like cryoprecipitate. This has been critically important during the COVID-19 pandemic time and immediately after the pandemic, when many hospitals could not access timely blood inventories to treat their patients in need. By continuous monitoring inventory levels, blood establishment and hospital transfusion services can optimize their operations and prevent understocking and define needs for appeal campaigns of blood donation, or more importantly, public awareness campaigns. This is especially important in trauma level 1 healthcare centers and nationally in identifying redundant systems aimed to support emergency preparedness. To track blood inventory levels effectively, blood establishments use specialized software systems that provide real-time visibility into inventory status, expiration dates, and product availability. These systems often integrate with other components of the blood supply chain, such as blood donation management, QC testing, and distribution, to ensure a seamless flow of blood products from donors to patients.

2. **Blood utilization rate.** Blood utilization rate is crucial to determine the following:

    (a) **Resource optimization**: Monitoring the Blood Utilization Rate (BUR) allows blood establishments to ensure that they are efficiently using their blood inventory. It helps prevent overstocking or understocking, which can lead to wastage or shortages, respectively.

    (b) **Cost-efficiency**: Efficient utilization of blood products can lead to cost savings for the healthcare facility. Minimizing wastage and maximizing use mean that the available resources are being put to the best possible use.

    (c) **Patient safety**: By understanding the demand for blood products through the utilization rate, blood establishments can ensure that they have an adequate supply to meet the needs of patients promptly. This supports timely and safe medical procedures that require supportive blood transfusions.

    (d) **Emergency preparedness**: A clear understanding of the utilization rate helps in planning for emergency and disaster situations where there might be a sudden surge in demand for blood products, ensuring preparedness for such scenarios.

    The Blood Utilization Rate is typically calculated as follows: Blood Utilization Rate (%) = (Number of Blood Units Issued/Total Number of Blood Units in Inventory) × 100.

    A high utilization rate indicates that a significant proportion of the blood inventory is being used, which can be a positive sign of efficiency and responsiveness to patient needs. However, very high utilization rates can also indicate a constant demand for blood and may require close monitoring to avoid potential shortages. On the other hand, a low utilization rate may suggest that blood units are not being used as effectively as they could be. This could be due to overstocking, which can lead to wastage if blood units expire before being used. Blood establishments and hospital transfusion services can use the Blood Utilization Rate to make data-driven decisions, such as adjusting inventory levels based on clinical demand patterns, optimizing blood product distribution, and planning blood drives to target specific blood types or products that are in higher demand. AI can help generate prediction models of clinical blood utilization that help anticipate logistical and resource demands to support specific seasonal shortages.

3. **Turnaround time**: Measuring the time it takes to process and distribute blood units from the time of donation to the time of issue, to assess efficiency. Turnaround time is a critical metric in blood banking that measures the efficiency of the process from the time of blood donation to the time the blood units are ready for issue to patients. This metric provides valuable insights into the speed and effectiveness of blood manufacturing operations, which directly impacts patient care and safety. The Turnaround Time is important for the following reasons:

   (a) **Patient safety**: Rapid turnaround time ensures that blood units are available promptly when needed for emergency transfusions or critical medical procedures. Quick access to blood products is crucial in situations where time is of essence.

   (b) **Optimal resource utilization**: Efficient turnaround time allows blood establishments to streamline their processes and maximize the utilization of available resources, including human resources, blood collections, QC testing, and inventory management.

   (c) **Blood product quality**: A shorter turnaround time means that blood products spend less time in storage, reducing the risk of deterioration and improving the quality and shelf life of the blood and blood product units.

   (d) **Patient satisfaction**: Faster turnaround time leads to improved patient satisfaction, as healthcare providers can provide timely transfusions, resulting in better patient outcomes.

   Turnaround time in blood banking is typically calculated as the time difference between the moment of blood donation (or collection) and the time the blood unit is ready for issue to patients. It typically includes the following: (a) Blood Donation Time (time of collection from donor); (b) Blood Testing and Processing Time (time taken to test and process the blood unit); (c) Inventory Storage Time (time the blood unit spends in storage awaiting issue); and (d) Time to issue to Patients (time until the blood or blood component unit is issued to the patient).

   The Turnaround Time can be calculated as the sum of the time spent in each stage: Turnaround Time = Time (Issue to Patients) − Time (Blood Donation). A shorter turnaround time suggests that the blood bank's operations are efficient, and blood units are quickly processed, QC tested, and made available for issue to patients. This indicates a well-managed blood supply chain with minimal delays. On the other hand, a longer turnaround time may signal potential bottlenecks or inefficiencies in the blood banking process. Identifying and addressing these issues can lead to improvements in overall efficiency and patient care.

   Identification and prediction of turnaround time data can help identify areas for improvement and streamline blood establishment operations. By analyzing the time spent in each stage of the blood banking process, they can pinpoint specific areas that require attention and optimization. Automation, improved testing processes (economy of scale), and better inventory management through AI/ML algorithms are current or future strategies that can help reduce turnaround time and enhance the overall efficiency of the blood banking system.

4. **Wastage rate**: Calculating the percentage of blood and blood product units that are discarded or wasted due to expiration or other reasons, to optimize inventory management. The Wastage Rate is a critical metric in blood banking that measures the percentage of blood units that are discarded or wasted due to various reasons, such as expiration, damage, or

other factors. Monitoring the wastage rate is essential for blood establishments and hospital transfusion services to optimize their inventory management and minimize unnecessary losses. Analysis and prediction of the wastage rate helps improve the following:

(a) **Cost-efficiency:** Minimizing blood wastage reduces unnecessary costs associated with the acquisition, QC testing, processing, and storage of blood units. Efficient inventory management helps allocate resources more effectively.

(b) **Resource conservation:** By reducing wastage, blood establishments can preserve a precious and limited resource. Blood donation is a voluntary process, and minimizing wastage ensures that every donated unit is put to good use.

(c) **Patient access:** Lower wastage rates mean more blood and blood product units are available for patients in need. This is particularly crucial for rare blood types or during times of increased demand.

(d) **Regulatory compliance:** Many regulatory agencies have guidelines on blood or blood product wastage. Maintaining a low wastage rate helps blood establishments adhere to these standards and ensure compliance with best practices.

The wastage rate is calculated as the percentage of blood and blood product units that are discarded or wasted within a specific period, usually a month, quarter of a year or a year, relative to the total number of blood and blood product units that were available during that period. The typical calculation is as follows: Wastage Rate (%) = (Number of Discarded Blood and Blood Product Units/Total Number of Blood and Blood Product Units Available) × 100.

A lower wastage rate indicates efficient inventory management and responsible use of blood and blood product units, reflecting a well-organized blood establishment that is closely managing expiration dates and minimizing losses due to damage or other factors. A higher wastage rate may indicate potential areas for improvement, such as enhancing inventory management practices, reviewing handling procedures, or optimizing blood product distribution.

By analyzing the wastage rate data and AI/ML algorithms, blood establishments can identify historical trends and patterns that lead to blood wastage and anticipate situations of potential wastage. This information can help them implement strategies to forecast anticipated wastage seasons through anticipation on blood donation programs, adapted inventory rotation and product handling, as well as closer monitoring of expiration dates. Implementing measures to minimize wastage can lead to cost savings, increased availability of blood and blood product units for patients, and a more sustainable and efficient blood banking system.

5. **Inventory days on hand**: Inventory Days on Hand is a critical metric in blood banking that indicates the number of days' worth of blood and blood product units available in inventory. It is a key measure of the organization's preparedness to handle emergencies, unexpected surges in demand, and fluctuations in blood supply. This KPI provides insight into how well a blood establishment is equipped to handle unforeseen emergencies or critical situations where there is an urgent demand for blood products; defines the blood supply chain and the level of adequate inventory needed to prevent shortages and ensure a consistent supply for routine and emergency medical sustainability of procedures; allows an adequate Inventory. Days on Hand allows blood establishments to respond quickly to fluctuations in demand, seasonal variations, or special events where blood supply requirements may change; helps minimize the wastage of blood and blood product units due to expiration; and together, an adequate number of Inventory Days on Hand reduces the risk of delays in critical clinical transfusion interventions, improving patient safety and care.

The number of Inventory Days on Hand is calculated by dividing the total number of blood units in inventory by the average daily usage of blood units, as follows: Inventory Days on Hand = Total Number of Blood and Blood Product Units in Inventory/Average Daily Usage of Blood and Blood Product Units.

A higher number of Inventory Days on Hand indicates a more significant reserve of blood and blood product units in inventory, which can be beneficial during emergencies or when faced with sudden surges in demand. However, excessively high inventory levels may lead to an increased risk of wastage due to units expiring before being used. Conversely, a lower number of Inventory Days on Hand could suggest a more efficient inventory management system but may increase the risk of shortages during times of increased demand. Blood establishments can use the Inventory Days on Hand metric to strike a balance between having sufficient blood and blood product units in reserve for emergencies and avoiding excessive wastage. Analyzing historical data and implementing AI/ML algorithms can help blood establishments forecast usage and optimize their inventory levels based on seasonal variations, expected demand, and any upcoming events that might impact blood usage.

6. **Out-of-Stock Incidents**: Measuring and monitoring the frequency of Out-of-Stock Incidents is a critical aspect of blood banking to assess the availability and accessibility of specific blood types and products. Out-of-Stock Incidents occur when the required blood types or products are not available in the inventory when needed, which can have significant implications for patient care and safety. The availability of specific blood types and products is crucial for patients requiring blood transfusions. Any situation of Out-of-Stock Incidents can lead to delays in critical medical interventions, compromising patient care and safety; it helps blood establishments assess their preparedness to handle emergencies and unexpected surges in demand for spe-

cific blood types, especially rare or uncommon ones; it provides warnings on the blood establishment's inventory management practices and through adjustments in inventory levels, this information can be used to adjust inventory levels, improve blood product rotation, and optimize supply chain logistics, improve quality of service, and comply with regulatory requirements.

Analyzing Out-of-Stock Incidents data helps blood establishments identify trends, patterns, and root causes of the unavailability of specific blood types or blood products. Its historical and trending analysis through AI/ML algorithms may identify patterns of repeated Out-of-Stock Incidents that were unappreciated by the blood establishment staff, helping optimize inventory management, and ensure a reliable and timely supply of blood products for patients in need.

7. **Adverse event (AE) rate**: Monitoring and recording AE related to blood transfusions is a critical aspect of blood banking to ensure patient safety and maintain quality control and assurance. AEs can occur during or after a blood transfusion, and keeping track of such incidents helps blood establishments and hospital transfusion services identify potential risks, improve safety protocols, and take appropriate measures to prevent similar events in the future. Monitoring AEs are important for the following reasons:

    (a) **Patient safety**: The primary concern in blood transfusion is patient safety. Monitoring adverse events allows blood establishments and hospital transfusion services to promptly identify any potential risks and take corrective actions to ensure the safety of patients receiving blood products.

    (b) **Quality control**: Recording adverse events is a crucial part of quality control and assurance, and risk management in blood banking. Analyzing the data can help identify trends, patterns, and root causes of adverse events, leading to process improvements and better patient outcomes.

(c) **Regulatory compliance**: Many regulatory bodies have strict guidelines regarding the reporting and management of adverse events in blood transfusions. Blood establishments and hospital transfusion services must adhere to these regulations to maintain their license and accreditation and ensure public trust.

(d) **Continuous Improvement**: Learning from adverse events enables blood establishments to implement continuous improvement strategies, enhance teaching and training programs, and update standard operating procedures to minimize the risk of future incidents.

(e) **Public confidence**: Transparently reporting and addressing adverse events foster public confidence in the blood system. This helps in maintaining a steady supply of blood through voluntary non-remunerated blood donations.

When adverse events occur during or after a blood transfusion, they need to be recorded in a systematic manner. This involves collecting relevant information about the patient, the blood product, and the circumstances surrounding the transfusion. The data may include details about the patient's medical history, the blood product's compatibility, the transfusion process, and any symptoms or reactions observed.

8. **Compliance with regulations**: Compliance with regulations is a critical aspect of blood banking operations to ensure the safety and quality of blood products. Blood establishments must adhere to various regulatory guidelines and standards set forth by national and international health authorities and their legislative framework. This compliance affects the following:

(a) **Licensing and accreditation**: Blood establishments and hospital transfusion services must obtain the necessary licenses and certifications to operate legally. In a growing number of countries, blood establishments need to be accredited by relevant regulatory bodies or accrediting agencies to ensure they meet specific quality and safety standards.

(b) **Good manufacturing practices (GMP)**: Blood banking facilities must adhere to current GMP guidelines, which outline the necessary procedures and controls for the design, monitoring, and maintenance of blood products' manufacturing processes.

(c) **Quality management systems (QMS)**: Implementing a robust QMS with its five key elements is essential to ensure that all processes, documentation, and personnel adhere to quality and technical standards and regulatory requirements.

(d) **Adherence to blood collection standards**: Proper collection of blood from healthy donors is crucial to ensure the safety of both donors and recipients. Compliance with guidelines for donor screening, blood collection techniques, and sample handling is necessary, preventing wrong blood in tube events.

(e) **Testing and screening protocols**: Blood establishments must implement appropriate testing and screening protocols for blood samples to detect infectious disease agents, genetic disorders, and other potential risks. These protocols are often mandated by national regulatory authorities (NRAs).

(f) **Storage and transportation requirements**: Blood products need to be stored and transported under specific conditions to maintain their integrity and prevent contamination. Adhering to regulatory guidelines ensures the proper handling of blood products throughout the supply chain.

(g) **Adverse event reporting**: Blood establishments and hospital transfusion services must report adverse events or reactions related to blood transfusions promptly, hemovigilance. This information is vital for monitoring and improving the safety of blood products.

(h) **Record-keeping and documentation**: Maintaining accurate and complete records of all blood banking activities, from donor screening to product distribution and transfusion, is crucial for compliance and traceability.

(i) **Regular audits and inspections**: Regulatory agencies may conduct regular audits and inspections to assess blood banking facilities' compliance with regulations. Blood establishments should be prepared for these assessments and demonstrate their adherence to guidelines and standards.

(j) **Continuous training and education**: Blood establishment and hospital transfusion service personnel should receive ongoing education and training to stay updated with the latest regulatory changes and best practices.

(k) **Risk management**: Implementing a risk management program helps identify and mitigate potential risks in blood banking operations and clinical transfusion practices, ensuring a safer environment for donors and recipients.

Monitoring compliance with regulations involves ongoing evaluation and improvement of processes and procedures. Regular internal audits and assessments using AI can help identify areas of noncompliance and ensure that corrective actions are taken promptly. By prioritizing compliance, blood establishments and hospital transfusion services can maintain public trust and uphold their critical role in providing safe and reliable blood products for patients in need.

5.7 Barriers to the Implementation of AI in Blood Banking and Clinical Transfusion Medicine

In April 2021, the European Commission proposed the first EU regulatory framework for AI [34]. It says that AI systems that can be used in different applications are analyzed and classified according to the risk they pose to users. The different risk levels will mean generation of specific regulatory frameworks. In June 2023, the European Parliament established the first regulation on AI in which all health care applications falling under the European Union's product safety legislation as well as all AI systems related to biometric identification and categorization of natural persons, access to and enjoyment of essential private services and public services and benefits were considered of "high risk."

The classification of high risk derives from several barriers and concerns that need to be addressed to ensure safe and ethical implementation of these technologies. Some of the major barriers include the following:

1. **Injuries and errors**: One of the primary risks associated with AI/ML in healthcare is the potential for errors, which could lead to patient injuries or adverse health outcomes. It is essential to thoroughly test and validate AI systems to minimize these risks and ensure that they are reliable and accurate in their predictions and recommendations.

2. **Data availability**: AI/ML algorithms require large amounts of high-quality data to be trained effectively. However, healthcare data are often fragmented across various systems, making it challenging to gather comprehensive, quality, and representative datasets. This fragmentation increases the risk of errors and limits the effectiveness of AI applications.

3. **Privacy concerns**: The collection and use of large datasets for AI training raise privacy concerns for patients. Developers must ensure that patient data is handled securely and in compliance with national privacy regulations. Patients should be informed about how their data will be used and have the option to opt out if they are uncomfortable with data sharing.

4. **Bias and Inequality**: AI systems can inherit biases present in the data they are trained on, leading to unequal treatment for certain patient populations. Developers must address bias in AI algorithms and ensure that they are fair and equitable across diverse patient groups.

5. **Professional realignment**: The widespread adoption of AI in healthcare may lead to shifts in medical professions, potentially reducing the human knowledge and expertise needed to catch and correct AI errors. Medical education and training must adapt to incorporate AI technology and equip healthcare providers to work effectively with AI systems.

To address these barriers and concerns, several possible solutions can be implemented:

1. **Data generation and availability**: Governments can play a role in providing infrastructural resources for quality data gathering and setting standards for electronic health records. Initiatives like All of Us in the United States [35] and BioBank in the U.K [36]. aim to collect comprehensive health data while ensuring effective privacy safeguards.

2. **Quality oversight**: Regulatory bodies like the Food and Drug Administration (FDA) in the USA can oversee the quality and safety of AI healthcare products. However, additional oversight efforts may be required for AI systems that fall outside the FDA's purview, such as back-end business or resource-allocation AI.

3. **Provider engagement and education**: Undergraduate and post-graduate medical education should include training to prepare healthcare providers to evaluate and interpret AI systems effectively. This will help them understand AI's role in healthcare including transfusion medicine and make informed decisions based on AI-generated recommendations.

4. **Ethical guidelines and standards**: Developing and adhering to comprehensive ethical guidelines and standards for AI implementation in healthcare and transfusion medicine can ensure that AI systems prioritize patient safety, privacy, and fairness.

5. **Regulatory framework**: As demonstrated by the European Commission's proposed regulatory framework for AI, establishing regulations specific to AI in healthcare including clinical transfusion medicine can help address risks and set standards for safety and privacy [34]. The European Parliament's regulation on AI in healthcare is a step towards achieving this.

By addressing these barriers and implementing appropriate solutions, healthcare organizations can leverage the full potential of AI/ML algorithms in blood management, while upholding patient safety, privacy, and ethical considerations. It is important to note that while AI/ML can greatly enhance donor matching and mobilization efforts, ethical considerations, privacy concerns, and regulatory guidelines must be carefully addressed. Ensuring the responsible use of data and protecting donor privacy is paramount in implementing AI-driven donor–patient matching systems.

By integrating AI and ML technologies into blood establishment management, organizations can enhance their operational efficiency, improve blood safety, and ultimately save more lives. It is crucial to ensure that these technologies are ethically implemented, protecting patient privacy, and adhering to regulatory guidelines surrounding blood donations and healthcare data.

5.8 Conclusion and Recommendations

Artificial Intelligence (AI) increasingly invades and concurs clinical medicine and transfusion medicine. Both the big data deep learning as well as the robotics and machine learning applications rapidly find their way in medicine. Problem, however, remains the need for quality and uniform or FAIR data, allowing precise and clean statistics and the creation of reliable and repeatable algorithms to be used. These shall be findable, accurate, interoperational, and reusable (FAIR). Stepwise application started in the blood establishments manufacturing blood products, contributing to more reliable safety and manufacturing procedures. This is followed by the clinical settings increasing patient safety, preventing mishaps, interpreting algorithms, and supporting prediction for which technical and human resources are needed, e.g., blood inventory levels, blood utilization rates (epidemiology of blood use), wastage rates, and adverse events.

There are, however, a number of barriers to the implementation of AI in transfusion medicine, both the manufacturing and the clinical use that need to be addressed to ensure safe and ethical implementation. These include among others injuries and errors or mishaps, FAIR data availability, ethical and privacy concerns, and a uniform professional alignment.

5.8.1 Recommendations

Several possible solutions have appeared to address these barriers:

- data generation and availability (FAIR data and a well-organized documentation system),
- a solid quality oversight (quality system and quality system management),
- provider engagement and continuous education (teaching and training),
- uniform ethical guidelines and standards (code of ethics),
- and not in the least, a competent regulatory framework (stewardship and governance).

That is only possible when the blood system at national level is well designed and based on a clear and patient (consumer)-oriented policy and a legislative and regulatory framework based on the principles of transfusion medic.

References

1. Smit Sibinga CT. Artificial intelligence in transfusion medicine and its impact on the quality concept. Transfus Apher Sci. 2020;59:103021.
2. van der Tuuk Adriani WP, Smit Sibinga CT. The pyramid model as a structured way of quality management. As J Transfus Sci. 2008;2(1):6–8.
3. Raicea R. Want to know how deep learning works? Here's a quick guide for everyone. 2017. https://medium.com/freecode-camp/want-to-know-how-deep-learning-works-heres-aquick-guide-for-everyone-1aedeca88076.
4. Du S, Lee J, Li H, Wang L, Zhai X. Gradient descent finds global minima of deep neural networks. In: International conference on machine learning. 2019. pp. 1675–85.
5. Frank SM, Waters JH. Patient blood management: multidisciplinary approaches to optimize care. Bethesda, MD: AABB Press; 2018.
6. Althoff FC, Neb H, Herrmann E, et al. Multimodal patient blood management program based on a three pillar strategy: a systematic review and meta-analysis. Ann Surg. 2019;269(5):794–804.
7. Smit Sibinga CT. Haemovigilance: an approach to risk management and control. In: Risk management in blood transfusion: the virtue of reality. Boston, MA: Springer; 1999.
8. De Vries RR, Faber JC, editors. Hemovigilance: an effective tool for improving transfusion safety. Hoboken, NJ: Wiley; 2012.
9. Abdella Y, Mataria A, Sajwani F, Pourfathollah AA, Sibinga CT. Ensuring effective financing of national blood systems in support of universal health coverage. EMHJ. 2019;25:371–3.
10. Mann D. Creating a lean culture: tools to sustain lean conversions. Productivity Press; 2005.
11. United Nations. Sustainable development goals. New York: United Nations; 2015. https://sustainabledevelopment.un.org/?menu=1300.
12. WHO Universal Health Coverage. http://www.who.int/universal_health_coverage/en/.
13. Smit Sibinga CT, Abdella YE, Seghatchian J. Poor economics-transforming challenges in transfusion medicine and science into opportunities. Transfus Apher Sci. 2020;59(2):102752.
14. Wilkinson MD, Dumontier M, Aalbersberg IJ, et al. The FAIR guiding principles for scientific data management and stewardship. Sci Data. 2016;2016(3):160018. https://doi.org/10.1038/sdata.2016.18. Erratum in: Sci Data. 2019 Mar 19;6(1):6.
15. Gaye A, Marcon Y, Isaeva J, LaFlamme P, et al. (2014). DataSHIELD: taking the analysis to the data, not the data to the analysis. Int J Epidemiol. 2014;43(6):1929–44. https://doi.org/10.1093/ije/dyu188. Epub Sept 26.
16. Eklund N, Andrianarisoa NH, van Enckevort E, et al. Extending the minimum information about BIobank data sharing terminology to describe samples, sample donors, and events. Biopreserv Biobank. 2020;18(3):155–64. https://doi.org/10.1089/bio.2019.0129. Epub 2020 Apr 17.
17. Merino-Martinez R, Norlin L, van Enckevort D, et al. Toward global Biobank integration by implementation of the minimum information about BIobank data sharing (MIABIS 2.0 Core). Biopreserv Biobank. 2016;2016:298–306. https://doi.org/10.1089/bio.2015.0070.
18. BBMRI-ERIC/miabis. https://github.com/BBMRI-ERIC/miabis.
19. Allysonlister. FAIRsharing.org: MIABIS CORE 2.0. 2022. https://doi.org/10.25504/FAIRsharing.20fed3. Accessed 26 Sept 2023.
20. Understanding GxP Regulations for Healthcare. https://www.cleardata.com/platform-services/gxp-

regulations/#:~:text=GxP%20is%20a%20collection%20of,%2C%20control%2C%20storage%20and%20distribution. Accessed 28 Sept 2023.

21. van der Velde KJ, Singh G, Kaliyaperumal R, et al. FAIR genomes metadata schema promoting next generation sequencing data reuse in Dutch healthcare and research. Sci Data. 2020;9:169. https://doi.org/10.1038/s41597-022-01265-x.

22. Bellman R. Dynamic programming. Princeton: Princeton University Press; 1957.

23. Haijema R, van Dijk N, van der Wal J, Smit Sibinga CT. Blood platelet production with breaks: optimization by SDP and simulation. Int J Prod Econ. 2009;121(2):464–73.

24. Van Dijk N, Haijema R, Van Der Wal J, Smit Sibinga CT. Blood platelet production: a novel approach for practical optimization. Transfusion. 2009;49(3):411–20.

25. Smit Sibinga CT. Artificial intelligence and the future of transfusion medicine. Neurosci Chron. 2021;2(2):25–30.

26. Levi R, Carli F, Arévalo AR, et al. Artificial intelligencebased prediction of transfusion in the intensive care unit in patients with gastrointestinal bleeding. BMJ Health Care Inform. 2021;28(1):e100245.

27. Walczak S, Velanovich V. Prediction of perioperative transfusions using an artificial neural network. PLoS One. 2020;15(2):e0229450.

28. Mitterecker A, Hofmann A, Trentino KM, et al. Machine learning–based prediction of transfusion. Transfusion. 2020;60(9):1977–86.

29. Guidance for Industry. Computerized Crossmatch (computerized analysis of the compatibility between the donor's cell type and the recipient's serum or plasma type). Washington, DC: US Dept. Health and Human Services, Food and Drug Administration, Center for Biologics Evaluation and Research; 2011. https://www.fda.gov/media/80857/download.

30. Doan M, Sebastian JA, Caicedo JC, et al. Objective assessment of stored blood quality by deep learning. Proc Natl Acad Sci USA. 2020;117(35):21381–90. https://doi.org/10.1073/pnas.2001227117. Epub 2020 Aug 24.

31. Knels R. Radio frequency identification (RFID): an experience in transfusion medicine. ISBT Sci Ser. 2006;1:238–41. https://doi.org/10.1111/j.1751-2824.2006.00039.x.

32. Holmberg J. The digital footprint in transfusion medicine and the potential for vein-to-vein management. Medic Labor Observer. 2018. https://www.mlo-online.com/information-technology/automation/article/13017030/the-digital-footprint-in-transfusion-medicine-and-the-potential-for-veintovein-management.

33. How to set SMART goals. https://www.kvk.nl/en/starting/how-to-set-smart-goals/. Accessed 1 Oct 2023.

34. EU AI Act: first regulation on artificial intelligence. 2023. https://www.europarl.europa.eu/news/en/headlines/society/20230601STO93804/eu-ai-act-first-regulation-on-artificial-intelligence?&at_campaign=20226-Digital&at_medium=Google_Ads&at_platform=Search&at_creation=RSA&at_goal=TR_G&at_advertiser=Webcomm&at_audience=ai%20eu&at_topic=Artificial_intelligence_Act&at_location=DK&gclid=CjwKCAjwseSoBhBXEiwA9iZtxnp8EGsVIroDG4PBFSBtnxocylrN-e2KN8h9Dsc0lOvvc1G_8pyfpBoCwh8QAvD_BwE.

35. What does AI mean to All of Us. https://www.bcg.com/capabilities/artificial-intelligence/ai-for-business-society-individuals. Accessed 1 Oct 2023.

36. UK BioBank. https://www.ukbiobank.ac.uk/. Accessed 1 Oct 2023.

The Importance of Digital Footprinting in Clinical Transfusion Medicine

Jerry A. Holmberg and Cees Th. Smit Sibinga

6.1 Introduction

6.1.1 Definition

A vein-to-vein (V2V) digital footprint extending from donor qualifications to blood product manufacturing and testing to distribution and finally to the patient receiving the blood components is needed to ensure both blood safety and availability in today's transfusion medicine (TM) services. Such digital footprints are robust records of all processes and data management of decisions and transactions associated with a transfusion event starting with donor mobilization. Once these events are captured and stored digitally in the cloud, the digital data footprint is potentially retained forever with the opportunity to evaluate "big data" for activities such as hemovigilance, process improvement, or clinical research using artificial intelligence (AI) [1–3].

A V2V digital footprint within transfusion medicine requires the presence of operational, well-analyzed, and well-documented primary and supportive processes, which may be facilitated by AI [4]. This spans the entire V2V blood chain including donor motivation, mobilization, and selection as well as data obtained during the collection process, manufacturing, testing, storage, and distribution of blood. Checks and balances among expected needs and supplies, as well as automation and robotic elements for greater efficiency, are envisioned in blood separation, quality testing using robotics, quarantine release, final labeling, storage, and distribution (cold chain logistics) to treatment centers. Quality and consistency of data determine the outcome of AI processes whether machine or deep learning. The processes in TM may have subprocesses and procedures to transform an input into an output. These primary processes are supported by secondary or supportive processes such as human resources, finance and administration, quality management, education, purchase of consumables and equipment, information and communication technology (ICT), public awareness campaigning, emergency preparedness, waste management, maintenance and repair, and domestic services. The supportive processes are elementary to the primary process operations and management and decisive for the implementation of the strategies initiated by the third layer or steering processes. The steering processes are based on the mission and vision statements or policies of the healthcare institution and blood establishment. Decisive in this chain or flow is data management—interrelated and interconnected documentation and archiving to achieve consistency, statistical evaluation of outcomes,

J. A. Holmberg
Maven Blood Consultants, Denver, NC, USA

C. T. Smit Sibinga (✉)
International Development of Transfusion Medicine, University of Groningen and IQM Consulting, Zuidhorn, Netherlands

© The Author(s), under exclusive license to Springer Nature Switzerland AG 2024
C. T. Smit Sibinga, Y. E. Abdella (eds.), *Clinical Use of Blood*,
https://doi.org/10.1007/978-3-031-67332-0_6

benchmarking and prediction of volume and changes in each of these processes and procedures [5].

None of these processes is stand-alone, they are all interconnected, forming a complex network of data and information from patient treatment outcomes to community awareness, motivation, and mobilization of potential voluntary donors. Today, data and documents are mostly stored in hardware and operated through hardware networks with appropriate restrictions (e.g., donor confidentiality, test results), to protect against unauthorized access.

A TM digital footprint helps management determine the data and access for other health care professionals, either in the same or other departments, for more comprehensive care. Industry acceptance of a blood availability and safety digital footprint depends on an integrated healthcare system and governance, through an open architecture based on common international standards of data elements for all essential V2V processes and procedures.

Blood product management, its labeling, and the blood samples for safety testing currently rely on human interaction or bar code data collection. However, the digital footprint could be improved by automating current manual processes with minimal human manual touch and errors through Radio Frequency Identification (RFID). For example, incorporating RFID into the digital footprint could automate processes to manage quality control, tubes for centrifugation, or whole blood delivered to a centrifuge and blood separator. While still in its infancy, RFID is estimated to reach a market size of $830 million (USD) with a compound annual growth rate (CAGR) of over 17.8% [6]. A digital footprint could even predict and streamline donor mobilization based on historical blood ordering and establish logistics for hospital inventory and delivery efficiency, ensuring the right blood at the right time to the correct location and patient; all while reducing technical manpower and human errors—identification, interpretation, transcription, documentation, and archiving [7].

When digitalizing TM from V2V, one needs to be aware of the risks e.g., cyber criminality, continuity, insufficient knowledge and skills, exchange of information, and access restriction. Originally, access to the internet could be gained only through a computer, but that has changed dramatically [8]. Now one can get access using smartphones, tablets, and some game consoles. Increasingly, other devices are becoming internet-linked as connectivity is extended to everyday objects such as televisions, radios, watches, and cars.

6.1.2 Concept of the V2V Chain and the Internet of Things (IoT)

The Internet of Things (IoT) is the interconnection of devices with sensors, data entry, and process transaction software to exchange data or processing checks through the connectivity of the internet. This requires well-designed interfaces to ensure safe firewall settings and access through a common software language.

The IoT promises a technological revolution. However, to work well, these "things" need to speak the same language and have common data elements [9]. Industry, however, tends to adopt common standards only after jostling between rival producers with competing systems. It was so for trains, televisions, video recorders, mobile phones, and the internet itself. It will be the same for connected devices, especially medical devices in the health care and blood system practices, as most personnel carry smartphones and cyber criminality has become a real challenge.

The V2V blood transfusion chain has two distinctly different operational and managerial parts: clinical or consumption and collection and manufacturing of the voluntarily donated source material [10].

The clinical or consumption part has three major primary processes:

1. **bedside**—diagnosis, indication, decision, informed consent, and ordering;
2. **laboratory/blood transfusion service**—immunohematology (ABO/RhD, alloantibodies), extended phenotype and genomic testing, selection of blood component, and compatibility testing;
3. **bedside**—patient identification, vital signs, matching with the prepared blood component,

transfusion, observation of outcome, and data collection of potential adverse events, and feedback to transfusion and donor services.

The collection and manufacturing of the source material, human blood, has six major aspects:

1. **community**: awareness and targeted motivation and mobilization;
2. **donor selection**: history and physical examination;
3. **blood collection**: identification, collection devices such as tubes and collection bags, mix-weighers, collection time, and data capture of any donor adverse events;
4. **processing**: manufacturing or separation of the source material into its cellular components and plasma and/or cryoprecipitate;
5. **laboratory/quality control**: testing of each collected unit for blood group and Transfusion Transmissible Infection agents or markers (TTIA), product specifications;
6. **storage and distribution**: quarantine release and labeling, inventory management, cold chain for storage, and transport/distribution to the hospitals; and feedback on product quality and disposition.

In the clinical transfusion and blood establishment, there are numerous procedures, medical devices, sensors, operators, and disposable supplies used in clinical transfusion medicine and in the manufacturing of blood products that may need to be digitalized and entered for process control. This may include data elements generated through primary, routine, and repetitive steps. The quality of these routinely generated data is of critical importance and therefore needs standardization and a commitment to ensure consistency of process operations and quality data generation.

6.2 Digital Footprint: Principles

No discussion on principles of the digital footprint in TM should occur outside the framework of the Quality System. This framework, as defined by AABB (Association for the Advancement of Blood and Biotherapies) and EDQM (European Directorate for the Quality of Medicine and HealthCare), includes key elements [11, 12]. These elements below apply also to TM digital footprint:

- Organization,
- Resources,
- Equipment,
- Suppliers and customer issues,
- Process control,
- Documents and records,
- Deviations, nonconformances, and adverse events,
- Assessments: internal and external,
- Process improvement through corrective action, and
- Facilities and safety.

The scope of this chapter is not a deep dive into all the key elements of the Quality System. Rather, it is to ensure that these elements are discussed in understanding the principles of the digital footprint in TM.

6.2.1 Transparency of Data

All data, including initial data or contributing data, must be transparent to the entire process for traceability and trackability (T&T) in the V2V chain. Transparency of data is the ability to access transfusion or product data related to a specific unit regardless of where it is located as well as the confidence that the data are true and come from official sources. This is critically important in TM procedures in current good manufacturing practices (cGMP) of blood component preparation and the clinical transfusion practice. This requires transparency of all material involved in the transfusion process that potentially could compromise the purity, potency, and efficacy of the blood product to achieve anticipated outcomes in the recipient patient (clinical efficacy). In order to accomplish this, there must be agreements and safeguards built into the data collection, storage, and access to ensure patient confidentiality and data integrity.

6.2.2 Firewalls and Cybersecurity

Protection from unauthorized access, use, manipulation, and disclosure of electronic data and assets is a principle of healthcare cybersecurity [13]. The goal of healthcare cybersecurity is confidentiality, integrity, and availability of data. HIMSS (Information and Management Systems Society) calls these goals the "CIA triad" [14, 15].

As with other databases, the TM digital footprint and associated databases must have sufficient gatekeepers which monitor access, that is, traffic both in and out of the data network. Software firewalls usually are simpler and protect a single computer while hardware firewalls protect the entire network and are more sophisticated to configure. This type of gatekeeping not only monitors but also blocks suspicious, malicious, and nefarious attacks. No country is exempt from these cyberattacks. A vendor agnostic survey of 5600 ICT professionals in 31 countries in 2022 indicated 66% of healthcare organizations surveyed experienced ransomware attacks in 2021, a rate up from 34% in 2020 [16]. Ransoms to recover encrypted data were more likely to be healthcare at 61% compared to a global average of 46%.

Precautionary steps should be implemented to identify potential risks and migration procedures to protect against cyber criminality and attacks [17]:

1. Risk assessment—draw and maintain a complete list of vulnerabilities in the ICT system;
2. Mitigation of risk:
    (a) Select a safe organization and settings of equipment to enhance efficient firewalls for software and internet connections;
    (b) Regular/frequent updates, and make sure there are functioning security updates in place;
    (c) Restrict access to data, software, and hardware, e.g., through frequently changing access codes and passwords;
    (d) Prevent virus infections and other malware using e.g., antivirus programs, personnel attitudes, the safety of app downloading, restricted software installation;
    (e) Ongoing audits to continually assess both the risks and the mitigations.

6.2.3 Data Integrity

Principles of data integrity ensure its accuracy including completeness and consistency as well as its security. Much of the management of data integrity relies on rules and internal processes that dictate data entry, storage, access, and transfer [18]. Some regulatory authorities, such as the European Union's General Data Protection Regulation (GDPR) went into effect in May 2018 and sets a legal framework for the use of personal data both within the European Union and outside [19]. The GDPR enables the general public to have more control over the collection, handling, and distribution of personal data. Types of data integrity errors include:

- **Human errors** are the most common type of risk to data integrity. This error occurs when processes or procedures are not followed or when data is incorrectly entered, duplicated, or deleted.
- **Transfer errors** can also compromise data integrity when data cannot be recognized and transferred from one database to another. For example, a transfer error can occur when data is incorrectly added to a destination table but was not in a relational database source table.
- **Bugs and viruses** from spyware and malware have the potential to alter, add, delete or unauthorized access or malicious use.
- **Compromised hardware** is a potential threat to data. Problems such as computer crashes or other failures can compromise hardware and ultimately data by altering, deleting, or rendering the data unusable.

6.3 Risk Management

As with any disruptive technology or a change in process, there will be a certain amount of risk that will be identified and assessed for severity. If

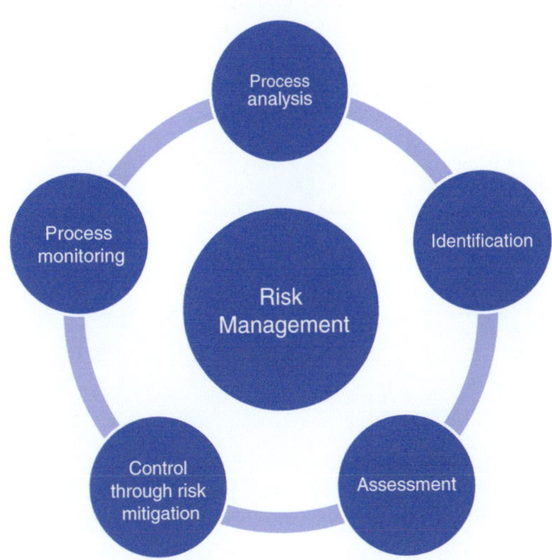

Fig. 6.1 Risk management process with analysis of the process, identification of the potential risk, assessment of the risk, control through mitigation, and monitoring the risk within the process

there is risk of an error, data corruption, or even a compromise to data integrity, a risk analysis with appropriate mitigations must be implemented (Fig. 6.1). To reduce the risk of error, logical data-driven decision steps must be well thought out, validated, and verified to ensure that errors are not made. Since humans are vulnerable to fatigue and distractions, computerization of the clinical transfusion medicine process with continuous checks is valuable to minimize potential risks. The future digital footprint must be highly reliant on computerized data collection, analysis, and decisions. This along with the automation of repetitive steps will in the future minimize human intervention.

6.3.1 Data Accountability

In the Quality System, an assessment step is fundamental to monitoring the entire process. The same is true in vein-to-vein TM digitalization. Of prime importance is not only an audit of the process and cybersecurity firewalls but also the accountability of the data. The principle of internal database audits is key to tracking the processes and systems for accountability of data, intrusion detection, protocol violations or overrides, performance, application errors, event reconstruction, and problem-solving. Reviews of internal audit trails as well as external reviews provide an opportunity for process improvement as well as ensuring data accountability.

6.4 The V2V Transfusion and Blood Consumption Chain

The concept of V2V digital footprint in TM tries to capture an entire system of meeting the patient's needs while ensuring that the appropriate donor is mobilized to provide the necessary blood component whether it is whole blood, red cells, plasma, platelets, plasma-derived medicinal products (PDMP), or biotherapies. This may be achieved efficiently if the blood collection is co-located within the same medical institution with common ICT systems. Unfortunately, in many locations in the world, the clinical care within the hospital is not physically or digitally connected with the blood collection establishment.

6.4.1 Data Transparency

Overcoming the traditional segregation of roles between clinicians and TM specialists as well as the data they share commonly has the potential of being resolved through data transparency of the TM digital footprint. In some organizations, the blood establishments are co-located or under the hospital organization. However, in some organizations, the blood establishment may be administered by the National Blood System or blood establishment outside the hospital organization. This separation of services needed for managed care and legal responsibility (product liability versus patient rights protection) emphasizes the critical communication requirements between clinical services, hospital TM, and either internal or external blood establishment (Fig. 6.2).

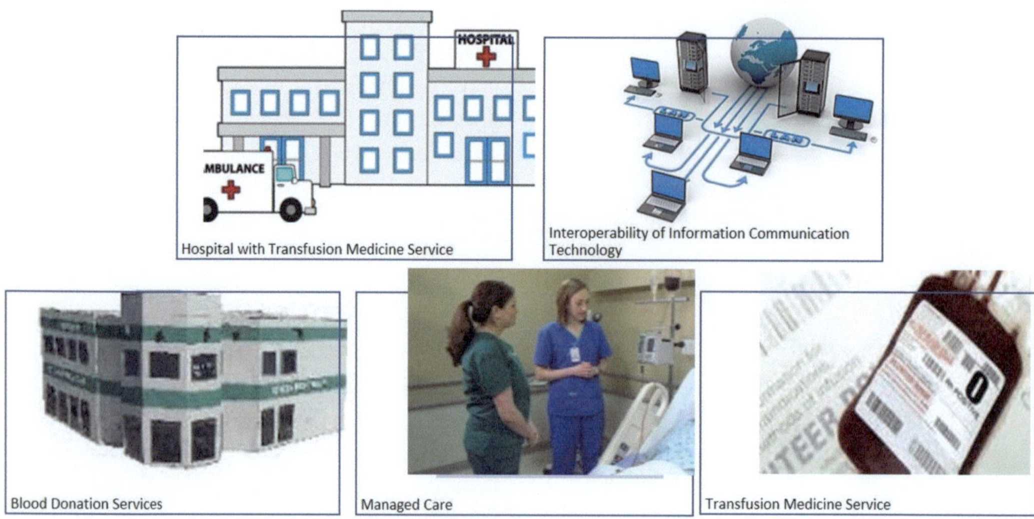

Fig. 6.2 Interoperability between TM and managed care requires data transparency between hospitals and blood donation services, without affecting legal responsibilities

Today's medical advances rely on precision medicine for the treatment of patients. Red cell phenotyping or even genotyping in the chronically transfused patient may need to be ordered early in the diagnosis of the disease to facilitate appropriate and compatible blood components. Such advances in blood genotyping have been extremely helpful in chronically transfused individuals suffering with Sickle Cell Disease, (SCD) Thalassemia β, or myeloproliferative disorders [20–23]. Patients undergoing advanced immunotherapy for treatment of certain cancers may interfere with transfusion medicine testing such as in the case of anti-CD38 and anti-CD47 therapies [24–28]. Communication of these special needs highlights the role that transparent data can have in obtaining the best blood components for the patient.

6.4.2 Process Map of V2V

To those unfamiliar with TM, the processes and procedures may be overwhelming with many steps from obtaining blood or blood products from a suitable donor to transfusion of those products needs of a patient. Figure 6.3 is a high-level overview of the various steps involved. As one can imagine the amount of data collected at each step either by oral questions or data gener-

ated by medical devices or laboratory instruments require collection, storage, and access to data for appropriate decision-making on the suitability of the blood product collected. The upper pathway in Fig. 6.3 identifies the steps for donor screening and collection including history and physical as well as diagnostic testing blood groups and infectious disease agents screening. The lower pathway in Fig. 6.3 identifies the steps required within the Transfusion Service to obtain the blood and ensure compatibility with the patient. The clinical pathway also includes the hand-off of the blood component from the Transfusion Service to the nursing staff for administration and monitoring.

As one can imagine with the many steps in Fig. 6.3 the digital footprint is expansive and data must be assessable for the management of not only blood critical for the patient but also critical for all the logistical supplies needed in the entire process. The ordering and management of supplies, disposable kits, test kits, quality control and labels must be managed to ensure there are no stock outages.

6.4.2.1 Supportive Digital Processes through Standard Data Elements

Over the last three decades, the transfusion community has been working globally to standardize

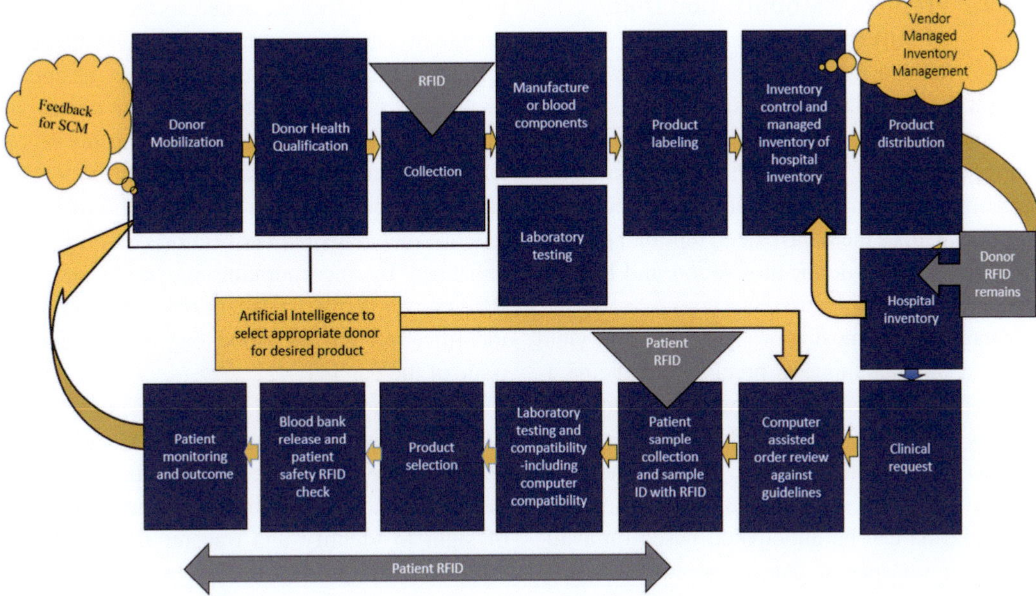

Fig. 6.3 Integrated pathways of steps involved in TM incorporating the procurement and the transfusion process. Data collected at every step either by manual data entry or medical device/instrument entry is critical to the decision of the blood product's suitability for transfusion. The diagram highlights the role that supply chain management (SCM) and vendor-managed inventory (VMI) have in the process

data elements to enhance interoperability through the digital footprint. This was first recognized as a global need during the first Gulf War in the early 1990s when North Atlantic Treaty Organization (NATO) members realized that data elements were not standardized such as donor identification numbers, blood product identification numbers, collection establishment identities, blood groups, anticoagulant, and associated product characteristics. In addition to the lack of standardization, the previous acceptable coding system for blood products was antiquated. Seeing this need, the blood community joined together to form a working group of the International Society of Blood Transfusion (ISBT). Outgrowing the working group, the International Committee on Commonality in Blood Bank Automation (ICCBBA) was formed [29]. ICCBBA is a global not-for-profit organization, a "non-state actor that manages, develops, and licenses ISBT 128, the international information standard for the terminology, coding, and labeling of medical products of human origin."

Supportive commonality through ISBT 128 established by ICCBBA is more than a digital identifier; it established commonality within TM. While bar codes using ISBT 128 code are only one means of transferring data elements from an item into an established ICT system, other formats exist. Formats such as RFID, using ISBT 128 common elements have advancing capabilities for progress, improving processes, reducing errors, and minimizing the human resource requirement within TM [30, 31].

6.4.2.2 Supportive Digital Process of Supply Chain Management

In TM the blood establishment provides the supply side for biological products while the clinical side creates the demand for such products. The digital footprint of supportive data through supply chain management (SCM) is key in managing the balance of supply and demand. Data either generated or created based on clinical demand subsequently drives the starting point for the entire V2V process ensuring that the appropriate donors with specific attributes (i.e., phenotype or genotype) are mobilized. Normalization of the data over time can, and through AI modeling, SCM can support difficult times in TM such as holidays, weekends, and emergencies [32].

6.4.2.3 Predictive Mobilization Data of Suitable Donor

Using available data, SCM, integrated with AI, can set the mobilization objectives to ensure the appropriate blood donor is mobilized at the most appropriate time. This predictive mobilization supported by the digital footprint is becoming more critical, as there have been reported generational changes in donor motivation and barriers to donation [33].

Obtaining the most appropriate donor to yield the best product supports precision medicine as TM expands in clinical treatments. For example, antigen negative red cell donors or specific Human Leukocyte Antigen (HLA) negative platelet donors or even immunoglobulin A deficient plasma can be anticipated based on availability of transparent data between the supply side and demand side of the digital footprint. This may mean reaching out to specific ethnic or racial panels or pools to mobilize the best donors [34–36].

6.4.2.4 Donor History and Physical Data

The introduction and regulatory approval of the uniform donor history questionnaire in many countries has added to the digital footprint in blood establishments [37–40]. In addition to the data obtained via the donor interview whether with an interviewer or through the computer, other measurements are also collected to determine the physical ability of donors. Such measurements as the hemoglobin, hematocrit, blood pressure, temperature, and pulse rate can all be electronically performed and data transferred into the donor's digital profile. Data based on the acceptance or deferral of donors can easily be deidentified and provide the blood establishment with critical health information on various donor populations. Such data can potentially improve the public health of the donor community served if it is extracted and confidentially available.

6.4.2.5 Collection and Process Control by RFID

It is at the collection stage that the greatest control can be achieved for T&T using lot numbers and expiration dates of disposable products (i.e., blood bags, test tubes, apheresis kits) linked to the facility, donor, personnel, and associated collected products. Data elements such as the doctor or medical personnel determining the donor eligibility, the donor assistant collecting the blood and testing samples as well as time the collection started can be tracked to ensure quality parameters are met. This data collection can be greatly enhanced by incorporating bar code entry or RFID such as employee identification, and tubing identification on the blood bag at the time of issue of the bag [41, 42].

The technology of RFID may also be referred to as automatic identification and data capture (AIDC). Like barcoding, RFID has the advantage that it does not have to be within the optical line of sight to identify and transfer data. Through radio waves, the object is identified and data associated with the object is transmitted to the reader or interrogator via radio waves. The interrogator converts the radio waves into usable data, which can be passed through a communication interface into a host computer system (Fig. 6.4).

Characteristics of various radio frequencies used in RFID are compared in Table 6.1. Low frequency (LF) has a very short reading range and minimal sensitivity to interference. In contrast, ultra-high frequency (UHF) has the largest range but is highly sensitive to interference. The high frequency (HF) is the range that is used most with medical products, per International Organization for Standardization (ISO 20909:2019(en)) standards for medical the radio frequency is 13.56 KHz, but asset management may be varied based on the read range [43].

The RFID tag associated with the object can be either passive or active. If it is active, the tag requires a battery source to continuously generate data for transmission back to the reader. The most common type of RFID tags is passive since they can be smaller and less expensive. With passive tags, the RFID reader/interrogator powers up the tag to activate radio waves that represent the data associated with the passive tag located on the object.

For blood products, the RFID is usually passive with the tag protected under the product label. This is important since passive RFID tags are only energized when activated by the inter-

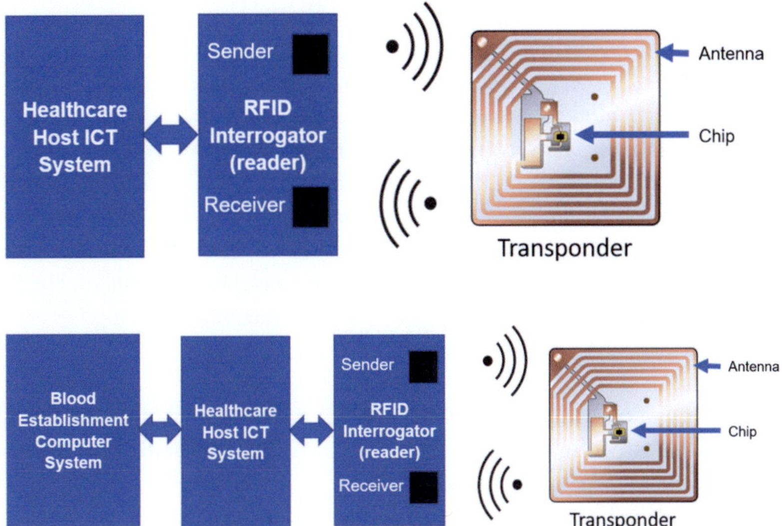

Fig. 6.4 The upper figure is an example of an RFID reader and a passive high-frequency (HF) tag. RFID reader (interrogator) sends a radio signal to the transponder and is picked up by a tag antenna. The transponder is "woke-up" and the chip sends requested data back to the interrogator via the antenna. The healthcare host ICT system can seek requests and obtain feedback through system interfaces. The lower figure is an example of integration into the blood supply affording the benefit of complete transparency

Table 6.1 Difference in bands and ranges used in RFID

Band	Band range	Read range	Read rate	Interference
Low frequency (LF)	30–300 KHz	10 cm	Slow	Low sensitivity
High frequency (HF)	3–30 KHz	10 cm to 1 m	Moderate	Moderate sensitivity
Ultra-high frequency (UHF)	300 MHz to 3 GHZ	12 m	Fast	High sensitivity

rogator. Further testing and laboratory data would be needed to demonstrate that active RFID would not warm the blood products such as represented by hemolysis or denaturation of proteins.

6.4.2.6 Donor Testing and Component Preparation with RFID

It is at this stage of donor sample testing and component preparation that processes and data must be orchestrated and all data generated or even associated with the testing must be captured. In the futuristic laboratory and blood processing laboratory, samples enter the system through delivery systems such as conveyor belts or other sample delivery mechanisms to the testing or component processing equipment. Decisions, based on validated and verified algorithms, decide on the appropriate sample and its condition (i.e., serum or anticoagulant plasma, whole blood mixed specimen, temperature,

detection of hemolysis). Test results are likewise scrutinized through verified and validated algorithms to determine acceptability.

Like the processing of donor sample testing, the futuristic component department obtains donated whole blood through automated delivery systems. Algorithms based on patient needs and donor blood group characteristics direct the blood product to stages such as centrifugation, leukocyte reduction, platelet preparation (buffy coat or platelet-rich plasma), plasma separation, and cryoprecipitate production. An example of the detail of optimized algorithms is the optimized use of O Rh D negative, antigen-negative red cells, and even restriction of plasma from multiparous women to reduce the risk of Transfusion Related Acute Lung Injury (TRALI). All these processes based on quality parameters and algorithms are monitored and data is captured via RFID for cGMP T&T.

6.4.2.7 Quarantine Release and Inventory Labeling with RFID

In the modern and futuristic blood donor service, culmination of required testing and component manufacturing must result in a decision of donor and components' acceptability, unacceptability, or need for further testing. Data collected through means such as RFID on the donor, products, and quality control, can be evaluated with computerized logic for critical decisions. The numerous data and process control checks are unlimited compared to time-consuming human evaluation. The digital footprint logically directs the product into the labeling process or a quarantine hold. If the data passes the established logic, the final process of labeling can occur. Labeling has always been a critical control step in blood processing. Before the implementation of a comprehensive digital footprint, this process would have required at least two human full-time equivalents to perform.

6.4.2.8 Digital Footprint in Inventory Management

One can quickly imagine how the digital footprint with the aid of RFID can assist in filling inventory requirements for shipment to the healthcare facility. The data management of blood products can assist in selecting the appropriate blood product to meet the hospital's specific order while at the same time tracking costs for reimbursement. Extending the digital footprint with the RFID, inventory management can locate the exact location of the blood product in refrigerators, room temperature agitators, and freezers. Extending the digital footprint of available blood products to the clinical facility can greatly assist the blood service in vendor-managed inventory management (VMI). This helps the blood service have product visibility to know where the product location is and its final disposition. If the product is available and not used in one clinical facility, it can be relocated to another clinical facility.

6.5 Digital Footprint in Clinical Transfusion Medicine

The digital footprint especially with the use of RFID cannot stop at the blood establishment but must be extended into the clinical transfusion practice at the healthcare facility. The donor testing results, including even special testings such as phenotyping and genotype, must remain embedded in the RFID and transported into the hospital blood bank information system for optimum effectiveness and decision-making.

As illustrated in Fig. 6.5, there are many steps and decision points within clinical transfusion medicine. Along with these process steps, data and decision steps must be collected within the patient's record. The digital footprint of decision algorithms and data is essential to be captured and is critical to transfusion-associated risk prevention. This includes positive identification of the patient and samples associated with the patient as well as the chain of custody of the sample and the blood product.

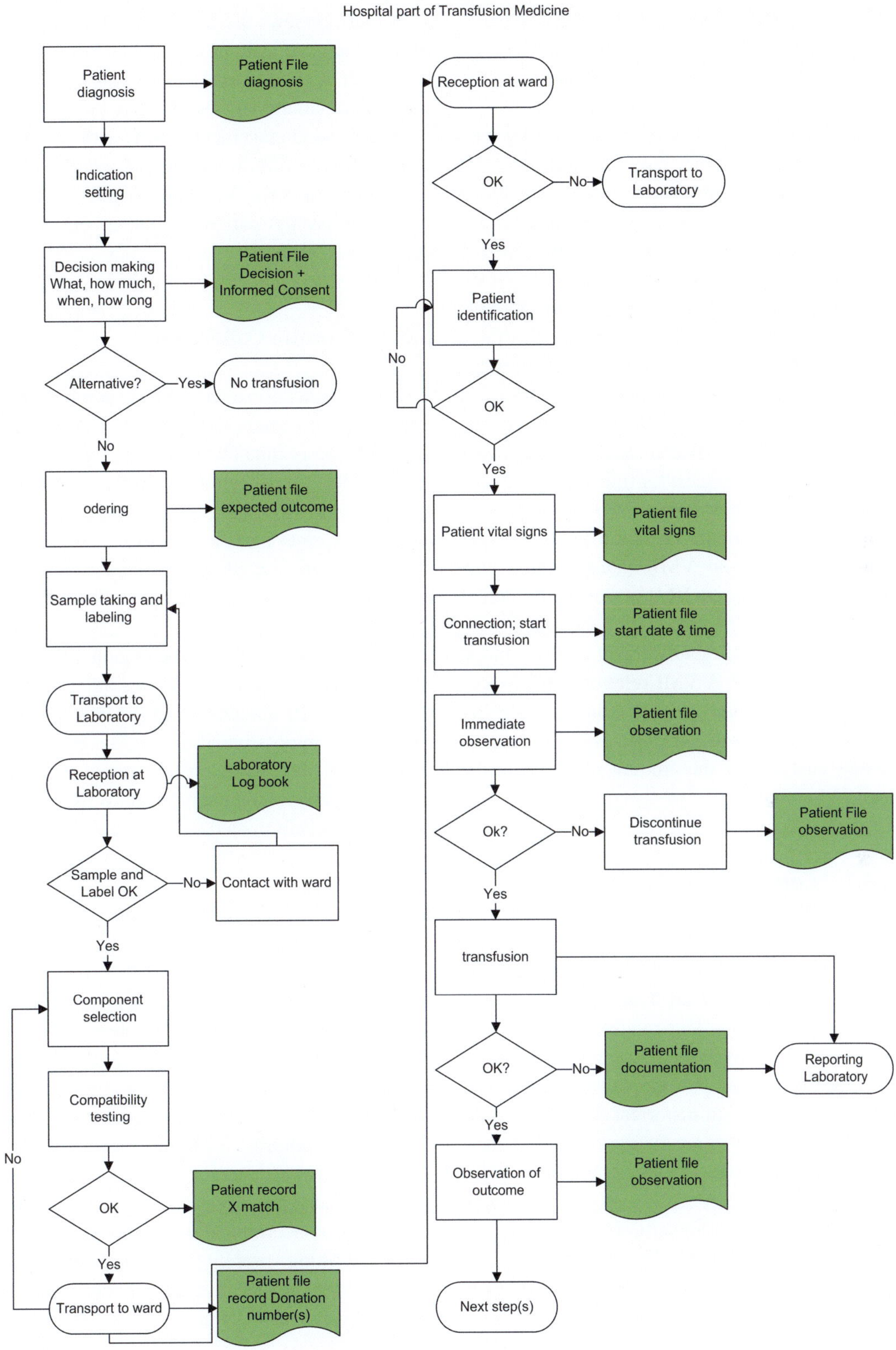

Hospital part of Transfusion Medicine

Patient diagnosis → Patient File diagnosis

Indication setting

Decision making What, how much, when, how long → Patient File Decision + Informed Consent

Alternative? —Yes→ No transfusion

No

odering → Patient file expected outcome

Sample taking and labeling

Transport to Laboratory

Reception at Laboratory → Laboratory Log book

Sample and Label OK —No→ Contact with ward

Yes

Component selection

Compatibility testing

OK → Patient record X match

Yes / No

Transport to ward → Patient file record Donation number(s)

Reception at ward

OK —No→ Transport to Laboratory

Yes

Patient identification

No

OK

Yes

Patient vital signs → Patient file vital signs

Connection; start transfusion → Patient file start date & time

Immediate observation → Patient file observation

Ok? —No→ Discontinue transfusion → Patient File observation

Yes

transfusion

OK? —No→ Patient file documentation → Reporting Laboratory

Yes

Observation of outcome → Patient file observation

Next step(s)

Fig. 6.5 Process flow chart of physician request and TM review. The left side of the flow chart represents processes related to TM and the technical staff of the medical facility's blood bank. The right-hand side identifies the healthcare providers' processes and data collection on the clinical ward

6.6 Vendor-Managed Inventory (VMI) Management in Transfusion Medicine

As mentioned previously the use of a fully integrated digital footprint with the assistance of RFID provides transparency between the blood establishment and clinical TM. Since RFID can have product/donor-associated data embedded, it is a redundant step between the blood establishment digital footprint and acts as a transportable interface with the clinical facility. As illustrated in Fig. 6.4, when incorporating this into the healthcare ICT host system and permission granted, the blood establishment can query the healthcare ICT host system and manage inventory as well as see request for impending patients. This facilitates fulfilling the TM ordering process and locating the optimum blood product, especially assisting with VMI management if the product is not utilized. VMI places the burden of accountability of the product and the cost associated with the blood establishment until the blood product is utilized. A VMI relationship between blood establishment and healthcare facility requires trust and security permissions in order to ensure visibility of the amount of blood in the total TM system.

6.6.1 Computer-Assisted Order Review

In the modern TM service, computer-assisted reviews are implemented based on verified and validated algorithms. This reduces the time commitment of the TM specialist in reviewing clinical requests and can provide valuable additional information based on historical data. For example, in a review of a transfusion-dependent therapy (TDT) for a Thalassemia patient, there might be evidence of the effectiveness of maintaining the hemoglobin level higher to reduce ineffective erythropoiesis (IE) [44]. The electronic review might identify previous alloantibodies or even the patient's red cell genotype.

If these reviews are based on validated algorithms, they can even prompt the ordering clinician with recommended justifications such as supportive laboratory testing and can support patient blood management (PBM) with initiation of supportive consultations for alternative therapy. Once an order has been justified, digital action can prompt patient sample collection and appropriate testing.

6.6.2 Sample Collection

Patient identification at the time of sample collection is also a critical point in the TM process. Wrong blood in tube (WBIT) or wrong name on tube (WNOT) has been noted in hemovigilance data as one of the major problems [45]. Effective digital footprints include checks to ensure both the correct patient is identified and a sample collected as well as the appropriate sample and sample identification.

On the patient side of the digital footprint, RFID on sample tubes can be instituted. While placing an RFID antenna on a tube may be difficult, it is not impossible. If the RFID is integrated into patient identification and sample labeling, the risk of patient identification and WBIT can be reduced if not eliminated.

6.6.3 Patient Record Review and Testing

As mentioned previously, patient record review should be performed during the justification of transfusion and prior to the collection of the patient sample. This is key for the laboratory, especially if the patient transfusion record is part of the digital footprint. Such information can provide historical evidence of blood group typing, genotype status, phenotype status, and significant information concerning allo- or auto-antibodies.

Reconfirming present antibody status and obtaining antigen-negative compatible blood is also within the reach of the digital footprint and tools such as RFID. Blood ordered from the blood supplier provider, if equipped with the data in the RFID can be helpful to find antigen negative blood that has been transferred to the hospital inventory.

6.7 Release of Blood to the Patient Care Team and Digital Footprint

In the past, TM's responsibilities stopped with the issuing of blood products since in many hospitals, the patient care team obtains the blood product from the hospital transfusion service and administers the blood. However, some countries and institutions have extended TM to administration and clinical follow-up of patient outcomes. This extended care from the laboratory to the bedside is greatly enhanced with the use of the digital footprint (Fig. 6.6).

The use of RFID can continue to collect data as the blood component is checked out of the transfusion service and transported to the patient's bedside. Data collection and checks such as confirmation of positive patient identification, transfusion administration sets, time out of the refrigerator, use of accessory devices (blood warmer), vital signs before and through-

out the transfusion, and essential critical outcomes are all possible through the RFID digital footprint.

6.8 Hemovigilance Data Collection and the RFID Digital Footprint

The vigilance of transfusion safety has gained its position of importance over the years. An outcome of the HIV crisis of the late twentieth century, hemovigilance is more developed in some countries than others. The digital footprint of TM using RFID provides increased transparency of blood and blood components not only within the blood establishment but also throughout the clinical setting. With the use of the RFID and its reader (responder) throughout the clinical facility, blood can be tracked and its status monitored in real time. This enables TM specialists to monitor several transfusions at one time in a different part of the clinical setting.

Extending this to the patient's bedside, critical control data such as temporary storage locations, temperature, patient identification, crossmatch reference to the specific blood component, and vital signs can all be collected to support hemovigilance data collection. Some clinical settings

Fig. 6.6 These pictures represent a system used in the Catalonian region of Spain. This is a representation of two RFID systems linked for transparency from the healthcare facility to the regional blood establishment. RFID beacons (readers) have been placed in key locations to enhance reception between the interrogator and the transponder. (Photos were taken by JA Holmberg)

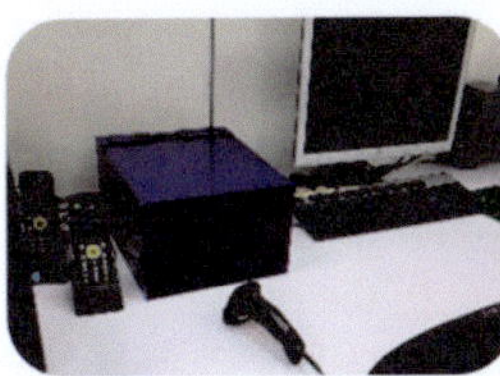

Reader interphase with healthcare ICT

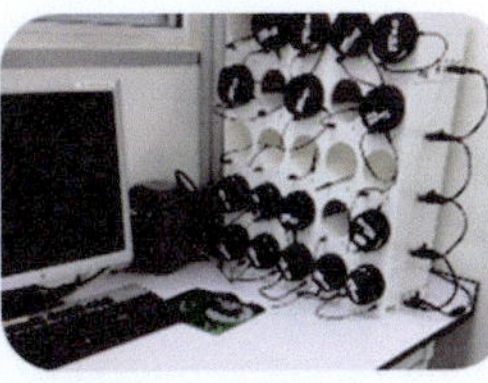

Transportation tubes with RFID for hospital tracking

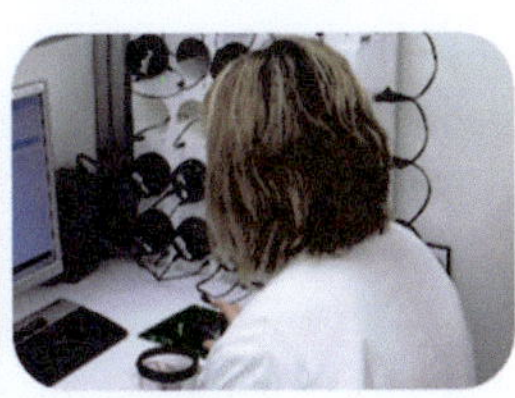

Transportation tubes linked to patient request

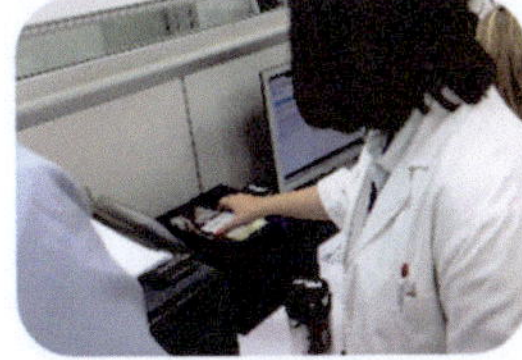

Blood unit RFID information from blood establishment read and associated with patient transportation tube

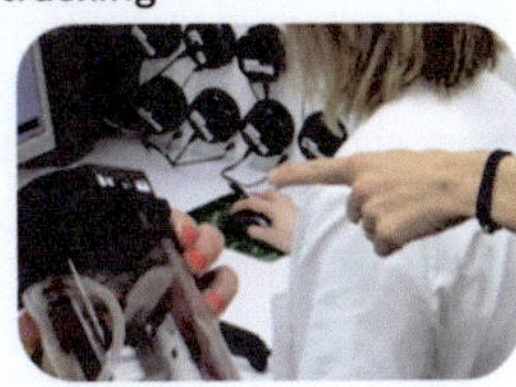

Blood unit is place into RFID transportation tube for delivery to patient

that have implemented RFID as a data collecting tool into their hemovigilance program have been able to have transparency and monitoring throughout the facility. One can see that with the collection of critical data and decisions at critical control points, hopefully, critical errors can be eliminated. In addition, adverse events can be quickly investigated to determine the route case.

6.9 Challenges, Benefits, and Recommendation for RFID Implementation

Over the years, there has been increased attention to patient safety benefits as well as the saving of time and expenses within the healthcare and supplier setting. As within most healthcare facilities, the implementation of RFID must face economic challenges as well as privacy, security, user acceptance, perceived value, improved workflow, and technical challenges.

6.9.1 Benefits of RFID

Correct identification of patients' specimen identification of blood, fluids, tissues, and biopsies directly affects results and appropriate medical decisions [46]. The ability to establish a chain of custody of a specimen linked to the correct patient is a requirement of good laboratory practices (GLP) and cGMP. This emphasizes the key essentials of patient safety; that is, to ensure the T&T of patient samples, environment conditions, and process monitoring of therapeutic interventions such as blood and blood component transfusions.

This ability to T&T medical device equipment can be beneficial if an RFID tag is associated with medical devices such as infusion pumps and blood warmers temporarily stored on the patient ward. The benefit would not only be the reduced time to locate collateral equipment, but assurance of maintenance, calibration, and the medical device linkage to the therapeutic intervention.

Once a therapeutic intervention is linked with RFID to the ICT, other devices such as those used for vital signs can also be linked through the IoT for monitoring and evaluation. The benefit of complete capture of T&T as well as monitoring and evaluation is risk avoidance and it has the advantage to contribute to the hemovigilance system, which can lead to patient care process improvement.

6.9.2 Barriers to RFID Implementation

The best ideas and concepts of improved safety in medical procedures can quickly be killed by barriers to acceptance. Most of the time it is associated with incomplete requirements identified for the workflow and processes in the blood establishment or healthcare facility.

In healthcare, the cost is usually the greatest barrier to the implementation of process improvement, even for safety. The initial investment in both RFID software and hardware can be a substantial barrier if not well thought out for total integration between the mobilization of the donor to blood collection through to patient sampling and medical therapeutic intervention and hemovigilance.

While the cost of the software will continually increase with new versions and additional data management, the cost of disposable RFID tags has come down over the years. The cost can be further reduced using recycled tags; however, process control of these recycled tags may require additional steps to erase previous data associated with the tag [46].

Realistic expectations such as ease of use and improved or reduced workforce requirements may also be a barrier. Setting the expectations through system requirements, pilot testing, and education can offset these barriers.

The main limitation of RFID in TM is the distance from the transponder to the reader (interrogator) based on the radiofrequency used. In the clinical setting, this has been the major reason for the lack of acceptance, especially if the RFID is tagged to a device. Expectations from healthcare staff that quick identification of the blood unit location in the delivery chain or the location of the peripheral equipment for administration was not realistic and wasted time. Many times, these problems highlighted the limitation of the HF reading distance of less than a meter from the beacon (interrogator). In these cases, based on the facility's requirement for a system, a secondary RFID system using UHF had to be incorporated into the overall system to be able to detect products in a secondary container up to 12 m away. Of course, the placement of an RFID beacon or even repeating beacons in strategic locations to ensure maximum transmission. Figure 6.6 is one example of how two systems were married together, the HF and UHF radio frequency. One for close work used in the blood establishment and transfusion medicine administration process and the other for intra-hospital transportation.

The temperature of storage can be another barrier to acceptance. Again, based on system requirements, the use of RFID must be well-identified. Radiofrequency can slow down based on ultra-cold temperatures. If RFID is attached to blood products like Frozen Fresh Plasma stored in the ultra-cold (-65 °C or colder), the electron movement and radio frequency will be impaired. This can often be overcome by removing the product from the ultra-cold freezer for a few minutes to regain the radio frequency.

6.10   Conclusion

While the risk of errors in TM is known, clerical errors and patient misidentification are still major concerns globally. Most of these errors are related to WBIT. Improving the digital footprint in all aspects of blood donation, processing, labeling, storage, and distribution to activities within the clinical transfusion medicine setting is greatly needed. In addition to error reduction to improve patient safety, a more integrated digital footprint can be beneficial in donor mobilization to ensure the right blood at the right time for clinical intervention. Using AI in TM to assist donor services in predicting the blood component needed, especially platelets with a limited shelf-life, continues to be developed with vari-

ous algorithms for consideration of holidays and other times when donors are not traditionally available. As with the application of AI, the IoT connectivity of electronic devices such as vital signs monitors, point-of-care testing, and electronic records is constantly being developed. These advances in the digital footprint emphasize the need for transparency with appropriate cybersecurity firewalls to reduce the risk while maintaining data integrity, data accessibility, and improving processes.

Capturing the processes on the clinical side as well as on the donor side can substantially be improved using tools like RFID. The critical step in using any data capturing tool is understanding the data to be collected and assigning recognized standardized data elements and understanding the story the data tell. Within TM and cell therapies, ICCBBA maintains a key position in data element management for different systems. Standardization of data elements is key as new data elements can be added with new advances but the core elements must be well accepted. As tools change, the data elements must remain stable as an industry standard.

One of the most exciting applications of the digital footprint and the use of various tools such as RFID is the availability of the data to review for advancing hemovigilance and process improvement. Requirements for the digital footprint including all applications and the use of RFID as a tool are clearly defined. As with any ICT system, poor requirements or not well-defined requirements add to the inefficiency of the ICT application and drive the cost up.

6.10.1   Recommendations for Implementation

Meeting and exceeding customer expectations for a successful implementation of an RFID-enhanced system can be achieved. Success requires careful and realistic planning as well as detailed customer requirements. The goal of capturing requirements is to provide the developers with details to enhance safety, improve user interaction, ease workflow, and enhance data collection. Clarity in system requirements can facilitate development and reduce the cost for modification later.

Establishing the requirements requires complete analysis both at the blood establishment and healthcare facility for workflow. During the workflow analysis, data collection and process decision points are identified. This is key to understanding how RFID, as a tool, can be of additional value. Once identified, the workflow analysis must be validated through observations of various users, compared to the standard operating procedures and the workflow supervisors. Relying on only one of these validation points can lead to inconsistencies and revision later in the process of implementation [47].

When using RFID as a tool within the blood establishment and healthcare ICT system, identification of data elements that will be stored within the RFID chip and requested by the ICT systems must be mapped out. Standardization of these data elements with the various systems is critical for accurate and efficient data transfers. If data elements are not standardized, an interface between systems may be required.

Based on the workflow analysis and transparent discussion between TM/blood establishment personnel, healthcare members, ICT managers, and administrators, requirements can be confirmed and established system by-in. These requirements are the blueprint that can also be used for not only system design but also the comparison of potential off-the-shelf (OTS) systems as well as cost analysis.

Cost analysis is needed to justify the incorporation of RFID as a tool in the transfusion process, in both blood establishments and healthcare facilities. Identification of workflow improvement of time and required personnel as well as improved reduction of errors all contribute to offsetting the system cost.

Once the system has been selected or designed, successful implementation must be planned with a step-wise approach before replacing the current process. The current process is the legacy process and must be retained as a backup throughout the process. An implementa-

tion team made up of key personnel in TM, ITC, patient care providers, and trainers is strongly recommended.

A step-wise or phased approach embraced with transparent communication and competency training can enhance successful implementation. A step-wise approach may start at the blood establishment with the incorporation of RFID in donor collection, blood processing, testing, labeling, and storage. Once this is successful, the implementation can be methodically incorporated into TM at the healthcare facility. Success at each step is essential, and if problems are encountered, corrective and documented actions must be implemented before moving to the next stage.

Moving from the TM service to the healthcare delivery team also should be done in a step-wise process. It is strongly recommended that implementation in the healthcare setting be done as a pilot in a manageable location such as a hematology clinic where transfusions are common. As mentioned before, training, monitoring, and detection of process improvement is essential. During the pilot process, the legacy system is dually maintained and is only replaced by the RFID system once all parties have signed off on acceptance. After acceptance of the pilot, full implementation can occur in that healthcare setting and the implementation team can move to another healthcare location that transfuses.

During and after full implementation, monitoring for process improvement is recommended. Key success factors and user feedback are vital to process improvement of the complete transfusion process. The documented areas of process improvement may include how the user interacts with the system including shortcuts or overrides to the system. These documented events can improve the safety of the system and potentially improve procedure time. If the events require changes in procedures, then the change process can be implemented. As with all functional systems, change control is needed as it supports process control.

Once the system has been implemented and initial monitoring indicates the system is meeting the requirements, it is recommended that best practices or areas of improvement be documented in a final written report. The report should include the workflow analysis, final requirements, system decisions, validation steps, implementation plans, training plans, monitoring plans, process improvement plans, and change control.

While this chapter is not exhaustive in covering all areas of the TM digital footprint, it is hoped that this will be an introduction to future advancement.

Key Points

- Humans make errors that could result in fatalities.
- Most human errors are related to administration, misinterpretation, and identification.
- Digital footprinting supported by radio frequency identification in the vein-to-vein transfusion medicine chain (manufacturing and clinical consumption) could prevent these errors and improve on quality and safety of clinical transfusion practice.
- Personnel involved in transfusion medicine need education, both knowledge and practice in implementing and operating a digital footprint in clinical transfusion medicine.

References

1. Smit Sibinga CT. Artificial intelligence in transfusion medicine and its impact on the quality concept. Transfus Apher Sci. 2020;59:103021. https://doi.org/10.1016/j.transci.2020.103021. Epub 2020 Nov 21.
2. Smit Sibinga CT. Chapter 8. Transfusion medicine: from AB0 to AI (artificial intelligence). In: Linwood SL, editor. Digital health. Brisbane, AU: Exon Publications; 2022. https://doi.org/10.36255/exon-publications-digital-health-transfusion-medicine.
3. Villamin C, Bates T, Mescher B, et al. Digitally enabled hemovigilance allows real-time response to transfusion reactions. Transfusion. 2022;62:1010–8. https://doi.org/10.1111/trf.16882.
4. Holmberg J. The digital footprint in transfusion medicine and the potential for vein-to-vein management. Medic Labor Observer. 2018. https://www.mlo-online.com/information-technology/automation/article/13017030/the-digital-footprint-in-transfusion-medicine-and-the-potential-for-veintovein-management.
5. van der Tuuk Adriani WPA, Smit Sibinga CT. The pyramid model as a structured way of quality management. Asian J Transf Sci. 2008;2:6–8.
6. HealthcareAnalyst, Inc. "Global RFID Blood Management Systems Market $830 M by 2029." 2022. www.ihealthcareanalyst.com/global-rfid-blood-management-systems-market/#:~:text=The%20global%20market%20for%20radiofrequency%20identification%20blood%20management,drugs%2C%20and%20elimination%20of%20trading%20of%20counterfeit%20drugs. Accessed 27 Feb 2023.
7. Taswell HF, Sonnenberg CL. Error analysis: types of errors in the blood bank. In: Smit Sibinga CT, Das PC, Taswell HF, editors. Quality assurance in blood banking and its clinical impact. The Hague, Dordrecht, Lancaster: Martinus Nijhoff Publ. Boston; 1984. p. 227–37.
8. Brown JS. Where have all the computers gone? Technol Rev. 2001:86–7.
9. Kallinikos J. The consequences of information. Northampton, MA: Institutional implications of technological change. Edward Elgar Publ; 2006.
10. Jansen van Galen JP, Smit Sibinga CT. Process management in the vein-to-vein chain. In: Smit Sibinga CT, editor. Quality Management in Transfusion Medicine. Nova Science Publ. New York; 2013. p. 131–85.
11. AABB standards for blood banks and transfusion services, current edition. Bethesda, MD: AABB Press.
12. Quality Indicators for Monitoring the Clinical Use of Blood. European Directorate for the Quality of medicines & HealthCare of the Council of Europe (EDQM). Council of Europe; 2015.
13. Cybersecurity in Healthcare. https://www.himss.org/resources/cybersecurity-healthcare. Accessed 9 Feb 2023.
14. Chai W. What is the CIA triad (confidentiality, integrity and availability)? https://media.techtarget.com/digitalguide/images/Misc/EA-Marketing/Eguides/Data_Security_Guide_Everything_You_Need_to_Know.pdf. Accessed 23 Feb 2022.
15. Fruhlinger J. The CIA triad: definition, components and examples. CSO; 2020. https://www.csoonline.com/article/3519908/the-cia-triad-definition-components-and-examples.html Accessed 23 Feb 2023.
16. The state of ransomware in healthcare 2022. Sophos white paper report 2022. sophos-state-of-ransomware-healthcare-2022-wp.pdf Accessed 9 Feb 2023.
17. Dutch Ministry of Economic Affairs and climate. Digital Trust Center; 2003. https://www.digitaltrustcenter.nl/de-5-basisprincipes-van-veilig-digitaal-ondernemen
18. Wrong-record, wrong-data errors with health IT systems. ECRI institute PSO navigator. 2015;7(2). https://www.ecri.org/Resources/In_the_News/PSONavigator_Data_Errors_in_Health_IT_Systems.pdf#:~:text=Data%20integrity%20failures%20can%20result%20in%20delayed%20or,must%20be%20corrected%20wherever%20it%20has%20been%20copied. Accessed 23 Feb 2023.

19. Frankenfield J. General data protection regulation (GDPR) definition and meaning. Investopedia. 2020. https://www.investopedia.com/terms/g/general-data-protection-regulation-gdpr.asp. Accessed 23 Feb 2023.
20. Miller S, Kim H-Y, Weiner DL, et al. Red blood cell alloimmunization in sickle cell disease: prevalence in 2010. Transfusion. 2013;53:704–9. https://doi.org/10.1111/j.1537-2995.2012.03796.x.
21. Ribeiro KR, Guarnieri MH, Da Costa DC, et al. DNA array analysis for red blood cell antigens facilitates the transfusion support with antigen-matched blood in patients with sickle cell disease. Vox Sang. 2009;97:147–52. https://doi.org/10.1111/j.1423-0410.2009.01185.x.
22. Cruz BR, de Souza Silva TC, de Souza Castro B, et al. Molecular matching for patients with haematological diseases expressing altered RHD-RHCE genotypes. Vox Sang. 2019;114:605–15. https://doi.org/10.1111/vox.12789.
23. Denomme GA, Fernandes BJ. Fetal blood group genotyping. Transfusion. 2007;47:64S–8S. https://doi.org/10.1111/j.1537-2995.2007.01313.x.
24. Krog GR, Rieneck K, Clausen FB, Steffensen R, Dziegiel MH. Blood group genotyping of blood donors: validation of a highly accurate routine method. Transfusion. 2019;59:3264–74. https://doi.org/10.1111/trf.15474.
25. Anani WQ, Marchan MG, Bensing KM, et al. Practical approaches and costs for provisioning safe transfusions during anti-CD38 therapy. Transfusion. 2019;57:1470–9. https://doi.org/10.1111/trf.14021.
26. De Vooght KMK, Oostendorp M, van Solinge WW. Dealing with anti-CD38 (daratumumab) interference in blood compatibility testing. Transfusion. 2016;56:778–9. https://doi.org/10.1111/trf.13474.
27. Velliquette RW, Aeschlimann J, Kirkegaard J, et al. Monoclonal anti-CD47 interference in red cell and platelet testing. Transfusion. 2019;59:730–7. https://doi.org/10.1111/trf.15033.
28. Kim TY, Yoon MS, Hustinx H, et al. Assessing and mitigating the interference of ALX148, a novel CD47 blocking agent, in pretransfusion compatibility testing. Transfusion. 2020;60:2399–407. https://doi.org/10.1111/trf.16009.
29. ICCBBA. https://www.iccbba.org. Accessed 10 Feb 2023.
30. Knels R. Radio frequency identification (RFID): an experience in transfusion medicine. ISBT Science Series 1:238 2006;1:238–41. https://doi.org/10.1111/j.1751-2824.2006.00039.x.
31. Gutierrez A, Levitt J, Reifert D, et al. Tracking blood products in hospitals using radio frequency identification: lessons from a pilot implementation. Vox Sang. 2013;8:65–9. https://doi.org/10.1111/voxs.12015.
32. Mitterecker A, Hofmann A, Trentino KM, et al. Machine learning-based prediction of transfusion. Transfusion. 2020;60:1977–86. https://doi.org/10.1111/trf.15935.
33. France CR, France JL, Ysidron DW, et al. Blood donation motivators and barriers reported by young, first-time whole blood donors: examining the association of reported motivators and barriers with subsequent donation behavior and potential sex, race, and ethnic group differences. Transfusion. 2022;62:2539–54. https://doi.org/10.1111/trf.17162.
34. Kreuger AL, Haasnoot GW, Somers JAE, et al. Ensuring HLA-matched platelet support requires an ethnic diverse donor population. Transfusion. 2020;60:940–6. https://doi.org/10.1111/trf.15728.
35. Allan D, Kiernan J, Gragert L, et al. Reducing ethnic disparity in access to high-quality HLA-matched cord blood units for transplantation: analysis of the Canadian Blood Services' cord blood Bank inventory. Transfusion. 2019;59:2382–8. https://doi.org/10.1111/trf.15313.
36. Yazer MH, Anani WQ, Denomme GA, et al. Trends in antigen-negative red blood cell distributions by racial or ethnic groups in the United States. Transfusion. 2018;58:145–50. https://doi.org/10.1111/trf.14376.
37. Zou S, Eder AF, Musavi F, et al. Implementation of the Uniform Donor History Questionnaire across the American Red Cross Blood Services: increased deferral among repeat presenters but no measurable impact on blood safety. Transfusion. 2007;47:1990–8. https://doi.org/10.1111/j.1537-2995.2007.01422.x.
38. Goldman M, Ram SS, Yi Q-L, Mazerall J, O'Brien SF. The donor health assessment questionnaire: potential for format change and computer-assisted self-interviews to improve donor attention. Transfusion. 2007;47:1595–600. https://doi.org/10.1111/j.1537-2995.2007.01329.x.
39. Sümnig A, Lembcke H, Weber H, et al. Evaluation of a new German blood donor questionnaire. Vox Sang. 2014;106:55–60. https://doi.org/10.1111/vox.12088.
40. Katz LM, Cumming PD, Wallace EL, Abrams PS. Audiovisual touch-screen computer-assisted self-interviewing for donor health histories: results from two years experience with the system. Transfusion. 2005;45:171–80. https://doi.org/10.1111/j.1537-2995.2004.04020.x.
41. Davis R, Geiger B, Gutierrez A, Heaser J, Veeramani D. Tracking blood products in blood centres using radio frequency identification: a comprehensive assessment. Vox Sang. 2009;97:50–60. https://doi.org/10.1111/j.1423-0410.2009.01174.x.
42. Guidelines for the use of RFID Technology in Transfusion Medicine. Vox Sang. 2010;98:1–24. https://doi.org/10.1111/j.1423-0410.2010.01324.x.
43. ISO 2009:19 Radio frequency identification (RFID) tyre tags. Downloaded April 24, 2023 from ISO 20909:2019 - Radio frequency identification (RFID) tyre tags.
44. Cappellini MD, Farmakis D, Porter J, Taher A, editors. Guidelines for the management of transfusion dependent thalassaemia (TDT). Nicosia, Cyprus: Thalassaemia International Federation; 2021. https://thalassaemia.org.cy/publications/tif-publications/guidelines-for-the-managementof-transfusion-

dependent-thalassaemia-4th-edition-2021-v2/. Accessed 22 Aug 2022.

45. Bolton-Maggs PH, Wood EM, Wiersum-Osselton JC. Wrong blood in tube—potential for serious outcomes: can it be prevented? Br J Haematol. 2015;168:3–13. https://doi.org/10.1111/bjh.13137. Epub 2014 Oct 4.

46. Seckman C, Bauer A, Moser T, Paaske S. Emerging Technologies. The Benefits and Barriers to RFID Technology in Healthcare. 2017. https://www.himss.org/resources/benefits-and-barriers-rfid-technology-healthcare#:~:text=Promising%20benefits%20related%20to%20the%20implementation%20of%20RFID,included%20economic%2C%20technical%2C%20organizational%2C%20privacy%2C%20and%20security%20challenges. Accessed 3 Apr 2022.

47. Profetto L, Gherardelli M, Iadanza E. Radio frequency identification (RFID) in health care: where are we? A scoping review. Health Technol (Berl). 2022;12:879–91. https://doi.org/10.1007/s12553-022-00696-1. Epub 2022 Aug 23.

Part III

Clinical Practice: Restrictive Versus Liberal Use of Blood and Blood Components

Arwa Z. Al-Riyami

Philip J. Crispin, Yashawi Dhiman,
Divjot Singh Lamba, and Arwa Z. Al-Riyami

7.1 Introduction

The term patient blood management (PBM) first appeared in 2005, distinguishing the systematic approach to optimizing and maintaining a patient's own blood from the management of blood transfusion supply chains [1]. PBM is a systematic, holistic, and multidisciplinary approach to optimize and conserve a patient's own blood. There have been a variety of definitions proposed, highlighting conflicting application and understanding of the term throughout the medical community. Common features of these definitions are that PBM describes a systematic approach rather than an intervention, it is patient-focused, and it is evidence-based.

Various organizations have differed significantly in whether they specifically reference transfusion within their proposed definitions:

1. The Association of Advancement of Blood and Biotherapies (AABB) specifically states that PBM strategies are targeted to patients who might need a transfusion [2].
2. The World Health Organization (WHO) includes the optimal management of transfused blood products within its definition, within a framework of improving overall patient outcomes [3, 4].
3. Others have focused on the goal of improving patient outcomes without specific reference to transfusion [5, 6].

Most recently, a consensus definition included patient safety and empowerment, in addition to improved patient outcomes as the goals of PBM [7].

The principles behind PBM have been present in the medical literature for a long time [8]. Transfusion developed historically when the demands for evidence of efficacy were significantly less than they are today. The lifesaving benefits of transfusion in some circumstances led to widespread adoption of transfusion as a preemptive or salvage therapy rather than focusing on the underlying cause for or the physiological

P. J. Crispin
Haematology Department, Canberra Hospital and College of Health and Medicine, Australian National University School of Psychology and Medicine, Canberra, Australia
e-mail: philip.crispin@anu.edu.au

Y. Dhiman
Department of Immunohaematology and Blood Transfusion, Himalayan Institute of Medical Sciences, Dehradun, Uttarakhand, India

D. S. Lamba
Department of Transfusion Medicine, Post Graduate Institute of Medical Education and Research, Chandigarh, India

A. Z. Al-Riyami (✉)
Department of Haematology, Sultan Qaboos University Hospital, Sultan Qaboos University, Muscat, Oman
e-mail: arwa@squ.edu.om

C. T. Smit Sibinga, Y. E. Abdella (eds.), *Clinical Use of Blood*,
https://doi.org/10.1007/978-3-031-67332-0_7

requirements of the patient [9]. The culture of medicine embraced opinion-based targets without sound scientific rationale [10]. Meanwhile, the adverse events of transfusion were frequently underestimated, a pattern that began with the very first human-to-human transfusions [11], until the formal development of hemovigilance systems [12]. The recognition of the overuse and potential harms associated with transfusion has certainly been a significant driver for PBM programs [13], but while reduction in blood transfusion and optimal use of the blood supply are expected outcomes, the focus of PBM is improved patient outcomes rather than transfusion avoidance [14].

This chapter will review PBM as a holistic approach to the care of patients' blood. It requires an understanding of the physiology of hematopoiesis and hemostasis, their changes during normal development, and their pathophysiology and responses to stress. The three pillars of PBM, optimizing the hemoglobin in anticipation of bleeding, maintaining hemostasis and preventing blood loss, and the tolerance of anemia rather than transfusion, will be outlined. Finally, practical approaches will be presented to the systematic introduction of PBM within organizations using quality improvement frameworks.

7.2 Normal Physiology

7.2.1 Hematopoiesis

Hematopoiesis is a continuous process involving the formation and turnover of blood cells to meet everyday demands and increased demand during acute blood loss, hemolysis, injury, or infections. On average, an adult human produces approximately one trillion blood cells every day, accounting for 45% of the blood, while the remaining 55% is plasma [15]. Hematopoiesis originates from hematopoietic stem cells (HSCs), which possess self-renewal and multipotent differentiation characteristics into various lineages with committed progenitors and mature blood including erythrocytes, platelets, lymphocytes, monocytes/macrophages, and granulocytes. This process of hematopoiesis occurs in two phases: *extra-embryonic/primitive hematopoiesis*, occurring in the blood islands of the yolk sac at approximately 21 days of gestation in humans, and *intra-embryonic definitive/adult hematopoiesis,* characterized by HSCs that arise from the mesoderm-derived aorta/gonad/mesonephros (AGM), a region that gives rise to the dorsal aorta, genital ridges, and mesonephros from the embryo proper, starting from day 27 post conception in humans [16–18].

Most of the cells generated during the *extra-embryonic/primitive hematopoiesis* phase are erythrocytes that are much larger than the red blood cells (RBCs) produced during the later stages of hematopoiesis. These cells retain their nucleus and continue their maturation in the bloodstream, with few myeloid cells and immature megakaryocytes, indicating that their primary function is to meet the rapidly increasing oxygen demands of the developing embryo. Primitive hematopoiesis is largely regulated by two transcription factors, Gata1 and Pu1, which exhibit a cross-inhibitory relationship to regulate primitive erythroid and myeloid fates [17].

During the *definitive/adult hematopoiesis* phase, AGM-derived HSCs migrate to the fetal liver, which is the primary site of intra-embryonic hematopoiesis until the sixth month of gestation when the bone marrow takes over and remains the site of hematopoiesis throughout life. Hematopoiesis mostly occurs in the red bone marrow found in the long bones of the arm (humerus) and thigh (femur), flat bones such as the sternum and cranial bones, and the vertebrae and pelvic bones. Multi-potent hematopoietic cells differentiate into several types of blood cells, with a multi-potent progenitor (MPP) cell identified with limited self-renewal capacity and short-term reconstituting ability, functionally indistinguishable from HSC (Fig. 7.1).

MPPs give rise to all blood cells that undergo lineage-restricted differentiation into committed hematopoietic progenitor cells (HPCs), known as

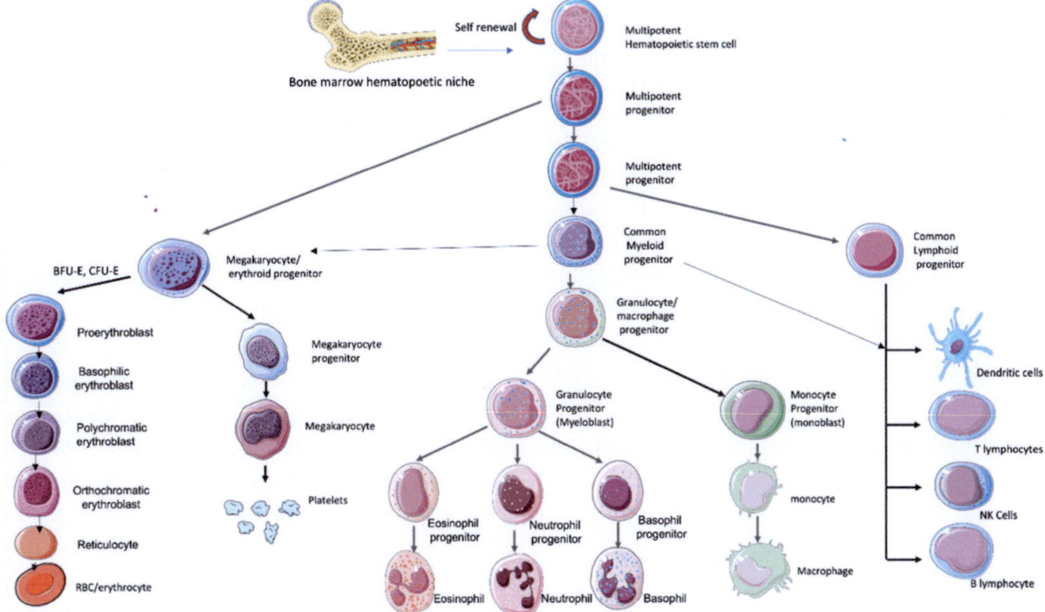

Fig. 7.1 Hematopoietic tree. *RBC* red blood cells; *BFU-E* burst-forming unit-erythroid; *CFU-E* colony-forming unit-erythroid; *NK* natural killer [19]

pluripotent cells, including common lymphoid progenitor, common myeloid progenitor, granulocyte–monocyte progenitor, and megakaryocyte–erythrocyte progenitor. Additionally, common myelo-lymphoid progenitor and common myelo-erythroid progenitor have been described, blurring the once strict demarcation between myeloid and lymphoid branches [19].

7.2.2 Erythropoiesis

Erythropoiesis is the process of RBC production that occurs in the yolk sac during early fetal development, and then in the bone marrow until the reticulocyte stage (Fig. 7.1).

Reticulocytes are irregularly shaped cells that are devoid of a nucleus and contain hemoglobin and organelles called the "reticulum." Once in the circulation, they mature into erythrocytes within 1–2 days. Via autophagy, they lose the reticulum and remodel their shape to form a discoid-shaped structure with a biconcave shape and called erythrocytes [20]. This biconcave discoid shape is owed to a well-regulated membrane surface area ($140 \ \mu^2$) to cytoplasmic volume (90 fL) ratio created by the geometric alignment of its membrane and sub-membrane cytoskeleton that gives them the ability to distort from their normal 7–8 μ diameter to a much smaller size to be able to pass through the narrow blood capillaries and endothelial slits in the red pulp of the splenic cords depending on viscosity of the cytoplasm [20]. The mechanical membrane stability or deformability of a RBC is evaluated as the maximum extent of deformation it can undergo and still recover its initial shape. Any further increase in deformation results in membrane failure and cell fragmentation.

The primary physiological role of RBCs is to transport gases (O_2, CO_2) from the lungs to the tissues and back, while also maintaining the acid-base balance of blood and tissues. In addition, RBCs are particularly well equipped with potent non-enzymatic and enzymatic antioxidant systems that maintain hemoglobin in a reduced oxygen binding form, limit oxidative modifications of membrane lipids, structural proteins, channels, and metabolic enzymes, and hence keep the cell functioning for its average life span of 120 days.

Besides their basic functions, RBCs are also known to contribute in nitric oxide (NO) metabolism (via scavenging, transporting, and releasing NO and its metabolites), are a systemic redox buffer contributing to maintaining systemic redox regulation, and transport and release vasoactive molecules [20]. Additionally, RBCs may control systemic hemodynamics by influencing blood rheological properties, and contribute to tissue protection and cardiovascular homeostasis [21–23].

7.2.3 Hemostasis

Hemostasis is a series of processes that involve carefully regulated blood clot formation at the site of vascular injury and the removal of the clot once healing is complete, and maintenance of blood in a fluid state. Hemostasis can be categorized into three concurrent processes: *primary hemostasis* (platelet plug formation), *secondary hemostasis* which results in a stabilized fibrin clot through the coagulation cascade; and *tertiary hemostasis*, which involves the formation of plasmin for breakdown of fibrin via fibrinolysis. The basic components involved in hemostasis include blood vessels, platelets, plasma coagulation factors, natural anticoagulants, and the fibrinolytic system.

When vascular injury occurs, reflex vasoconstriction is the first response, and platelets form a monolayer by adhering to the exposed subendothelial myofibrils with the help of glycoprotein-I-b (GPIb) and von Willebrand factor (vWF), as well as GPIa/IX complex with the exposed collagen. This further exposes GpIIb/IIIa complex on the platelet surface, which binds

to vWF and activates the platelets, releasing its granular contents, including calcium. The negatively charged phospholipids relocate from within the platelets to the outer surface, and phospholipase pathway is activated, which changes the platelet shape from disc to sphere. This is followed by platelet aggregation mediated by thromboxane A2 (TXA2), ADP, collagen and thrombin, forming an initial loose platelet plug marking the completion of *primary hemostasis* [24].

Secondary hemostasis begins with platelet procoagulant activity that involves binding of vitamin K-dependent coagulation factors (II,VII,IX,X) to the exposed negatively charged phospholipids (phosphatidylserine) on the platelet surface, activation of the coagulation cascade and formation of a stabilized fibrin clot involving two types of cells, platelets and cells bearing tissue factor (TF) (Fig. 7.2) [24].

The formation of a stabilized clot indicates the end of secondary hemostasis and the beginning of the tertiary phase, during which this coagulation process needs to be terminated to maintain a balance. Several inhibitory pathways are activated by the coagulation cascade, including protein C and protein S pathway, serine protease inhibitors (particularly antithrombin) and tissue factor pathway inhibitor (TFPI) [25]. Fibrinolysis is initiated during fibrin formation to remove the fibrin clot after the vasculature is repaired. Tissue plasminogen activator (tPA) converts plasminogen into plasmin, which in turn, lyses the fibrin, forming fibrin degradation products (FDPs), including D-dimer. The rate of fibrinolysis is controlled by the concentration of active tPA in blood which in turn is regulated by plasminogen activator inhibitor-1 (PAI-1) released from endothelial cells and platelets. The formation of FDPs marks the end of all three stages of hemostasis, establishing a balance to maintain hemodynamic stability in the circulatory system [26].

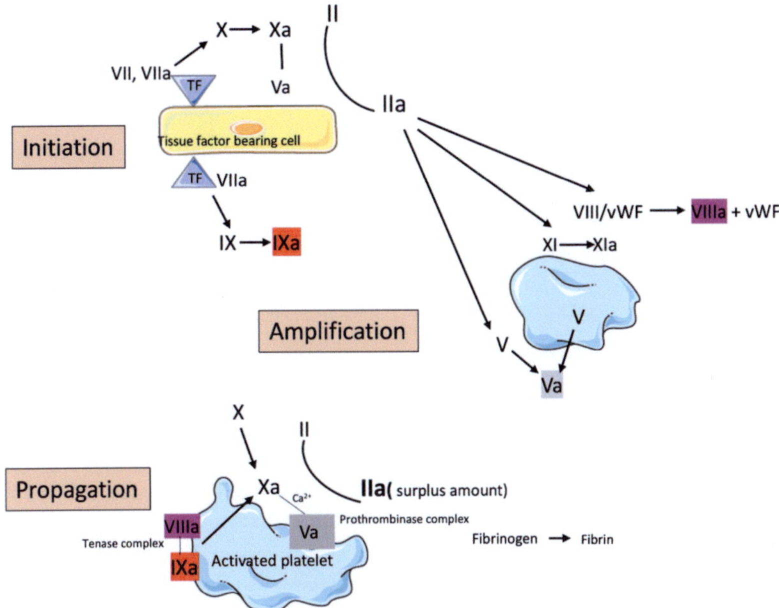

Fig. 7.2 Cell-based model of coagulation. **Initiation phase**: Tissue factor (TF) bearing cells complexes with active and inactive factor VII. TF/factor VIIa then catalyses activation of factors X and IX. Factor Xa on the TF-bearing cells complexes with factor Va to catalyze the production of a small amount of thrombin (IIa). **Amplification phase**: This thrombin diffuses away from the TF-bearing cell and is available for activation of platelets that have leaked from the vasculature at the site of injury, cleaves FXI to FXIa and activates FV to FVa on the platelet surface. Thrombin also cleaves von Willebrand factor from FVIII releasing it to mediate platelet adhesion and aggregation. FVIII is subsequently activated into FVIIIa. **Propagation phase**: The propagation phase occurs on the surface of these few activated platelets. Activated platelets increase the negatively charged phospholipids on their membrane surfaces leading to platelet aggregation and facilitate the assembly of tenase and prothrombinase complexes. Factor IXa (from initiation phase) binds to FVIIIa (from amplification phase) on the activated platelet forming the tenase complex and generating FXa on the platelet. This FXa generated on platelets rapidly binds to FVa (generated by thrombin in the amplification phase) along with calcium forming the prothrombinase complex and cleaves prothrombin to thrombin. This prothrombinase activity results in a burst of thrombin generation leading to cleavage of fibrinopeptide A from fibrinogen forming fibrin. When enough thrombin is generated with enough speed to result in a critical mass of fibrin, these soluble fibrin molecules will spontaneously polymerize into fibrin strands, by crosslinks formed by factor XIII resulting in an insoluble fibrin matrix forming a stabilized clot. (Image credited to Y. Dhiman)

7.3 Physiological Responses

7.3.1 Physiological Response to Anemia and Thrombocytopenia

Anemia is characterized by a reduction in the number of RBCs or the hemoglobin level, resulting in a reduced oxygen-carrying and release capacity of the blood. Anemia results from a decrease, defect, or loss of RBCs due to blood loss, inefficient erythropoiesis, hemoglobinopathy or hemolysis. Manifestations of anemia include fatigue, weakness, pallor, shortness of breath due to reduced oxygen supply to the lungs and the body's increased demand for oxygen, and dizziness due to the reduced oxygen supply to the brain.

The physiological response to anemia is complex and aims to compensate for the reduced oxygen-carrying capacity of the blood. While these compensatory mechanisms can help to maintain oxygen supply to the tissues, they can also cause a range of signs and symptoms, particularly in cases of severe or prolonged anemia such as increased heart and respiratory rates.

Thrombocytopenia is characterized by low platelet count in the blood. Thrombocytopenia can cause increased bleeding, which may manifest as nose bleeds, gum bleeding, or easy bruising. In this setting, the body responds in several ways to minimize bleeding and maintain clotting. These include increased platelet and clotting factor production and blood vessel constriction.

7.3.2 Physiological Response to Bleeding

The body's response to bleeding is a complex process that involves a variety of mechanisms to stop the bleeding, repair the damaged blood vessel, and maintain adequate blood flow and oxygen delivery to the body's tissues.

The first response to bleeding is the constriction of blood vessels at the site of injury, which helps to slow down or stop the bleeding. Platelets begin to clump together at the site of injury to form a temporary plug that helps to further reduce blood loss. Once the platelet plug is in place, the coagulation cascade gets activated to form a stable blood clot at the site of injury (see Hemostasis). The blood clot helps to seal the wound and prevent further blood loss.

In addition to the local response at the site of injury, a systemic response also gets initiated, including the release of epinephrine and norepinephrine, to increase heart rate and blood pressure and improve blood flow to the injured area. The body also produces more RBCs to replace the lost blood volume and maintain adequate oxygen delivery to the tissues.

7.3.3 Physiological Response to Pregnancy

Pregnancy is a complex physiological process that involves significant changes to support the growth and development of the fetus. Hemostatic changes in pregnancy are essential for maintaining a healthy pregnancy and ensuring a safe delivery. The changes that occur in the hemostatic system during pregnancy are necessary to prevent excessive bleeding and thrombosis, which can be life-threatening for the mother and the fetus.

One of the key hemostatic changes during pregnancy is an increase in clotting factors, such as fibrinogen and factors VII, VIII, IX, and X. This increase in clotting factors helps to prevent excessive bleeding during delivery. The increase in clotting factors is thought to be an adaptive response to the increased risk of bleeding during delivery.

Another important hemostatic change during pregnancy is the decrease in natural anticoagulants, such as protein S and antithrombin III. This decrease is thought to be a compensatory mechanism to prevent excessive bleeding during delivery. It is also believed to be necessary to support the formation of the placenta, which requires adequate blood supply and the prevention of excessive bleeding. Fibrinolysis is increased during pregnancy to prevent thrombosis in the placenta.

7.4 Pillars of Patient Blood Management

PBM is underscored by the growing acknowledgment and endorsement by numerous national and international societies and organizations with the aim of enhancing patient outcomes [27]. Evidence suggests that blood transfusion is associated with high morbidity rates, longer hospital stays, increased mortality rates, and higher overall hospitalization costs. Frequent transfusion emerges as an independent risk factor associated with poorer outcomes [28]. In order to achieve optimal PBM, it is important to adhere to a restrictive transfusion strategy that is supported by evidence [29]. Additionally, it is crucial to examine instances of inappropriate transfusion practices and identify areas of noncompliance. Such efforts can help mitigate blood shortages, prevent unnecessary transfusions, reduce adverse outcomes, and generate significant cost savings to the healthcare systems [7, 30].

The concept of PBM has evolved over time to ensure blood safety, optimize blood utilization, and explore alternatives to transfusion [31]. To develop a successful PBM program, healthcare

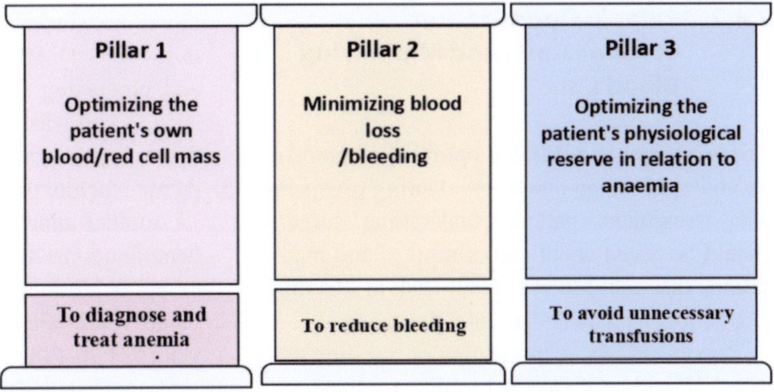

Fig. 7.3 Pillars of patient blood management. (Image credited to Y. Dhiman)

programs and systems need well-defined principles that guide their framework and recommendations.

These principles can be enumerated to include (Fig. 7.3):

1. **Anemia correction**: identifying anemia, determining its cause, using pharmaceuticals to stimulate hematopoiesis (e.g., erythropoietin), reducing oxygen consumption, and transfusing blood products when clinically necessary.
2. **Optimization of hemostasis and minimizing bleeding**: reducing iatrogenic blood loss (e.g., reduce laboratory draws), utilizing surgical techniques that minimize blood loss, promptly identifying and stopping ongoing blood loss, and utilizing transfusion methods that minimize allogeneic transfusion (e.g., autologous transfusion, intraoperative red cell salvage, normovolemic hemodilution). This includes properly assessing coagulopathy/hemostasis, determining the underlying cause of coagulopathy, treating coagulopathy with specific medications.
3. **Restrictive transfusion** and rational and guideline-appropriate use of allogenic blood components.

7.4.1 Pillar 1: Anemia Correction

Hemoglobin optimization is a crucial component of PBM. Blood conservation is a key aspect of PBM, emphasizing the importance of preserving and safeguarding a patient's own blood whenever possible to reduce the need for allogeneic transfusions. By prioritizing the optimization of hemoglobin levels, PBM strives to reduce the reliance on blood transfusions, and mitigate the potential risks and complications associated with it. This is achieved through evidence-based practices such as managing anemia and utilizing appropriate pharmaceutical interventions.

Anemia affects approximately one-third of the global population, making it a prevalent condition worldwide. Studies report that anemia impacts 25–50% of hospitalized patients, with its occurrence influenced by factors such as comorbidities, demographics (such as age and gender), and the progression of care (e.g., procedural blood loss and phlebotomies). Notably, anemia has been identified as an independent risk factor for adverse outcomes, including an increased risk of hospitalization or readmission, extended length of hospital stays, increased morbidity, and mortality [32–34].

Making a definitive diagnosis of the underlying cause of anemia is of utmost importance. The diagnostic tests for anemia encompass blood cell count, blood film, serum ferritin, serum iron, transferrin, and iron binding capacity measurements. Of these, the combined assessment of serum ferritin and transferrin saturation (Tsat) are effective in detecting iron deficiency, a leading cause of anemia [35]. Early intervention to promote erythropoiesis to restore the red cell volume may be indicated, such as by the use of replacement iron and erythropoietic agents [36].

7.4.2 Pillar 2: Optimization of Hemostasis and Minimizing Blood Loss

The second pillar of PBM is optimizing hemostasis and minimizing blood loss. During preoperative assessment, patients undergoing surgery should be asked about comorbidities, and medications that could increase their risk of bleeding (e.g., anticoagulant and antiplatelets agents).

Perioperatively, identification of bleeding tendency should be performed to direct transfusion therapy. Point-of-Care Testing (POCT), such as using thromboelastography (TEG) and rotational thromboelastometry (ROTEM), is applied to direct transfusion therapy in many scenarios including surgeries and massive transfusion. Effective PBM through POCT improves medical and surgical care by supporting the use of directed transfusion therapies. Blood sampling for diagnostic purpose should be reduced as much as possible to minimize iatrogenic blood loss.

Intraoperatively, proactive management of bleeding sources, such as the use of appropriate surgical techniques and the judicious use of hemostatic agents play a crucial to optimize hemostasis and minimize bleeding. Examples of these techniques are as follows:

1. **Minimally Invasive Surgical Approaches**

   Whenever possible, minimally invasive surgical techniques, such as laparoscopic or radiologic interventions, should be considered, especially for high-risk patients. These techniques help reduce blood loss and improve treatment outcomes.

2. **Cell Salvage**

   Cell salvage (autologous blood recovery) involves collecting and reinfusing the patients' own blood intra- and postoperatively. Studies have shown that autologous blood cell salvage can reduce the need for allogenic blood transfusions in various surgical procedures, especially cardiovascular and orthopedic [37]. Postoperative cell salvage demonstrated its utility in reducing perioperative blood loss, maintaining higher postoperative hemoglobin level, and reducing the rates of allogenic blood transfusion in major surgical procedures [28]. Different strategies for collecting and processing the blood before reinfusion, such as cell washing and filtration autotransfusion systems, are available [38].

3. **Acute Normovolemic Hemodilution (ANH)**

   Another approach is acute normovolemic hemodilution (ANH), where crystalloid and/or colloidal solutions are used to maintain blood volume, typically reaching hematocrit values of 20–30%. Meta-analyses of randomized controlled studies on ANH in lowering allogenic blood transfusion have shown a modest decrease in the need for transfusions compared to standard therapy [39, 40].

4. **Antifibrinolytic Medications**

   Antifibrinolytic medicines (hemostatic agents) are commonly used to reduce blood loss and the need for transfusions during surgical procedures. Antifibrinolytics (e.g., tranexamic acid) have been shown to significantly reduce perioperative blood loss in major orthopedic and cardiovascular procedures, as well as liver transplants. However, there are risks of thrombo-embolic events that should be considered when using these agents [41].

7.4.3 Pillar 3: Optimizing Physiological Tolerance of Anemia

There are several guidelines [42–46] and resources available to inform and guide transfusion practices. Transfusion triggers should be followed judiciously, using single unit transfusions instead of two for non-bleeding patients [47]. A decision to transfuse should consider various clinical factors and should only be made when there is detrimental reduction in the tissue oxygenation. The most efficient and cost-effective approach to reduce unnecessary RBC transfusions is to adhere to the recommended restrictive transfusion triggers. Optimizing the patient's physiological reserve to handle anemia is crucial to tolerate it. This can be achieved by identifying and treating underlying comorbidities [48].

7.5 Developing Patient Blood Management Programs

7.5.1 Overview

PBM as described by the three pillars requires the optimization of care pathways to value patients' own blood. In an ideal world it should be the standard of care. However, it is evident that this is not yet universal practice. Organizations and clinicians have different approaches to how the patient is perceived and managed, with the historical paradigm of relying on transfusion rather than seeking to optimize and preserve patient's own blood still pervasive. In order to shift to more appropriate care, organizations need to consider the practicalities of implementing the three pillars of PBM in their own care pathways, aided by principles of practice improvement and implementation science.

Practice improvement can be difficult, particularly if there exists little desire for change. Utilizing practice improvement teams already established within the institution, including people with expertise in practice improvement methodology and utilizing practice improvement tools should be considered. There are numerous frameworks to guide practice improvement with the common features being to: Identify the evidence base; adapt it to local needs; identify barriers to implementation; introduce changes; monitor the clinical processes; evaluate outcomes and embed practice change [49]. These have been developed into toolkits, which can help with practice change [50–52].

Where there are multiple similar sites with the same aim, collaborative methodology may be used to try different improvement strategies simultaneously with the aim of adopting the most successful approaches [53, 54]. While short term project teams may be used to implement change, strategies should wherever possible include structural, organizational, and permanent process change. Education is essential but when used alone may result in only transient improvements [55].

Hospitals have their own environments and cultures and these need to be understood and leveraged to effect change. Leaders are critical, especially from within the organization and craft groups [55, 56]. Executive leadership is important to support and advocate for an effective place for PBM within the hospital. Respected clinical leaders are the most valuable assets to focus the attention of clinicians on the evidence base and the need for practice change. Identifying clinical champions within affected craft groups should be considered early. A PBM or transfusion committee embedded within and integral part of hospital governance can bring together key stakeholders with permanent oversight and demonstrate institutional commitment to PBM. Transfusion practitioners have often had a leading role in implementing PBM, beyond previously narrow role delineations restricted to transfusion. Involvement of local clinicians and patients are vital to co-design projects to ensure applicability to a particular setting and maximize the chance of success [57]. In developing project teams, consideration should also be given to engaging non-clinical stakeholders whenever they may be affected by changed processes. Involvement of patients or community representatives ensures that changes keep patients at the center of care, an accepted principle in PBM as in all models of care.

The practice changes used to implement PBM should have well defined goals. It is important to identify what can be achieved. Smaller incremental gains are often easier to attain than large sweeping changes and small successes can incentivize continued engagement [55]. Successive small improvements sum to major changes. Goals should therefore be discrete and measurable.

Quality improvement aims to implement safe, effective and efficient care. Measurement should be adequate to establish these outcomes and the temptation to collect large datasets typically required to establish efficacy should be avoided. Surrogate markers rather than patient-centered outcomes may be appropriate goals, although it is important to be able to associate the success of the proposed improvement intervention with patient-centered quality outcomes, such as from prior studies. For example, showing improved compliance with preoperative anemia screening should be considered a successful result of a quality improvement intervention, whereas it would require much larger numbers to demonstrate an impact on hemoglobin or transfusion rates and larger still to prove an impact on patient symptoms [58]. Considering each stage within clinical care allows interventions to target where barriers exist. Statistical process controls (SPC), run charts and even individual case discussions (particular where unanticipated negative impacts are identified) are the data management tools of quality improvement [59].

The three pillars appear purpose-built for the perioperative setting, particularly when elective, as the development of PBM has some roots in efforts to achieve bloodless surgery [60]. Patients requiring emergency surgery have fewer opportunities to optimize care preoperatively, but there is still much that can be achieved through standardized multidisciplinary approaches, even in the critical bleeding setting [61, 62]. Pregnancy, with an expected confinement posing a potential risk of bleeding has also been a site for implementation of PBM strategies. Involvement of all maternity care providers is important to integrate PBM into all phases of care and ensure buy-in from stakeholders. This may include obstetricians, primary care medical practitioners, midwives and other health care workers. Involvement of mothers and expectant mothers will also help to design PBM programs fit for the community they serve. Models for pregnancy care vary between and within cultures and locations.

While perioperative and obstetric PBM will be considered here, readers should not be limited to these circumstances. Optimizing the blood should be considered for all the challenges facing patients and as a rule of thumb, if there is a likelihood of transfusion, then a PBM approach should be considered. Implementation of PBM in a particular setting will involve understanding the models within that setting and the people involved in delivering that care.

7.5.2 Perioperative PBM

7.5.2.1 Anemia Correction

In the elective setting, there are *ample* opportunities for preoperative optimization. Unfortunately, there is still too little attention given to preoperative optimization even in hospitals and jurisdictions with long histories embracing PBM [63, 64]. Detection and management of anemia in the preoperative setting should start when a surgical procedure is being contemplated (Fig. 7.4). This may start at the time of initial surgical referral, with the referrer beginning to ask whether the patient is currently fit for surgery and what more can be done to optimize their condition. In many health services though, this step is beyond their reach, with patients being referred in for surgical assessment or pre-admission anesthetic assessment, each providing shorter timeframes for intervention.

Iron deficiency anemia is commonly seen in the lead up to surgery [65, 66]. This may be expected due to the association of the underlying condition with blood loss, such as gastrointestinal and gynecological procedures. However, iron deficiency is relatively common in the community and so a proportion of patients presenting for procedures unrelated to blood loss will have iron deficiency. Identifying this group early is important as it may allow assessment of the need for further investigations for iron deficiency. Early identification of all iron deficient patients allows consideration of oral iron therapy, which takes longer to restore marrow iron stores than intravenous (IV) iron [67], but is more efficient in terms of pharmaceutical costs and health professional time when tolerated. Anemia of chronic disease is also common in patients requiring surgery. It is more complex to manage than iron deficiency as it requires optimization of the underlying inflammatory disorder first, then consideration of the merits of erythropoietin receptor agonists and IV iron therapy where functional iron deficiency anemia exists [68–70]. End stage renal failure is another circumstance where optimization of hemoglobin using erythropoietic agents has proven benefits, with increasing risks once the hemoglobin concentration rises above 12 g/dL

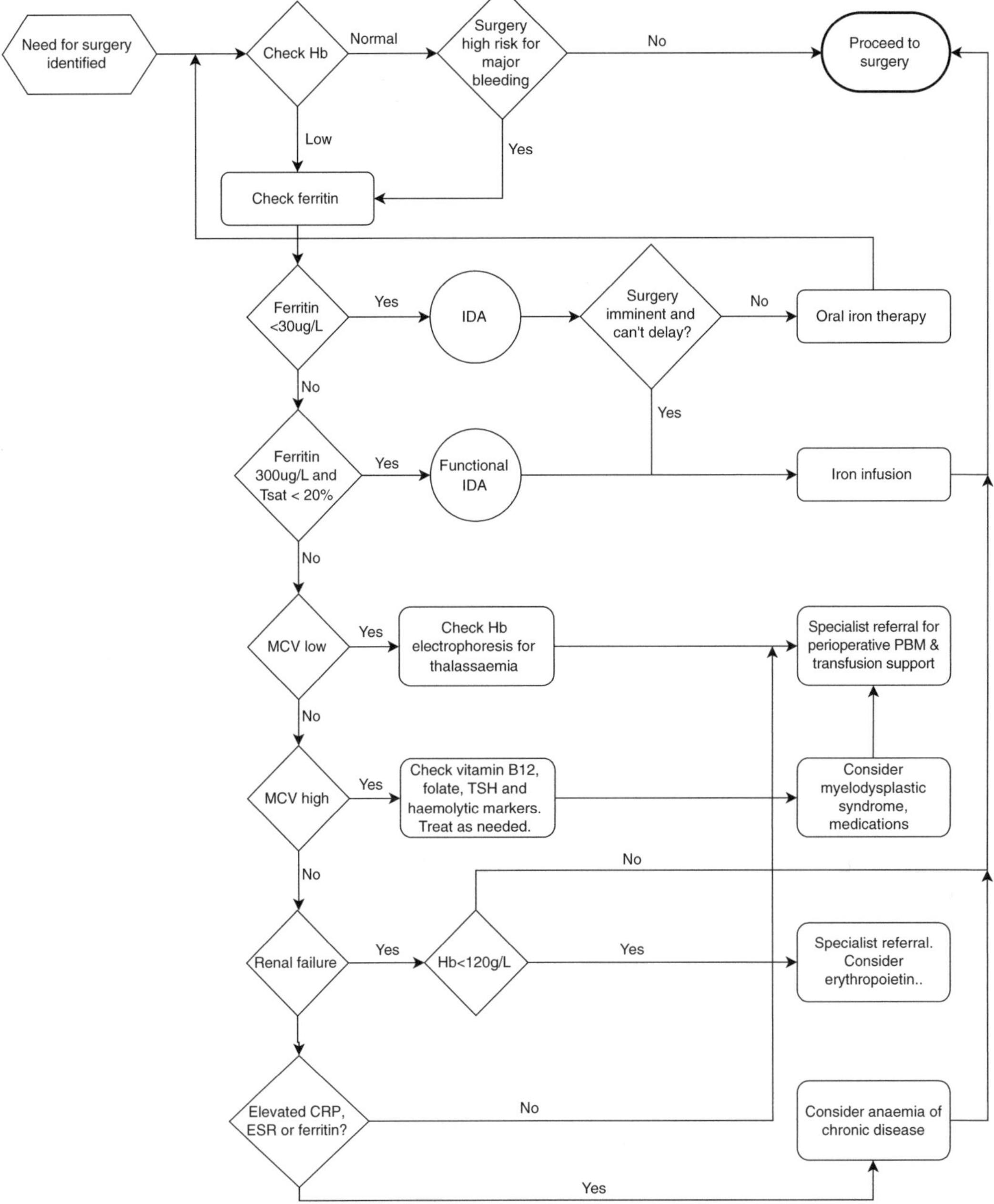

Fig. 7.4 A suggested approach to preoperative anemia management. *CRP* C-reactive protein; *ESR* erythrocyte sedimentation rate; *Hb* hemoglobin

[71, 72]. Where major bleeding is anticipated during surgery, the relative risks and benefits of higher hemoglobin targets should be considered. Early attention to PBM also allows identification, investigation and management of other causes of anemia, some of which have special perioperative considerations. The particular management of sickle cell disease (SCD) for example is beyond the scope of this chapter and recent evidence and guidance should be considered when developing strategies for managing this patient group [73, 74].

There are fewer studies on non-anemic iron deficiency. Many studies performed for non-anemic iron deficiency have been undertaken in mostly healthy young women with fatigue and the applicability of this to the perioperative setting is uncertain [75]. There are good data showing an improvement in functional state following iron infusion for non-anemic iron deficiency in congestive cardiac failure [76, 77]. Optimizing iron stores should therefore be considered at least in this population.

The timing and nature of anemia screening has been controversial. While anemia screening has been recommended in numerous guidelines [3, 78, 79] there have been few randomized trials on anemia screening and iron therapy [80]. A small single centre study showed that blood transfusions were reduced through the use of anemia screening and IV iron therapy in the 14 days prior to major surgery [81]. Another single center study showed the combination of iron infusion, erythropoietin, vitamin B12 and folate reduced transfusion following next-day cardiac surgery [70]. By contrast, the large multicentre PREVENTT study did not find a reduction in transfusion or length of stay [82]. Similarly, a large cluster randomized trial of collaborative methodology did show enhanced uptake of preoperative anemia screening, but no reduction in transfusion rates [54]. The authors of this latter study pointed to other variables that may impact on the rates of transfusion, and the lack of a defined transfusion protocol in the PREVENTT study may have contributed to this observed lack of effect despite the improvement in hemoglobin concentration at all time points after treatment allocation [83]. PREVENTT showed that the improvement in hemoglobin was significantly higher even at 8 weeks and 6 months, and despite showing no improvement in overall quality of life, the magnitude of the difference has been associated with clinically meaningful symptom-specific improvements in other settings [84]. The study also showed a reduction in readmission rates in the treatment arm.

Unfortunately, pre-admission assessments may be the first time that hospitals are able to implement meaningful practice change. These combined data suggest that when surgery is imminent, the difference of an additional hospital attendance for iron treatment only a few days earlier may be small and intraoperative or immediately postoperative iron may be an alternative [81, 85, 86].

7.5.2.2 Optimization of Hemostasis

Preoperative optimization should also consider hemostasis. This should include a targeted bleeding history. The use of prothrombin time and activated partial thromboplastin time have no role in routine perioperative bleeding risk assessment [87, 88]. When there is concern in the clinical history, appropriately targeted investigations and specialist consultation are required.

Patients with known bleeding disorders should have perioperative management plans including the use of transfusion, factor replacement and other supportive care, as well as plans for monitoring and supervision, which may require the surgery to be performed in centers where this is routinely managed. The author's experience includes patients with bleeding disorders, even Hemophilia, still come to pre-admission without adequate specialist input.

The hemostasis plan preoperatively should include a plan to manage anticoagulation where appropriate. In most cases bridging to heparin is not required as it has limited efficacy, is difficult to accomplish, both for the patient and institution and in many cases increases bleeding [89, 90]. Nevertheless, specific plans to manage anticoagulation and anti-platelet therapy should be personalized to the patient, taking into account local guidelines, the patient's risk factors with thromboembolism, renal failure, and the nature of the procedure.

The hemostasis plan should consider the role of platelets and plasma and plasma-derived medicinal products (PDMP) where appropriate. Evidence based guidelines should be used to develop individual patient plans and protocols for the management of unexpected excessive surgical bleeding. Often, transfusion decisions are based on fixed ratios. Whole blood viscoelastic testing has been used to identify balanced reductions in natural anticoagulants and can show hypercoagulable states despite prolonged prothrombin time (PT), for example, in liver disease [91–93]. These may be used to obtain a more balanced view of hemostasis. There is no uniform consensus on the appropriate transfusion algorithms based on viscoelastic test results. Hospitals introducing these tests should therefore identify suitable protocols to direct blood product use based on the results [94]. Since much of transfusion practice has been based on opinion and assertions, the introduction of a new technology is a good way to focus attention of a clinical group on the hemostasis, reviewing the current evidence and guidelines and updating practice. In this process, it is essential to have input from transfusion specialists who understand the composition and limitations of the products available locally.

7.5.2.3 Minimizing Bleeding

Controlling bleeding is largely an intraoperative PBM role. Surgical engagement is critical since intraoperative blood loss will depend on the surgical techniques and tolerance for bleeding [87, 95]. Cell salvage may be used where larger blood losses are anticipated. While used in many large centers, it may not be suitable for all. Instrument costs and staff training overheads will require hospitals to consider whether the demand warrants the investment, particularly in smaller institutions [96], and where there are other concurrent surgical and anaesthetic techniques being implemented to reduce blood loss.

Specific anesthetic techniques to minimize blood loss may include acute normovolemic hemodilution and permissive hypotension [97]. Avoiding acidosis and maintaining normothermia will maintain the ideal conditions for hemostasis. Tranexamic acid has been shown to reduce bleeding in major cardiac and noncardiac surgery and should be included in all patients at risk of major bleeding [98–101]. Finally, in the postoperative setting, controlling blood loss and preventing thrombosis need to be balanced through the appropriate timing and dosing of anticoagulation reintroduction or prophylaxis.

7.5.2.4 Transfusion

The role of transfusion triggers will be dealt with in subsequent chapters. In general, restrictive red cell transfusion strategies based on hemoglobin alone show no benefits over liberal strategies, based on the triggers used in various large randomized trials. However, while it is widely used, the hemoglobin concentration should be considered a surrogate marker. The aim of hemoglobin is to deliver oxygen to the tissues [102], and performance correlates with the total red cell mass. Tissue oxygenation and thread of organ failure have been used to guide transfusion, particularly in intensive care, neonatology and major surgery [103]. While there is no consensus approach, using alternative techniques such as tissue oxygen sensing may be useful to show that a cardiovascularly stable patient is adequately delivering oxygen to the tissues and therefore is unlikely to benefit from transfusion.

In the absence of a good proven clinical marker for the need for RBC transfusion, clinicians will need to rely on clinical features. In doing so, decision-makers rely on their experience of moderate anemia, which may be limited in environments where liberal transfusion practice has been accepted dogma [10, 104]. Once the evidence base for the safety of restrictive transfusion has been reviewed, and surgical buy-in achieved, sharing data on transfusion rates and comparing pre and post transfusion hemoglobin values has been shown to be an effective way to reduce red cell use and gets surgeons driving PBM on their own patients [105–107]. While this may require setting up data analytics, it can be a sound investment given the significant savings to be made with blood products and improved patient outcomes [108].

7.5.2.5 Obstetric Patient Blood Management

The role of PBM in obstetrics, particularly during antenatal care, is vastly underutilized. Iron deficiency is common in young women coming into pregnancy. The expansion of maternal red cell mass during pregnancy and the demands of the growing fetus deplete storage iron so anemia may develop in women with borderline iron stores and normal hemoglobin prior to pregnancy. Delivery creates a hemostatic challenge and despite the procoagulant state created by pregnancy, hemorrhage remains the most common single cause of pregnancy-related death.

7.5.2.6 Anemia Correction

The WHO recommends iron replacement for all pregnant women, with lower doses recommended in regions with a lower [prevalence of anemia [109]. Others have recommended targeted therapy based on screening based on antenatal hemoglobin [110] or with serum ferritin [50, 111, 112]. The approach will depend on anemia prevalence, resources and antenatal care pathways. Women with adequate iron stores in early pregnancy as measured by serum ferritin are unlikely to benefit from iron therapy, whereas in late pregnancy, a low ferritin is expected and measuring it is likely to add little to measuring the hemoglobin [113].

Screening for anemia should begin as early as the first antenatal visit (Fig. 7.5). Iron therapy is best given orally. For proven iron deficiency a dose of 100–200 mg of elemental iron is recommended. Gastrointestinal side effects may limit therapy in some women. Daily dosing may improve tolerance and iron polymaltose may also be better tolerated than other effective preparations [114]. There are many products available containing much smaller doses of iron and these are often popular due to lower side effects. In the community, all iron may be considered equal, but oral iron therapy should not be considered ineffective until there has been at least a 2-week trial of effective dose iron and no improvement in hemoglobin [110]. Specifically identifying or prescribing adequately dosed iron tablets will help women identify appropriate formulations from amongst the multitude of options [112].

For women unable to tolerate or who do not see an improvement in hemoglobin with oral iron, intravenous iron is recommended [50, 112, 115]. A single dose is usually adequate to enable restoration of hemoglobin, however in severely anemic women, a second dose may be required. Significant improvement in hemoglobin occurs quickly; most will respond with an increment of at least 20 g/dL within 3 weeks, with a lower baseline hemoglobin predicting a more rapid response and inflammatory comorbidities a

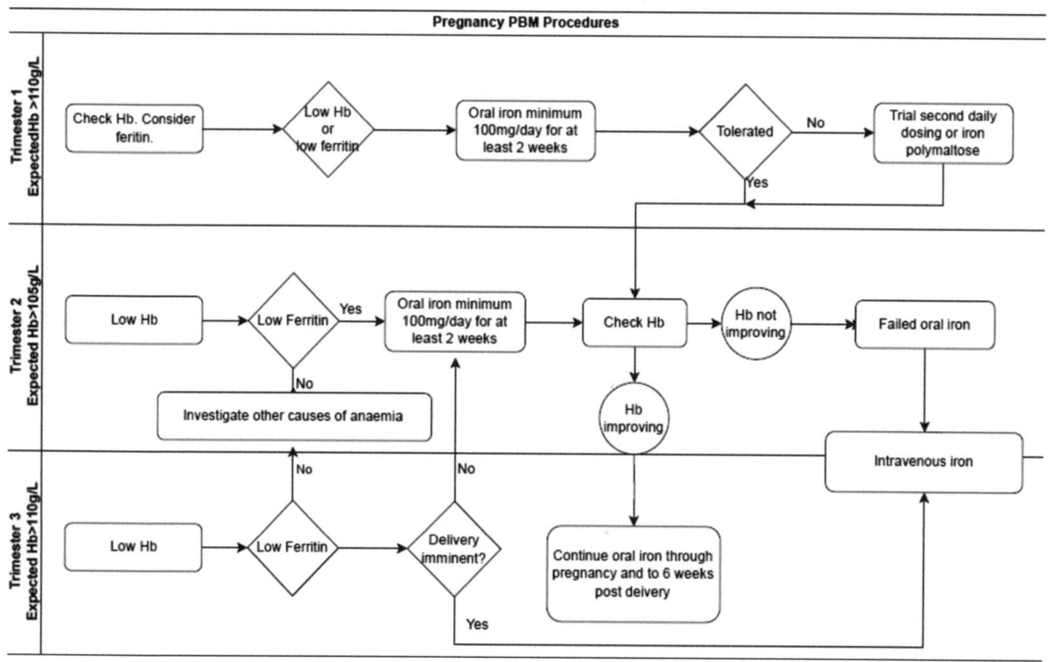

Fig. 7.5 Pathway for iron management during pregnancy. *Hb* hemoglobin

slower response [116, 117]. Iron carboxymaltose has a maximum dose of 1000 mg. Ferric derisomaltose can be given at higher single dose infusions [118]. Neither has adequate safety data for use in the first trimester. Anaphylactoid reactions seen with former versions of IV iron are rare with most modern iron carbohydrate complexes, but it is important to ensure that adequate staff and facilities are available to initiate urgent treatment. Intramuscular iron is generally not preferred, as it requires many doses and is painful.

Anemia not due to iron deficiency may be a signal to investigate other causes. Theses may reveal issues such as thyroid disease that may impact on pregnancy outcomes or inherited anemias, particularly hemoglobinopathies that will be of relevance to fetal and neonatal welfare. Iron deficiency anemia screening programs should therefore have access to more specialized hematology input as required.

Maternal antibody screens are a standard aspect of antenatal care. These do not impact on a woman's risk of anemia, but can have a severe impact on the fetus. Identifying a pregnancy that may be complicated by hemolytic disease of the fetus and newborn will help lay plans for the management of the baby's blood. Antenatal prophylaxis with anti-D immunoglobulin for RhD negative women to prevent RhD alloimmunization is routine practice in many countries. Prioritization of the scarce resource to pregnancies with an RhD positive baby through the use of noninvasive prenatal testing for fetal RHD genes in maternal blood is being increasingly offered.

7.5.2.7 Optimization of Hemostasis

Consideration should also be given to hemostasis planning during pregnancy. Thromboembolism is a significant cause of maternal morbidity and mortality and for affected women anticoagulation plans should include managing anticoagulation in the peripartum period. Women with bleeding disorders should have preemptive plans, although the most common bleeding disorder, type I von Willebrand disorder is not usually associated with an increased risk of post-partum bleeding due to the increased von Willebrand factor levels during pregnancy [119]. Clinicians experienced in the management of bleeding disorders should be involved in developing plans for delivery and able to provide advice in the event of excessive bleeding.

Active management of the third stage of labor reduces the risk of significant postpartum hemorrhage. This involves administration of uterotonic agents, cord clamping and controlled cord traction to encourage placental delivery rather than waiting for passive [placental separation [120]. Whether this should be used in women at low risk of postpartum hemorrhage is uncertain, however, uterotonic agents should be used with excessive bleeding after delivery.

7.5.2.8 Transfusion

Postpartum hemorrhage may at times be very rapid in onset and catastrophic in outcome [121]. Preparing in advance so that there is a plan on how to manage critical bleeding in pregnancy and in the puerperium is critical to success. This is sometimes predictable, such as with placenta accreta, and in these cases planning delivery in centers with surgical and supportive care expertise, neonatal intensive care and transfusion services may be lifesaving. Interventions to stop bleeding including hysterectomy, suturing perineal tears or embolization should be considered early when the need becomes apparent and implemented quickly. Cell salvage should be considered where large blood losses are anticipated. Concerns about recirculating amniotic fluid are unfounded when red cells are washed prior to transfusion, as is standard practice, and safety has been shown [122]. Tranexamic acid should be used in major postpartum hemorrhage as it improves survival [123]. Diffuse intravascular coagulation (DIC) may be catastrophic and rapid in obstetric bleeding. Rapid interrupting the excessive thrombin formation, and immediate fibrinogen replacement should be available, however, surgical procedures to obtain hemostasis should not be delayed while trying to improve hemostatic parameters if there is uncontrolled bleeding [111, 124].

7.5.2.9 Postpartum

Postpartum fatigue is common and anemia is only one contributor. Most healthy young women are able to tolerate a significant degree of anemia.

Ensuring iron stores are repleted enables rapid improvement in hemoglobin concentration [111]. While RBC transfusion leads to a more rapid improvement, the benefit from this in terms of quality of life is minimal compared with intravenous iron [125]. Anemia is often assumed to be the major cause for fatigue when it is present postpartum. Not surprisingly, fatigue is common after delivery and more severe after postpartum hemorrhage. Irrespective of anemia or its treatment, and improvement in fatigue is seen during the first few days post-delivery as the trauma associated with delivery and postpartum hemorrhage subsides. Once bleeding has stabilized, red cell transfusion should be carefully considered and avoided when possible. Single unit transfusions then reassessing until symptom control is adequate are all that is usually required [111, 126].

Implementing restrictive transfusion triggers in this setting can be difficult. Clinicians may have been taught to fear anemia and that transfusion is mandatory below certain arbitrary thresholds. Paradoxically, clinicians dealing with older myelodysplastic patients may have learned that patients are able to tolerate much lower levels of anemia than clinicians who are managing women encountering moderate to severe anemia for the first time in conjunction with the stressors of delivery and postpartum hemorrhage. Transferring experience from one setting to another may be a helpful tool to encourage clinicians to trial lower transfusion thresholds, particularly when led by respected peers. This will give confidence to practise transfusion guided more by the signs and symptoms than the numbers.

The postpartum setting may also be a time to start PBM for the next pregnancy. Advice on healthy diets and iron rich foods, and providing iron therapy where appropriate may be helpful in many young women, but especially where another pregnancy is planned. Focusing on active anemia management may assist in reducing fatigue and postpartum depression [127], valuable aims in a patient-focused program. This is especially important when another pregnancy may be planned [128]. In that circumstance, a discussion on longer inter-pregnancy intervals may also be appropriate, or the role of iron therapy when this is not preferred.

7.6 Conclusion

PBM is a comprehensive approach that focuses on optimizing patient outcomes by using strategies such as optimizing red blood cell mass, minimizing blood loss, and rationalizing the use of blood transfusions. Implementing PBM practices in healthcare organizations is essential for several reasons:

1. It improves patient safety and clinical outcomes by reducing the risks associated with unnecessary transfusions, including transfusion reactions and infections.
2. PBM helps conserve valuable blood resources and reduces the financial burden on healthcare systems. By minimizing the need for allogeneic blood transfusions, organizations can enhance cost-effectiveness and allocate resources more efficiently.
3. PBM promotes evidence-based, patient-centred care, ensuring that transfusion decisions are made based on individual patient needs, laboratory findings, and clinical evaluation. Overall, embracing PBM is crucial for organizations to enhance patient care, optimize resource utilization, and improve healthcare outcomes.

Key Points
- Hematopoiesis forms the basic fundamental process for red blood cell formation whose pathological loss or defect causes anemia amounting to a global healthcare burden that is efficiently addressed by PBM.
- Minimizing blood loss and maintaining normal hemostasis by providing optimal blood and blood components to replenish clotting factors and cellular components forms an essential element of PBM.
- PBM has a patient focus, with improved patient outcomes rather than decreased blood component use as its goal.
- PBM is characterized by the three pillars of optimizing hemoglobin, reducing blood loss and harnessing physiological tolerance for anemia.
- Implementing PBM programs include consideration of local quality improvement

resources, understanding local care pathways, and engagement with key clinical leaders for successful outcomes.

References

1. Isbister JP. Why should health professionals be concerned about blood management and blood conservation? Blood Conserv Transfus Alt. 2005;2:3–7.
2. AABB. Definitions and Concepts in Patient Blood Management. 2019. http://www.aabb.org/pbm/Pages/definitionsconcepts.aspx. Accessed 7 Oct 2019.
3. World Health Organisation. The urgent need to implement patient blood management: policy brief. Geneva: World Health Organisation; 2021. https://apps.who.int/iris/handle/10665/346655. Accessed 23 Mar 2023
4. World Health Organization. Concept paper. Global forum for blood safety: patient blood management. Dubai: World Health Organization; 2011.
5. Society for the Advancement of Blood Management. SABM, Who are we? SABM; 2019. https://www.sabm.org/who-we-are/. Accessed 7 Oct 2019.
6. National Blood Authority. Patient Blood Management Companion 1. In: National Blood Authority, editor. Canberra: Commonwealth of Australia; 2019.
7. Shander A, Hardy JF, Ozawa S, et al. A global definition of patient blood management. Anesth Analg. 2022;135:476–88.
8. Crosby WH. Misuse of blood transfusion. Blood. 1958;13:1198–200.
9. Greenburg AG. A physiologic basis for red blood cell transfusion decisions. Am J Surg. 1995;170:S44–S8.
10. Gombotz H, Rehak PH, Shander A, et al. Blood use in elective surgery: the Austrian benchmark study. Transfusion. 2007;47:1468–80.
11. Crispin P. Transfusion reactions hidden from history. Hektoen Int. 2014. https://hekint.org/2017/01/28/transfusion-reactions-hidden-from-history/. Accessed 23 Mar 2023.
12. McClelland B, Love E, Scott S, et al. Haemovigilance: concept, Europe and UK initiatives. Vox Sang. 1998;74(Suppl 2):431–9.
13. Alter HJ, Klein HG. The hazards of blood transfusion in historical perspective. Blood. 2008;112:2617–26.
14. Hofmann A, Farmer S, Shander A. Five drivers shifting the paradigm from product-focused transfusion practice to patient blood management. Oncologist. 2011;16(Suppl 3):3–11.
15. Kelly EB. Stem Cells. Santa Barbara: Greenwood Press; 2007. p. 57–64.
16. Jagannathan-Bogdan M, Zon LI. Haematopoiesis. Development. 2013;140:2463–7.
17. Wertheim G, Bagg A. Normal Haematopoiesis. In: McManus LM, Mitchell RN, editors. Pathobiology of human disease. San Diego: Academic Press; 2014. p. 1628–43.
18. Kawahara R. Haematopoiesis. In: Enna SJ, Bylund DB, editors. xPharm: the comprehensive pharmacology reference. New York: Elsevier; 2007. p. 1–5.
19. Hoggatt J, Pelus LM. Haematopoiesis. In: Maloy S, Hughes K, editors. Brenner's encyclopedia of genetics. San Diego: Academic Press; 2013. p. 418–21.
20. Moras M, Lefevre SD, Ostuni MA. From erythroblasts to mature red blood cells: organelle clearance in mammals. Front Physiol Line. 2017;8:1076.
21. Gorressen S, Stern M, van de Sandt AM, et al. Circulating NOS3 modulates left ventricular remodeling following reperfused myocardial infarction. PLoS One. 2015;10:e0120961.
22. Horn P, Cortese-Krott MM, Keymel S, et al. Nitric oxide influences red blood cell velocity independently of changes in the vascular tone. Free Radic Res. 2011;45(6):653–61.
23. Kuhn V, Diederich L, Keller TCS, et al. Red blood cell function and dysfunction: redox regulation, nitric oxide metabolism. Anemia Antioxid Redox Signal. 2017;26(13):718–42.
24. Abshire TC, Jobe SM. Chapter 88—Overview of the coagulation system. In: Shaz BH, Hillyer CD, Roshal M, Abrams CS, editors. Transfusion medicine and Haemostasis. San Diego: Elsevier; 2013. p. 587–92.
25. Rogers HJ, Nakashima MO, Kottke-Marchant K. Chapter 2—Haemostasis and thrombosis. In: Hsi ED, editor. Haematopathology. Philadelphia: Elsevier; 2018. p. 57–105.e4.
26. Hellstern P, Composition of plasma. In: Solheim BG, Snyder EL, McCullough J, Strauss RG, Simon TL, editors. Rossi's principles of transfusion medicine. Wiley; 2016. p. 286–94.
27. Goodnough LT, Shander A. Patient blood management. Anesthesiology. 2012;116(6):1367–76.
28. Shander A, Javidroozi M, Ozawa S, et al. What is really dangerous: anaemia or transfusion? Br J Anaesth. 2011;107(Suppl 1):i41–59.
29. Friedman MT. Patient blood management in haematology and oncology: AABB. 2020. https://www.aabb.org/docs/default-source/default-document-library/resources/pbm-in-haematology-and-oncology.pdf?sfvrsn=21725df9_2. Accessed 1 July 2023.
30. Althoff FC, Neb H, Herrmann E, et al. Multimodal patient blood management program based on a three-pillar strategy: a systematic review and meta-analysis. Ann Surg. 2019;269:794–804.
31. Goodnough LT, Shander A, Brecher ME. Transfusion medicine: looking to the future. Lancet. 2013;361:161–9.
32. Hayden SJ, Albert TJ, Watkins TR, et al. Anemia in critical illness: insights into etiology, consequences, and management. Am J Respir Crit Care Med. 2012;185:1049–57.

33. Migone De Amicis M, Poggiali E, Motta I, et al. Anemia in elderly hospitalized patients: prevalence and clinical impact. Intern Emerg Med. 2015;10:581–6.

34. Caughey MC, Avery CL, Ni H, et al. Outcomes of patients with anemia and acute decompensated heart failure with preserved versus reduced ejection fraction (from the ARIC study community surveillance). Am J Cardiol. 2014;114:1850–4.

35. Cappellini MD, Comin-Colet J, de Francisco A, et al. Iron deficiency across chronic inflammatory conditions: international expert opinion on definition, diagnosis, and management. Am J Haematol. 2017;92(10):1068–78.

36. Meier J, Gombotz H. Pillar III—optimisation of anaemia tolerance. Best Pract Res Clin Anaesthesiol. 2013;27:111–9.

37. Carless PA, Henry DA, Moxey AJ, et al. Cell salvage for minimising perioperative allogeneic blood transfusion. Cochrane Database Syst Rev. (4):Cd001888. 2003:CD001888.

38. Bisbe E, Moltó L. Pillar 2: minimising bleeding and blood loss. Best Pract Res Clin Anaesthesiol. 2013;27(1):99–110.

39. Carless P, Moxey A, O'Connell D, et al. Autologous transfusion techniques: a systematic review of their efficacy. Transfus Med. 2004;4:123–44.

40. Virmani S, Tempe DK, Pandey BC, et al. Acute normovolemic haemodilution is not beneficial in patients undergoing primary elective valve surgery. Ann Card Anaesth. 2010;13:34–8.

41. Henry DA, Carless PA, Moxey AJ, et al. Antifibrinolytic use for minimising perioperative allogeneic blood transfusion. Cochrane Database Syst Rev. 2011; (3):Cd001886

42. Goel R, Cushing MM, Tobian AA. Pediatric patient blood management programs: not just transfusing little adults. Transfus Med Rev. 2016;30:235–41.

43. Crighton GL, New HV, Liley HG, et al. Patient blood management, what does this actually mean for neonates and infants? Transfus Med. 2018;28:117–31.

44. Steinbicker AU, Wittenmeier E, Goobie SM. Pediatric non-red cell blood product transfusion practices: what's the evidence to guide transfusion of the 'yellow' blood products? Curr Opin Anaesthesiol. 2020;33:259–67.

45. McCormick M, Delaney M. Transfusion support: considerations in pediatric populations. Semin Haematol. 2020;57:65–72.

46. World Health Organisation. Educational modules on clinical use of blood. Geneva: World Health Organisation; 2021. https://apps.who.int/iris/handle/10665/350246. Accessed 26 July 2023.

47. Delaforce A, Duff J, Munday J, et al. Overcoming barriers to evidence-based patient blood management: a restricted review. Implement Sci. 2020; 15:6.

48. Hare GM. Tolerance of anemia: understanding the adaptive physiological mechanisms which promote survival. Transfus Apher Sci. 2014;50:10–2.

49. Graham ID, Logan J, Harrison MB, et al. Lost in knowledge translation: time for a map? J Contin Educ Heal Prof. 2006;26:13–24.

50. Abdulrehman J, Lausman A, Tang GH, et al. Development and implementation of a quality improvement toolkit, iron deficiency in pregnancy with maternal IRON optimization (IRON MOM): a before-and-after study. PLoS Med. 2019;16:e1002867.

51. Barac R, Stein S, Bruce B, et al. Scoping review of toolkits as a knowledge translation strategy in health. BMC Med Inform Decis Mak Line. 2014;14:121.

52. Hempel S, O'Hanlon C, Lim YW, et al. Spread tools: a systematic review of components, uptake, and effectiveness of quality improvement toolkits. Implement Sci. Line. 2019;14:83.

53. Nadeem E, Olin SS, Hill LC, et al. Understanding the components of quality improvement Collaboratives: a systematic literature review. The Milbank Q. 2013;91:354–94.

54. Scrimshire AB, Booth A, Fairhurst C, et al. Scaling up quality improvement for surgical teams (QIST)-avoiding surgical site infection and anaemia at the time of surgery: a cluster randomised cntrolled trial of the effectiveness of quality improvement collaboratives to introduce change in the NHS. Implement Sci Line. 2022;17:22.

55. Hughes R. Tools and strategies for quality improvement and patient safety. In: Hughes R, editor. PatientSafety and quality: an evidence-based handbook for nurses. Rockville: Agency for Healthcare Research and Quality; 2008. p. 3-1–3-39.

56. McNett M, Gorsuch PF, Gallagher-Ford L, et al. Development and evaluation of the Fuld institute evidence-based implementation and sustainability toolkit for health care settings. Nurs Adm Q. 2023;47:161–72.

57. Batalden P. Getting more health from healthcare: quality improvement must acknowledge patient coproduction—an essay by Paul Batalden. BMJ. 2018;362:k3617.

58. Delaforce A, Farmer S, Duff J, et al. Results from a type two hybrid-effectiveness study to implement a preoperative anemia and iron deficiency screening, evaluation, and management pathway. Transfusion. 2023;63(4):724–36.

59. Marang-van de Mheen PJ, Woodcock T. Grand rounds in methodology: four critical decision points in statistical process control evaluations of quality improvement initiatives. BMJ Qual Saf. 2023;32:47–54.

60. Spence RK, Erhard J. History of patient blood management. Best Pract Res Clin Anaesthesiol. 2013;27:11–5.

61. Consunji R, Elseed A, El-Menyar A, et al. The effect of massive transfusion protocol implementation on the survival of trauma patients: a systematic review and meta-analysis. Blood Transfus. 2020;18:434–45.

62. Paganini M, Abowali H, Bosco G, et al. Quality improvement project of a massive transfusion protocol (MTP) to reduce wastage of blood components. Int J Environ Res Public Health. 2021;18:274.

63. POSTVenTT Study Collaborative. The management of peri-operative anaemia in patients undergoing major abdominal surgery in Australia and New Zealand: a prospective cohort study. Med J Aust. 2022;17:487–93.

64. Van der Linden P, Hardy JF. Implementation of patient blood management remains extremely variable in Europe and Canada: the NATA benchmark project: an observational study. Eur J Anaesthesiol. 2016;33:913–21.

65. Abraham J, Sinha R, Robinson K, et al. Aetiology of preoperative anaemia in patients undergoing elective cardiac surgery-the challenge of pillar one of patient blood management. Anaesth Intensive Care. 2017;45:46–51.

66. Kearney B, To J, Southam K, et al. Anaemia in elective orthopaedic surgery—Royal Adelaide Hospital. Australia Intern Med J. 2016;46:96–101.

67. Keeler BD, Simpson JA, Ng O, et al. Randomized clinical trial of preoperative oral versus intravenous iron in anaemic patients with colorectal cancer. Br J Surg. 2017;104:214–21.

68. Menkis AH, Martin J, Cheng DC, et al. Drug, devices, technologies, and techniques for blood management in minimally invasive and conventional cardiothoracic surgery: a consensus statement from the International Society for Minimally Invasive Cardiothoracic Surgery (ISMICS) 2011. Innovations (Phila). 2012;7:229–41.

69. Spahn DR, Schoenrath F, Spahn GH, et al. Effect of ultra-short-term treatment of patients with iron deficiency or anaemia undergoing cardiac surgery: a prospective randomised trial. Lancet. 2019;393:2201–12.

70. Kaufner L, von Heymann C, Henkelmann A, et al. Erythropoietin plus iron versus control treatment including placebo or iron for preoperative anaemic adults undergoing non-cardiac surgery. Cochrane Database Syst Rev. 2020;8:Cd012451.

71. Metra M, Cannella G, La Canna G, et al. Improvement in exercise capacity after correction of anemia in patients with end-stage renal failure. Am J Cardiol. 1991;68:1060–6.

72. Mikhail A, Brown C, Williams JA, et al. Renaclinical practice guideline on Anaemia of chronic kidney disease. BMC Nephrol. 2017;18:345.

73. Estcourt LJ, Kimber C, Trivella M, et al. Preoperative blood transfusions for sickle cell disease. Cochrane Database Syst Rev. 2020;7:Cd003149.

74. Salvi PS, Solomon DG, Cowles RA. Preoperative transfusion and surgical outcomes for children with sickle cell disease. J Am Coll Surg. 2022;235:530–8.

75. Dugan C, Cabolis K, Miles LF, et al. Systematic review and meta-analysis of intravenous iron therapy for adults with nonanaemic iron deficiency: an abridged Cochrane review. J Cachexia Sarcopenia Muscle. 2022;13:2637–49.

76. Alnuwaysir RIS, Hoes MF, van Veldhuisen DJ, et al. Iron deficiency in heart failure: mechanisms and pathophysiology. J Clin Med 2021 Dec 27;11(1):123.

77. Anker SD, Comin Colet J, Filippatos G, et al. Ferric carboxymaltose in patients with heart failure and iron deficiency. N Engl J Med. 2009;361(25):2436–48.

78. National Blood Authority. Patient blood management guidelines. module 2: perioperative. Canberra: National Blood Authority; 2012. https://www.blood.gov.au/pbm-module-2. Accessed 26 July 2023.

79. Meybohm P, Froessler B, Goodnough LT, et al. "Simplified international recommendations for the implementation of patient blood management" (SIR4PBM). Perioper Med (Lond). 2017;6:5.

80. Mueller MM, Van Remoortel H, Meybohm P, et al. Patient blood management: recommendations from the 2018 Frankfurt Consensus Conference. JAMA. 2019;321:983–97.

81. Froessler B, Palm P, Weber I, et al. The important role for intravenous iron in perioperative patient blood Management in Major Abdominal Surgery: a randomized controlled trial. Ann Surg. 2016;264:41–6.

82. Richards T, Baikady RR, Clevenger B, et al. Preoperative intravenous iron to treat anaemia before major abdominal surgery (PREVENTT): a randomised, double-blind, controlled trial. Lancet. 2020;396:1353–61.

83. Keegan A, Crispin P, Ormerod A, et al. Iron deficiency in PREVENTT. Lancet. 2021;397(10275):669.

84. St. Lezin E, Karafin MS, Bruhn R, et al. Therapeutic impact of red blood cell transfusion on anemic outpatients: the RETRO study. Transfusion. 2019;59:1934–43.

85. Richards T, Miles LF, Clevenger B, et al. The association between iron deficiency and outcomes: a secondary analysis of the intravenous iron therapy to treat iron deficiency anaemia in patients undergoing major abdominal surgery (PREVENTT) trial. Anaesthesia. 2023;8:320–9.

86. Browning RM, Alakeson N, O'Loughlin EJ. Efficacy and safety of ultra rapid iron polymaltose infusion during general anaesthesia. Anaesth Intensive Care. 2017;45:320–52.

87. Hasan RA, Hess AS, Hess JR. Preoperative coagulation testing and patient blood management. Transfusion. 2022;62:2155–7.

88. Chee YL, Crawford JC, Watson HG, et al. Guidelines on the assessment of bleeding risk prior to surgery or invasive procedures. British Committee for Standards in Haematology. Br J Haematol. 2008;140:496–504.

89. Yong JW, Yang LX, Ohene BE, et al. Periprocedural heparin bridging in patients receiving oral anticoagulation: a systematic review and meta-analysis. BMC Cardiovasc Disord. 2017;17:295.

90. Bontinis V, Theodosiadis E, Bontinis A, et al. A systematic review and meta-analysis of periprocedural bridging for patients with mechanical heart valves undergoing non-cardiac interventions. Thromb Res. 2022;218:18130–7.

91. Andersen MG, Hvas CL, Tønnesen E, et al. Thromboelastometry as a supplementary tool for evaluation of haemostasis in severe sepsis and septic shock. Acta Anaesthesiol Scand. 2014;58:525–33.

92. Barton JS, Riha GM, Differding JA, et al. Coagulopathy after a liver resection: is it over diagnosed and over treated? HPB (Oxford). 2013;15:865–71.

93. De Pietri L, Bianchini M, Montalti R, et al. Thrombelastography-guided blood product use before invasive procedures in cirrhosis with severe coagulopathy: a randomized, controlled trial. Hepatology (Baltimore, Md). 2016;63:566–73.

94. Theusinger OM, Stein P, Levy JH. Point of care and factor concentrate-based coagulation algorithms. Transfus Med Haemother. 2015;42:115–21.

95. Bennett-Guerrero E, Zhao Y, O'Brien SM, et al. Variation in use of blood transfusion in coronary artery bypass graft surgery. JAMA. 2010;304:1568–75.

96. Klein AA, Bailey CR, Charlton AJ, et al. Association of Anaesthetists guidelines: cell salvage for perioperative blood conservation 2018. Anaesthesia. 2018;73:1141–50.

97. Shapira Y, Gurman G, Artru AA, et al. Combined haemodilution and hypotension monitored with jugular bulb oxygen saturation, EEG, and ECG decreases transfusion volume and length of ICU stay for major orthopedic surgery. J Clin Anesth. 1997;9:643–9.

98. Luo X, Huang H, Tang X. Efficacy and safety of tranexamic acid for reducing blood loss in elderly patients with intertrochanteric fracture treated with intramedullary fixation surgery: a meta-analysis of randomized controlled trials. Acta Orthop Traumatol Turc. 2020;54:4–14.

99. Sun L, An H, Feng Y. Intravenous tranexamic acid decreases blood transfusion in off-pump coronary artery bypass surgery: a meta-analysis. Heart Surg Forum. 2020;23:E039–e49.

100. Shi J, Zhou C, Pan W, et al. Effect of high- vs low-dose tranexamic acid infusion on need for red blood cell transfusion and adverse events in patients undergoing cardiac surgery: the OPTIMAL randomized clinical trial. JAMA. 2022;328:336–47.

101. Fowler H, Law J, Tham SM, et al. Impact on blood loss and transfusion rates following administration of tranexamic acid in major oncological abdominal and pelvic surgery: a systematic review and meta-analysis. J Surg Oncol. 2022;126:609–21.

102. Dzik WH. The air we breathe: three vital respiratory gases and the red blood cell: oxygen, nitric oxide, and carbon dioxide. Transfusion. 2011;51:676–85.

103. Crispin P, Forwood K. Near infrared spectroscopy in anemia detection and management: a systematic review. Transfus Med Rev. 2021;35:22–8.

104. Crispin PJ, Crowe BJ, McDonald AM. Blood transfusion prescribing in the ACT: an insight into clinical decision making. Aust Health Rev. 2005;29:240–6. https://doi.org/10.1071/ah050240.

105. Cohn CS, Welbig J, Bowman R, et al. A data-driven approach to patient blood management. Transfusion. 2014;54:316–22.

106. Gjata I, Olivieri L, Baghirzada L, et al. The effectiveness of a multifaceted, group-facilitated audit and feedback intervention to increase tranexamic acid use during total joint arthroplasty. Can J Anaesth. 2022;69:1129–38.

107. Trentino KM, Swain SG, Geelhoed GC, et al. Interactive patient blood management dashboards used in Western Australia. Transfusion. 2016;56:3140–1.

108. Leahy MF, Hofmann A, Towler S, et al. Improved outcomes and reduced costs associated with a health-system-wide patient blood management program: a retrospective observational study in four major adult tertiary-care hospitals. Transfusion. 2017;57:1347–58.

109. World Health Organisation. WHO recommendations on antenatal care for a positive pregnancy experience. Geneva: World Health Organisation; 2016. https://www.who.int/publications/i/item/9789241549912. Accessed 27 July 2023.

110. Pavord S, Daru J, Prasannan N, et al. UK guidelines on the management of iron deficiency in pregnancy. Br J Haematol. 2020;188(6):819–30.

111. National Blood Authority. Patient blood management guidelines: module 5-obstetrics and maternity. Canberra: National Blood Authority; 2015. https://www.blood.gov.au/pbm-module-5. Accessed 27 July 2023.

112. Flores CJ, Sethna F, Stephens B, et al. Improving patient blood management in obstetrics: snapshots of a practice improvement partnership. BMJ Qual Improv Rep. 2017;6(1):e000009.

113. Crispin P, Stephens B, McArthur E, et al. First trimester ferritin screening for pre-delivery anaemia as a patient blood management strategy. Transfus Apher Sci. 2019;58(1):50–7.

114. Ortiz R, Toblli JE, Romero JD, et al. Efficacy and safety of oral iron(III) polymaltose complex versus ferrous sulfate in pregnant women with iron-deficiency anemia: a multicenter, randomized, controlled study. J Matern Fetal Neonatal Med. 2011;24(11):1347–52.

115. Khalafallah A, Dennis A, Bates J, et al. A prospective randomized, controlled trial of intravenous versus oral iron for moderate iron deficiency anaemia of pregnancy. J Intern Med. 2010;268(3):286–95.

116. Hull J, Bloch E, Ingram C, et al. Slower response to treatment of iron-deficiency anaemia in pregnant women infected with HIV: a prospective cohort study. BJOG. 2021;128(10):1674–81.

117. Derman R, Roman E, Modiano MR, et al. A randomized trial of iron isomaltoside versus iron sucrose in patients with iron deficiency anemia. Am J Haematol. 2017;92(3):286–91.

118. Hansen R, Sommer VM, Pinborg A, et al. Intravenous ferric derisomaltose versus oral iron for persistent

iron deficient pregnant women: a randomised controlled trial. Arch Gynecol Obstet. 2022;308:1165. https://doi.org/10.1007/s00404-022-06768-x.

119. Pierce-Williams RAM, Makhamreh MM, Blakey-Cheung S, et al. Postpartum Haemorrhage in patients with type 1 von Willebrand disease: a systematic review. Semin Thromb Haemost. 2022;48(2):219–28.

120. Begley CM, Gyte GM, Devane D, et al. Active versus expectant management for women in the third stage of labour. Cochrane Database Syst Rev. 2019;2(2):Cd007412.

121. Say L, Chou D, Gemmill A, et al. Global causes of maternal death: a WHO systematic analysis. Lancet Glob Health. 2014;2(6):e323–e33.

122. Rong X, Guo X, Zeng H, et al. The safty profile of blood salvage applied for collected blood with amniotic fluid during cesarean section. BMC Pregnancy Childbirth. 2022;22(1):160.

123. Woman Trial Collaborators. Effect of early tranexamic acid administration on mortality, hysterectomy, and other morbidities in women with postpartum haemorrhage (WOMAN): an international, randomised, double-blind, placebo-controlled trial. Lancet. 2017;389:2105–16.

124. Neb H, Zacharowski K, Meybohm P. Strategies to reduce blood product utilization in obstetric practice. Curr Opin Anaesthesiol. 2017;30(3):294–9.

125. Prick BW, Jansen AJG, Steegers EAP, et al. Transfusion policy after severe postpartum haemorrhage: a randomised non-inferiority trial. BJOG. 2014;121:1005–14.

126. Shih AW, Liu A, Elsharawi R, et al. Systematic reviews of guidelines and studies for single versus multiple unit transfusion strategies. Transfusion. 2018;58(12):2841–60.

127. Wassef A, Nguyen QD, St-Andre M. Anaemia and depletion of iron stores as risk factors for postpartum depression: a literature review. J Psychosom Obstet Gynaecol. 2018;40:1–10.

128. Breymann C, Honegger C, Hösli I, et al. Diagnosis and treatment of iron-deficiency anaemia in preg. 2017;296(6):1229–34.

Kamini Khillan [iD], Flavia M. Bandeira [iD],
Tomohiko Sato [iD], and Katerina Pavenski

8.1 Platelet Transfusion

Platelets play a vital role in maintaining vascular integrity and hemostasis through adhesion, activation, and aggregation following blood vessel endothelial disruption. The platelet count is influenced by various factors that regulate production in the bone marrow, sequestration in the liver and spleen, and removal by reticuloendothelial system [1]. This complex process involves thrombopoietin regulatory feedback mechanism [2]. In cases of hypoproliferative thrombocytopenia, the prolonged bleeding time follows a nearly linear pattern as platelet counts decrease from 100×10^9/L to approximately 20×10^9/L [3].

K. Khillan (✉)
Department of Blood Transfusion Medicine, Sir
Ganga Ram Hospital, New Delhi, India
e-mail: kamini.khillan@sgrh.com

F. M. Bandeira
Blood Bank and Transfusion Medicine Department,
Rio de Janeiro State University, Pedro Ernesto
University Hospital, Rio de Janeiro, Brazil

T. Sato
Division of Transfusion Medicine and Cell Therapy,
The Jikei University Hospital, Tokyo, Japan
e-mail: tomosatou@jikei.ac.jp

K. Pavenski
Division Transfusion Medicine, St. Michael's
Hospital, Unity Health Toronto, Toronto, ON, Canada
e-mail: katerina.pavenski@unityhealth.to

Based on this correlation and considering splenic pooling, it is estimated that a fixed platelet amount of 7.1×10^9/L or about 18% of the normal platelet turnover rate is necessary to maintain vessel wall integrity for normal hemostasis [4, 5].

Thrombocytopenia can be categorized as mild (platelet count of 100 to 150×10^9/L), moderate (50–100×10^9/L), and severe ($<50 \times 10^9$/L). Clinically, in the absence of platelet dysfunction, thrombocytopenia is usually not detected until the platelet count falls below 100×10^9/L [6]. Platelet survival in thrombocytopenic patients is directly correlated with platelet count, with a significant reduction in lifespan once the count falls below 5×10^9/L. Notably, a significant spontaneous bleeding through an intact vascular system does not occur until the platelet count is 5×10^9/L or below [7, 8].

Platelet transfusions in clinical settings serve either therapeutic purposes to halt acute hemorrhage or prophylactic purposes to prevent bleeding before invasive procedures or when the platelet count falls below a certain threshold [9].

8.1.1 ABO and RhD Selection for Platelet Transfusion

Ideally, platelet transfusions should be ABO and Rh identical; however, limited resources and short shelf life of platelets make this challenging, and the reported overall impact on morbidity or survival among recipients of ABO nonidentical platelets has not been significant [10]. ABO matching is preferred but not required. Rh matching is preferred in RhD-negative recipients who are females of childbearing potential to reduce the risk of alloimmunization (Table 8.1).

Transfusing platelets that are plasma incompatible with recipient (major incompatibility, e.g., group O platelets to group A recipient) may cause hemolysis. Transfusing ABO-incompatible platelets (minor incompatibility, e.g., group A platelets to group O recipient) may lead to initial accelerated platelet clearance, resulting in slightly lower posttransfusion platelet increments and decreased platelet transfusion interval [11]. ABO-incompatible platelet concentrate can lead to formation of high-molecular-weight immune complexes in the recipient [12]. These have been speculated to cause inflammation, immune modulation, thrombocytopenia, increased rate of platelet destruction, and transfusion refractoriness [13–15]. Reports of platelets from group O donors with high-titer anti-A antibodies causing hemolysis have been documented [16, 17]. Risk mitigation approaches include screening titers for group O platelets [18], limiting the transfusion to group O recipients [19], restricting the allowable volume of incompatible plasma [20], use of platelet additive solution (PAS) [21], as well as employing volume reduction and washed platelets as component modification strategies.

RhD-negative females of childbearing potential are recommended to receive a standard 300 µg dose of Rh immune globulin (RhIg) for prophylaxis when transfused with platelets obtained from RhD-positive donors [22, 23]. RhIg half-life of 3 weeks provides protection for multiple transfusions of platelets obtained from RhD-positive donors over a 2–4-week period, as the volume of RBCs in each platelet dose is quite small. Some centers use platelets without consideration of RhD status and without RhIg prophylaxis due to the low risk involved [24, 25].

8.1.2 Platelet Transfusion Refractoriness

Platelet transfusion refractoriness (PTR) is characterized by a significantly lower platelet response than expected to at least two consecutive platelet transfusions [26]. It is commonly observed in patients with hematological malignancies who require repeated platelet transfusions [27–30]. The prevalence of PTR varies depending on the patient population, with reports indicating occurrence in 30–70% of multi-transfused patients [31–33]. PTR can have both nonimmune causes (fever/sepsis, splenomegaly, disseminated intravascular coagulation [DIC]) and immune causes (alloantibodies to platelet antigens) (Table 8.2).

Table 8.1 ABO group selection for platelet transfusion

Recipient ABO blood group	Choice of platelet blood group			
	First choice	Second choice	Third choice	Fourth choice
A	A	AB[a]	B[b]	O[b]
B	B	AB[a]	A[b]	O[b]
AB	AB	A[b]	B[b]	O[b]
O	O	A	B	AB[a]
Recipient Rh(D) type				
RhD positive	RhD positive	RhD negative		
RhD negative	RhD negative	RhD positive[c]		

[a] If readily available
[b] Components tested negative for high-titer anti-A and/or anti-B are recommended
[c] Consider administering Rh immune globulin for recipients who are children and females with childbearing potential

Table 8.2 Conditions causing platelet refractoriness

Immune	Nonimmune
HLA alloantibodies	Splenomegaly
Platelet alloantibodies	Medications
Autoantibodies	Sepsis
	Active bleeding
	DIC
	Fever

DIC disseminated intravascular coagulation

One-third of refractory cases are classified as immune PTR. Alloantibodies are directed against human leukocyte antigens (HLAs), typically HLA-A and HLA-B. Less commonly, alloantibodies against human platelet antigens (HPAs) and CD36 isoantigen or isoagglutinin to ABO antigens may be responsible. Alloimmunization to these antigens can result from previous transfusion, pregnancy, or transplantation; nonimmune and immune causes can often coexist [28, 34, 35]. To assess suspected PTR cases, the corrected count increment (CCI) is used measuring platelet recovery based on the amount of platelets transfused compared to the recipient body surface area. For assessing suspected PTR cases, measurement of CCI 10 min to 1 h posttransfusion (CCI-1 h) as well as CCI 24 h posttransfusion (CCI-24 h) is encouraged. Nonimmune PTR cases typically show CCI-1 h above 7.5×10^9/L and CCI-24 h below 4.5×10^9/L, indicating normal platelet recovery but reduced platelet survival. In contrast, immune PTR cases present with CCI-1 h below 7.5×10^9/L and CCI-24 h below 4.5×10^9/L, reflecting reduced platelet recovery almost immediately after transfusion [33, 36].

Appropriate assessment of PTR is critical, as poor response to platelet transfusion is associated with inferior survival, longer hospitalization, and higher hospitalization costs [37–39]. When PTR is suspected, nonimmune causes should be evaluated prior to investigating immune causes. Preventative measures for immune PTR include avoiding unnecessary transfusions and pre-storage leukoreduction. For patients with nonimmune PTR, addressing the underlying cause is crucial. Patients with immune PTR due to anti-HLA antibodies may require HLA-matched platelets, HLA antigen exclusion platelet units, or crossmatched platelet units [40]. For those without anti-HLA antibodies, anti-HPA antibodies should be investigated, and antigen-negative platelets can be transfused if necessary.

8.1.2.1 Corrected Count Increment Calculation

Clinically, the effectiveness of platelet transfusion is confirmed by reduction/control of bleeding. The CCI is a laboratory evaluation of the effectiveness of platelet transfusion and is calculated by the following formula [41]. Height and weight of the patient are needed. A CCI of $>7.5 \times 10^9$/L at 1 h and $>4.5 \times 10^9$/L at 20–24 h is considered to be a successful transfusion.

$$\text{Corrected Count Increment}\,(\text{CCI}) = \frac{\begin{bmatrix}(\text{post-transfusion platelet count}\,/\,\mu L) \\ -(\text{pre-transfusion platelet count}\,/\,\mu L)\end{bmatrix}}{(\text{number of platelets transfused} \times 10^{11}\,/\,\mu L).} \times (\text{body surface area in m}^2)$$

Body surface area (BSA) can be calculated using a nomogram or Mosteller formula as below:

$$\text{Body Surface Area}\left(\text{m}^2\right) = \sqrt{\text{height}\left(\text{cm}\right) \times \text{weight}\left(\text{kg}\right) / 3600}$$

8.1.2.2 Example

Patient BSA = 1.5 m²; platelet count: 3000/μL; post-count: 30,000/μL; and platelet transfused: 4.0×10^{11}:

$$CCI = \frac{\left(30,000 - 3000\right)}{4} \times 1.5$$
$$= 10,125 / \mu L \sim 10.1 \times 10^9 / L$$

8.2 Adult Platelet Transfusion

8.2.1 Prophylactic Platelet Transfusion

Prophylactic platelet transfusion thresholds have been a topic of interest for many years. Two randomized controlled trials (RCTs) challenged the necessity of providing prophylactic platelet transfusions. One study by Wandt et al. [42] randomized 391 AML and transplant patients to receive or not receive prophylactic platelet transfusions at a platelet threshold of 10×10^9/L or below. The trial reported significantly lower World Health Organization (WHO) Grade 2 or higher bleeding in the prophylaxis arm vs. the non-prophylaxis arm (19% vs. 42%, respectively, $p < 0.0001$). The risk of bleeding was much higher among patients receiving chemotherapy for acute myeloid leukemia (AML) compared to the autologous hematopoietic stem cell transplant (HSCT) patients. In the Trial of Prophylactic Platelets (TOPPS) study, 600 patients receiving chemotherapy or autologous HSCT were randomized to receive prophylactic platelet transfusion or none at a morning platelet threshold of 10×10^9/L. The results showed that prophylactic platelet transfusions reduced the occurrence of WHO Grade 2 bleeding in patients who received prophylaxis (43% vs. 50%, $p < 0.06$ for non-inferiority) [43, 44].

These two RCTs concluded that providing platelet prophylaxis in the setting of hypoproliferative thrombocytopenia is associated with a reduction in Grade 2 or higher bleeding [45]. A systematic review with a meta-analysis by Anthon et al. [46] analyzed seven RCTs [42, 44, 47–50] in 1642 hospitalized patients with hematological malignancies and thrombocytopenia. The trial revealed that prophylactic transfusions reduced clinically important bleeding (risk ratio (RR), 0.75; 95% confidence interval (CI), 0.64–0.87) but did not significantly reduce all-cause mortality (RR, 0.99; 95% CI, 0.58–1.68), with the overall certainty of evidence being low or very low. However, the trials included were conducted over 37 years with substantial heterogeneity with respect to patient populations, interventions, timing of outcome measurement, and definitions, assessments, and grading of clinically important bleeding.

The persistent controversies on prophylactic platelet transfusion relate to the threshold/trigger (platelet count below which transfusion is performed) and target value (platelet count to meet or exceed through transfusion). Various RCTs reviewed over the years have shown a high level of evidence favoring "trigger" over "target" transfusion [51]. Targeted approach will lead to an increased dose of platelet transfusion. Studies comparing prophylactic platelet transfusion triggers of 10×10^9/L versus 20×10^9/L showed no significant differences in hemorrhagic risks [52]. A significant reduction in hemorrhage-related mortality has been shown in thrombocytopenic patients, adults [8], and pediatric patients [53] with acute leukemia at a platelet threshold of 20×10^9/L. A meta-analysis showed that prophylactic transfusions reduced clinically important bleeding (RR, 0.75; 95% CI, 0.64–0.87), but did not significantly reduce all-cause mortality in hospitalized patients with hematological malignancies [46]. For non-hematological indications, such as disseminated intravascular coagulation (DIC), massive transfusion, and thrombocytopenia in patients undergoing minor invasive procedures or major surgery, there are no RCTs, and guidelines are based on expert opinions [54, 55].

Table 8.3 Prophylactic platelet transfusion thresholds according to different guidelines (all values represent platelet count $\times 10^9$/L)

Indication/procedure	AABB [60]	ASCO [62]	BSH [57]	SIMT [63]	JSTMCT [51]
Major surgery	<50 (WR)	<40–50 (WR)	<50 (WR)	>50	>50 (2D)
CNS or ophthalmic surgery	NR	NR	<100 (WR)	>100	>100
Central venous catheter placement	<20 (WR)	NR	<20 (SR)	>50	>20 (2D)
Lumbar puncture	<50 (WR)	NR	<40 (WR)	>50	≥50 (2D)
Epidural or spinal anesthesia	NR	NR	<80 (WR)	>50	Evidence is limited, no proposal
Bone marrow aspirate or trephine biopsy	NR	NR	Not indicated (SR)	NR	NR
Percutaneous liver biopsy	NR	NR	<50	>50	NR

AABB Association for the Advancement of Blood & Biotherapies; *ASCO* American Society of Clinical Oncology; *BSH* British Society for Hematology; *SIMTI* Italian Society of Transfusion Medicine and Immunohematology; *JSTMCT* Japan Society of Transfusion Medicine and Cell Therapy; *CNS* central nervous system; *NR* no recommendation is provided; *SR* strong recommendation; *WR* weak recommendation; *2D*-2* weakly recommended; *D (very weak)* confidence in the estimate of the effect

Guidelines generally recommend a prophylactic platelet threshold of 10×10^9/L for hypoproliferative thrombocytopenic patients [56–60], which can be increased to 20×10^9/L with additional bleeding risks. However, recommendations for prophylactic platelet transfusion vary in the presence of other risk factors such as bleeding and sepsis [57, 61, 62]. Table 8.3 summarizes recommendation from different guidelines [51, 57, 60, 62, 63].

8.2.2 Platelet Dosing

The standardization of platelet doses, whether given in large/infrequent or small/frequent strategies, also remains a subject of controversy. Deciding on the appropriate dose ideally involves considering body weight, desired posttransfusion platelet increment, and underlying medical condition. Thrombocytopenic patients experience a direct relationship between lower platelet counts and shorter platelet lifespan in the circulation [4], leading to a more rapid platelet consumption, particularly when platelet counts fall below 100×10^9/L. In adults, one unit of apheresis platelets, equivalent of four to six units of random donor platelets, contains approximately $3–4 \times 10^{11}$ platelets [60], which can increase platelet counts by $30–50 \times 10^9$/L. The Association for the Advancement of Blood & Biothera-pies (AABB) recommends transfusions of up to a single standard-dose apheresis unit of platelets or the equivalent [60]. However, in cases of therapeutic platelet transfusion, higher doses or more frequent platelet transfusions may be necessary, particularly for patients with active bleeding or those preparing for an invasive procedure.

In the context of prophylactic transfusion, two large trials have evaluated higher or lower platelet doses in patients with hypoproliferative thrombocytopenia due to bone marrow suppression by hematological malignancy, hematopoietic stem cell transplant (HSCT), or chemotherapy. However, these trials showed conflicting results. The PLADO trial included 1272 patients with thrombocytopenia due to chemotherapy or HSCT, randomized to receive standard-dose (2.2×10^{11} platelets/m^2), lower dose (1.1×10^{11}/m^2), or higher dose (4.4×10^{11}/m^2) platelet transfusions. The primary endpoint of prolonged mucosal or deep bleeding did not differ significantly among all groups, occurring in approximately 70% of patients [64]. On the other hand, in the STOP trial, randomized patients with hypoproliferative thrombocytopenia received standard-dose ($3–6 \times 10^{11}$) or lower dose ($1.5–3 \times 10^{11}$) platelet transfusion when platelet counts were below a trigger value of 10×10^9/L [65]. Because of life-threatening bleeding or bleeding requiring transfusion in the lower dose group, the trial was halted prematurely.

The Platelet Dose study [64] demonstrated that adult patients with hematological malignancies receiving low-dose prophylactic platelet transfusions for a morning platelet count of 10×10^9/L or less had the same bleeding risk as patients receiving standard- or high-dose platelets. Therefore, high-dose prophylactic platelet transfusions have not been shown to provide additional benefits. It is considered safe to provide low-dose platelet prophylaxis to patients with therapy-induced hypoproliferative thrombocytopenia, especially in light of the Platelet Dose study findings.

8.2.3 Special Indications

8.2.3.1 Hypoproliferative Thrombocytopenia

Patients with leukemia, or those being treated with cytotoxic chemotherapy or undergoing HSCT, have a suppressed bone marrow. The current evidence from various RCTs and meta-analyses supports the prophylactic platelet transfusion strategy for these patients [66, 67]. The current recommendation for prophylactic platelet transfusions in these cases is to maintain a platelet count threshold of 10×10^9/L to reduce the risk of spontaneous bleeding [60]. Implementing platelet transfusion for these patients has been shown to significantly decrease bleeding complications [44, 68].

In the management of coagulopathy, aggressive platelet transfusion to maintain platelet counts above $30–50 \times 10^9$/L is encouraged, until all clinical and laboratory signs of coagulopathy disappear [69, 70]. Additionally, hematological patients with fever, infection, or inflammation may require platelet transfusions with a higher-than-usual platelet threshold of $15–20 \times 10^9$/L due to the increased risk of bleeding [9].

8.2.3.2 Platelet Dysfunction Disorders

Qualitative platelet function disorders can be either inherited or acquired and may be associated with thrombocytopenia or a normal platelet count. In these settings, platelet transfusion is typically reserved for bleeding manifestations.

Examples of inherited cases of impaired platelet function are Glanzmann thrombasthenia and Bernard-Soulier syndrome. Acquired disorders, on the other hand, are caused by platelet-extrinsic factors that result in platelet dysfunction. Drug-induced platelet dysfunction can be triggered by antiplatelet drugs such as aspirin or P2Y12 inhibitors, or it may occur as an unwanted side effect of medications, such as selective serotonin reuptake inhibitors or tyrosine kinase inhibitors, or following cardiopulmonary bypass [71].

Despite the risk of alloimmunization, platelet transfusion remains a common first-line treatment for major bleeding or prophylaxis in patients with congenital disorders. In the case of Bernard-Soulier syndrome, where platelets have both platelet dysfunction and thrombocytopenia, platelet transfusion in combination with anti-fibrinolytic agents can effectively prevent bleeding [71]. Conversely, patients with Glanzmann thrombasthenia usually have platelet counts within the reference range, but are at risk of major hemorrhage. Therefore, platelet transfusions are often administered either prophylactically before invasive procedures or therapeutically to treat bleeding. However, it is still of debate that competition between the endogenous dysfunctional platelets and normal transfused platelets may reduce the therapeutic benefit of transfusion [71, 72].

Patients on single- or dual-antiplatelet therapy (with aspirin and a P2Y12 inhibitor) face an increased risk for various types of bleeding, including gastrointestinal bleeding, intracranial hemorrhage, and periprocedural bleeding (e.g., during coronary artery bypass grafting surgery) [71]. As residual antiplatelet effects have been linked to perioperative bleeding and transfusion [73], delaying operative timing should be considered along with possible platelet function testing. When surgery must proceed before the disappearance of antiplatelet effects, platelet transfusions should be carefully indicated; some studies regarding cardiac surgery suggest that platelet transfusion may help in a dose-dependent fashion [72, 74, 75], while studies in the setting of gastrointestinal bleeding and intracranial hemorrhage showed worse clinical outcomes related to platelet transfusions [76, 77].

8.2.3.3 Massive Blood Loss

In the setting of massive blood loss, the decrease in platelet count is strongly associated with mortality. Therefore, the idea of early and aggressive platelet transfusion has been considered beneficial [78]. The PROPPR trial [79] examined the impact of early transfusion using different but consistent ratios in patients predicted to receive a massive blood transfusion. Among the 680 patients in the trial who received plasma, platelets, and red blood cells in a 1:1:1 or 1:1:2 ratio, there was no significant differences in overall mortality at 24 h or 30 days. However, more patients achieved hemostasis in the 1:1:1 group, and fewer patients died due to exsanguinations. Interestingly, in the subgroup of patients who were effectively randomized to get either one or zero units of apheresis platelets, those who received platelets had significantly decreased 24-h and 30-day mortality, had a greater likelihood of hemostasis, and were less likely to die by exsanguination [80]. The findings of the PROMMTT study strongly support the early use of a 1:1:1 transfusion ratio in patients experiencing rapid bleeding. As per the American College of Surgeons Trauma Quality Improvement Program, a recommended transfusion ratio of red cells and platelets is a 1:1 ratio (one unit of apheresis platelets for every six units of RBCs) [81]. In the setting of severe trauma requiring massive transfusion, as fibrinogen levels can reach the critical level earliest among routine coagulation parameters including platelet counts [82], rapid fibrinogen supplementation by transfusion of fresh frozen plasma, cryoprecipitate, and fibrinogen concentrate should be prioritized.

8.2.3.4 Obstetrics

In cases of obstetric hemorrhage, platelet transfusions may be necessary when a massive transfusion is required (defined as transfusion of ten or more units of red blood cells within 24 h or four units of red blood cells within 1 h). However, specific recommendations for optimal blood product replacement therapy and timing of transfusion in obstetric patients have been mostly relied on consensus opinions [83]. The use of 1:1:1 ratios of red cells, plasma, and platelets is suggested until resuscitation can be guided by a laboratory-driven algorithm.

In non-bleeding pregnant women approaching delivery or undergoing a procedure, the platelet count threshold should be based on the expected mode of delivery or type of procedure. The risk of severe bleeding due to thrombocytopenia substantially increases only when platelet counts are below $10–20 \times 10^9$/L [65]. If pregnant women have platelet counts below 20×10^9/L and are at risk of severe bleeding, platelet transfusion should be administered immediately, regardless of the underlying cause of thrombocytopenia.

While platelet products should match the ABO and RhD group, inventories of RhD-negative platelet may not always be sufficient to support RhD-negative patients [84]. In RhD-negative females of childbearing potential who require platelet transfusions, there is a risk of alloimmunization to RBC antigens since platelet products contain small volumes of RBCs, leading to a risk for hemolytic disease of the fetus and newborn (HDFN) if the fetus is RhD positive. To prevent anti-D alloimmunization, administering Rh immunoglobulin is a well-established practice for RhD-negative pregnant women.

8.2.3.5 Preoperative Prophylactic Platelet Transfusion

8.2.3.5.1 Central Venous Catheter Placement, Lumbar Punctures, and Epidural Anesthesia

Three guidelines recommended a platelet count of more than 20×10^9/L for inserting central venous catheters [56, 57, 60]. For lumbar puncture procedure, a platelet count of more than $40–50 \times 10^9$/L is recommended by two related guidelines [57, 60]. When it comes to epidural anesthesia, it is recommended to have a platelet count of more than 80×10^9/L, provided that there are no additional risk factors for spinal hematomas, such as the use of anticoagulants, antiplatelet agents, and other acquired or congenital coagulopathies/platelet function defects. Rapidly falling platelet counts should also be taken into consideration in this context [85].

8.2.3.5.2 Biopsies

Platelet transfusion is not recommended before bone marrow aspirate or trephine biopsy, as the risk of significant bleeding is very low, less than 0.1%. If bleeding does occur during the biopsy, it can typically be stopped by applying pressure at the biopsy site [57].

8.2.3.5.3 Surgery

A Cochrane review has found insufficient evidence to recommend a specific platelet threshold for prophylactic platelet transfusions prior to minor surgery for people with a low platelet count due to insufficient related evidence [86]. However, for major elective non-neuraxial surgery, the AABB guideline suggests a platelet count of more than 50×10^9/L [60]. For surgeries involving the central nervous system, platelets are usually transfused prophylactically if the pre-procedure platelet count is less than $80–100 \times 10^9$/L, although the data supporting this threshold are of a low quality [60].

8.2.3.5.4 Vaginal Delivery vs. Caesarean Section

In the context of vaginal delivery versus caesarean section for patients with immune thrombocytopenia (ITP), the American Society of Anesthesiologists states that vaginal deliveries may be performed at a platelet count less than 50×10^9/L and that platelet therapy may be indicated for patients with platelet counts between 50 and 100×10^9/L [87]. The safety of these thresholds is supported by data from a review of 119 pregnancies associated with ITP [88]; 15% (17 out of 110) patients had platelet counts less than 50×10^9/L at delivery; however, hemorrhagic complications were uncommon and did not correlate with the platelet count. None of the patients with platelet counts less than 50×10^9/L had over 1 L of blood loss.

8.3 Neonatal and Pediatric Platelet Transfusion

8.3.1 Prophylactic Platelet Transfusion

Platelets begin to appear in the human fetus' circulation around 5 weeks after conception, and their numbers increase up to the 22nd week of gestation [89, 90]. Thrombocytopenia, defined as platelet count below 150×10^9/L, occurs in 1% of the general neonatal population [90]. It is frequently observed in neonatal intensive care units, with incidences reaching as high as 40% [91], estimated at 70% in newborns born at a weight <1000 g [92].

Neonatologists are particularly concerned about bleeding events, especially intracranial hemorrhage (ICH), as it increases the risk of death and poses challenges to neurodevelopment [93]. The causes of thrombocytopenia in neonates could be categorized as common and rare, also based on the time of onset (early onset ≤72 h after birth and late-onset ≥72 h after birth) and whether it occurs in a sick or in a well-appearing newborn [93]. Table 8.4 summarizes some causes of neonatal thrombocytopenia according to the time of onset and clinical presentation.

Platelets are commonly used to prevent bleeding in vulnerable patients such as neonates, as the occurrence of bleeding rises as gestational age decreases. However, there is a lack of good-quality evidence and evidence-based guidelines

Table 8.4 Causes of neonatal thrombocytopenia based on the time of onset and clinical presentation

Early (≤72 h)	Late (≥72 h)
Ill-appearing:	**Ill-appearing:**
Sepsis (bacterial, viral)	Sepsis (bacterial, viral, fungal)
TORCH[a]	Necrotizing enterocolitis (NEC)
Birth asphyxia	Inborn error of metabolism
Well-appearing:	**Well-appearing:**
Placental insufficiency	Drug-induced thrombocytopenia
Genetic disorders[b]	Thrombosis
Autoimmune	Fanconi anemia[c]
Neonatal alloimmune thrombocytopenia (NAIT)	

[a] Toxoplasma, rubella, cytomegalovirus, herpes simplex virus
[b] Trisomy 13, 18, 21; Turner syndrome; May-Hegglin anomaly; Bernard-Soulier syndrome; Wiskott-Aldrich syndrome; thrombocytopenia and absent radii; propionic acidemia, methylmalonic acidemia
[c] Most familial thrombocytopenias are present at birth except for Fanconi anemia, which usually does not appear until childhood

on when and to whom platelet transfusion should be given, leading to variation in recommendations and clinical practice [94, 95].

Recently, there has been a trend to more restrictive transfusion threshold (<25 × 10⁹/L) as compared to liberal threshold (<50 × 10⁹/L), as the latter has not proven to be more effective and in some cases was associated with increased risks of mortality and morbidity. The Platelets for Neonatal Thrombocytopenia (PlaNeT-2) trial demonstrated that a platelet count threshold of 50 × 10⁹/L for prophylactic platelet transfusion increased the risk of a composite major outcome of bleeding and/or death, when compared with a lower threshold of 25 × 10⁹/L (odds ratio [OR], 1.57; 95% CI, 1.06–2.32) [95].

Another study investigated whether groups of neonates experienced more or less benefit from the low transfusion threshold in the PlaNeT-2 trial. It was found that 25 × 10⁹/L threshold was beneficial compared with the 50 × 10⁹/L threshold in all subgroups of predicted baseline risk, although the absolute benefit varied. The authors suggested considering of a 25 × 10⁹/L transfusion threshold in all preterm neonates, including those with a high predicted risk of major bleeding and/or mortality [95, 96]. Additionally, a study involving 660 neonates from the PlaNeT-2/MATISSE (Platelets for Neonatal Transfusion-2/Management of Thrombocytopenia in Special Subgroup) showed that infants randomized to a higher platelet transfusion threshold of 50 × 10⁹/L compared with 25 × 10⁹/L also had a higher composite rate of death or adverse neu-

rodevelopmental outcome at a corrected age of 2 years, as well as a higher incidence of bronchopulmonary dysplasia developed at 36 weeks of corrected age [95–97].

For older children, chemotherapy and radiation are very common causes of thrombocytopenia, requiring prophylactic transfusions. Various conditions may necessitate platelet transfusions such as myelodysplasia, marrow infiltrative processes, bone marrow failure syndromes, congenital platelet disorders, and aplastic anemia [98]. The cause and severity of bleeding will guide platelet transfusion. For instance, bleeding during surgery or extracorporeal membrane oxygenation (ECMO) should trigger platelet transfusion when platelet count is 50–100 × 10⁹/L. Table 8.5 summarizes the thresholds for prophylactic platelet transfusion in children.

8.3.2 Platelet Dosing

A recent paper by Sola-Visner et al. [99] called the attention for a few characteristics that should be considered when ordering platelets for neonates, including heterogeneity in the type of product used, platelets inventory, and limited shelf life. Donor characteristics such as age and effects of donor-specific factors such as platelet function, ABO compatibility [100], and risk of ICH with the use of non-ABO-compatible platelets are still unanswered questions [101].

Platelet transfusions and the increased bleeding and mortality risk observed in neonatal ran-

Table 8.5 Thresholds for prophylactic platelet transfusion in children

Indication	Platelet transfusion threshold
Hypoproliferative thrombocytopenia	10 × 10⁹/L (15–20 × 10⁹/L for HSCT)
Line placement	20 × 10⁹/L
Lumbar puncture	30–50 × 10⁹/L (higher threshold considered when circulating blasts present)
CNS bleeding in children with sickle cell disease undergoing transplantation	30–50 × 10⁹/L
Major surgery	50 × 10⁹/L
CNS surgery	<100 × 10⁹/L
Platelet dysfunction with bleeding and/or in need of an invasive procedure	Not applicable

ECMO extracorporeal membrane oxygenation; *CNS* central nervous system; *HSCT* hematopoietic stem cell transplantation

domized trials highlight the need for a change in prophylactic platelet transfusion practices. The relationship between the severity of thrombocytopenia and its risk of bleeding, particularly ICH, is not well established [102, 103]. Neonates have hypofunctional platelets but normal primary hemostasis due to other compensatory factors, such as enhanced coagulation proteins, high hematocrit, high mean corpuscular volume, high von Willebrand factor levels, and predominance of ultralong von Willebrand factor polymers [99, 104, 105]. Concerns arise regarding the potential harm of transfusing adult-derived platelets into neonates with underlying inflammatory conditions and endothelial activation, as adult platelets may trigger or enhance microvascular thrombosis in neonates.

Additionally, platelets play various non-hemostatic platelet roles such as angiogenesis, tumor growth and metastasis, wound healing, immunity, and inflammation, further highlighting the need for cautious platelet transfusion practices [99]. Immature platelet count (IPC) and thrombopoietin (Tpo) concentrations in thrombocytopenic and non-thrombocytopenic very-low-birth weight (VLBW) infants and healthy term infants have been studied; however, further studies are warranted [106, 107].

The response to platelet transfusion is measured by the CCI, which should be above 20% of the pre-transfusion platelet count if measured within 10–60 min post-platelet transfusion and higher than 10% if measured within 24 h post-transfusion [108]. The typical dose is one unit of platelet transfusion per 10 kg, aiming to increase platelet count by 35–50 $\times$ 10^9/L and by 7–11 $\times$ 10^9/L/m^2 of body surface area (BSA). For neonates and infants, a platelet dose of 5–10 mL/kg should increase the platelet count by 50–100 $\times$ 10^9/L [108].

8.3.3 Special Indications

8.3.3.1 Fetal and Neonatal Alloimmune Thrombocytopenia (FNAIT)

In FNAIT, maternal IgG class antibodies cross the placenta and target human-platelet antigens (HPAs) causing immune-mediated thrombocytopenia. The majority of FNAIT cases involve anti-HPA-1a (79%), anti-HPA-5b (9%), HPA-3a (2%), and HPA-1b (4%) antibodies [109]. In most cases, the mothers are asymptomatic, and the disease spectrum ranges from mild asymptomatic thrombocytopenia to severe bleeding, including ICH, though extracranial hemorrhage is rare [110].

The treatment of choice for FNAIT is ideally to transfuse HPA-matched platelets, depending on the severity of thrombocytopenia and clinical symptoms. Random donor platelet transfusions do not typically lead to sustained increases in platelet counts but may be used to reduce the risk of ICH. Maternal platelets could be used; however, they should be antigen negative, leukoreduced, and irradiated. Intravenous immunoglobulin (IVIg) may be considered when multiple or long-term transfusions are necessary [93]. In a systematic review on postnatal management of FNAIT, the use of selected platelets or unselected platelets, as well as use of IVIg on platelet increments, hemorrhage, and mortality, showed that the use of selected platelets resulted in higher increments and longer response [111]. Unselected platelets were able to increase platelets above 30 $\times$ 10^9/L avoiding ICH or life-threatening bleeding. IVIg did not seem to improve platelet increments. A systematic review by Lieberman et al. presents evidence-based recommendations from a panel of experts considering the antenatal and postnatal periods, delivery, and maternal HPA screening. The paper also emphasizes unmet needs, such as further research on FNAIT, studies on biomarkers to guide the antenatal approach, studies on affected families' quality of life, reduction in mortality and morbidity associated with FNAIT, and screening algorithms [112].

8.3.3.2 Intrauterine Platelet Transfusion

Intrauterine transfusion (IUT) described by Liley in 1963 [113] has evolved and saved many lives. FNAIT is the most common indication for a platelet IUT. Platelets for IUT should be HPA compatible, irradiated, and cytomegalovirus (CMV) safe, making leukoreduction necessary.

The unit should be warmed to 37 °C before transfusion, and the infusion should be administered slowly [114].

Key Points
- Platelet dosing remains a subject of significant controversy, and there is no universally accepted "standard platelet dose." Close monitoring of patients' responses to platelet transfusions is crucial to identify those with poor responses, prompting further clinical and laboratory investigations to determine the underlying cause and the most appropriate management approach.
- Multiple medical societies' platelet transfusion guidelines align in strongly recommending prophylactic platelet transfusions for cases of severe hypoproliferative thrombocytopenia (platelet count less than 10×10^9/L).
- Decisions regarding platelet transfusions, whether for prophylactic or therapeutic purposes, should take into account the potential risks of adverse transfusion reactions, refractoriness, contraindications in specific clinical settings, and availability of platelet products.

References

1. Michelson AD. Platelets. Elsevier Science; 2013.
2. Grozovsky R, Begonja AJ, Liu K, Visner G, Hartwig JH, Falet H, et al. The Ashwell-Morell receptor regulates hepatic thrombopoietin production via JAK2-STAT3 signaling. Nat Med. 2015;21(1):47–54.
3. Harker LA, Slichter SJ. The bleeding time as a screening test for evaluation of platelet function. N Engl J Med. 1972;287(4):155–9.
4. Hanson SR, Slichter SJ. Platelet kinetics in patients with bone marrow hypoplasia: evidence for a fixed platelet requirement. Blood. 1985;66(5):1105–9.
5. Aursnes I. Blood platelet production and red cell leakage to lymph during thrombocytopenia. Scand J Hematol. 1974;13(3):184–95.
6. Mehmet Ali Erkurt EK, Berber I, Koroglu M, Kuku I. Thrombocytopenia in adults: review article. J Hematol. 2012;1(2–3):44–53.
7. Slichter SJ, Harker LA. Thrombocytopenia: mechanisms and management of defects in platelet production. Clin Hematol. 1978;7(3):523–39.
8. Gaydos LA, Freireich EJ, Mantel N. The quantitative relation between platelet count and hemorrhage in patients with acute leukemia. N Engl J Med. 1962;266:905–9.
9. Yuan S, Otrock ZK. Platelet transfusion: an update on indications and guidelines. Clin Lab Med. 2021;41(4):621–34.
10. Solves P, Carpio N, Balaguer A, Romero S, Iacoboni G, Gomez I, et al. Transfusion of ABO non-identical platelets does not influence the clinical outcome of patients undergoing autologous hematopoietic stem cell transplantation. Blood Transfus. 2015;13(3):411–6.
11. Triulzi DJ, Assmann SF, Strauss RG, Ness PM, Hess JR, Kaufman RM, et al. The impact of platelet transfusion characteristics on posttransfusion platelet increments and clinical bleeding in patients with hypoproliferative thrombocytopenia. Blood. 2012;119(23):5553–62.
12. Heal JM, Masel D, Rowe JM, Blumberg N. Circulating immune complexes involving the ABO system after platelet transfusion. Br J Hematol. 1993;85(3):566–72.
13. Heal JM, Masel D, Blumberg N. Interaction of platelet fc and complement receptors with circulating immune complexes involving the AB0 system. Vox Sang. 1996;71(4):205–11.
14. Heal JM, Rowe JM, Blumberg N. ABO and platelet transfusion revisited. Ann Hematol. 1993;66(6):309–14.
15. Heal JM, Rowe JM, McMican A, Masel D, Finke C, Blumberg N. The role of ABO matching in platelet transfusion. Eur J Hematol. 1993;50(2):110–7.
16. Moinuddin IA, Millward P, Fletcher CH. Acute intravascular hemolysis following an ABO non-identical platelet transfusion: a case report and literature review. Am J Case Rep. 2019;20:1075–9.
17. Berseus O, Boman K, Nessen SC, Westerberg LA. Risks of hemolysis due to anti-A and anti-B caused by the transfusion of blood or blood components containing ABO-incompatible plasma. Transfusion. 2013;53(Suppl 1):114S–23S.
18. Fung MK, Downes KA, Shulman IA. Transfusion of platelets containing ABO-incompatible plasma: a survey of 3156 north American laboratories. Arch Pathol Lab Med. 2007;131(6):909–16.
19. Quillen K, Sheldon SL, Daniel-Johnson JA, Lee-Stroka AH, Flegel WA. A practical strategy to reduce the risk of passive hemolysis by screening plateletpheresis donors for high-titer ABO antibodies. Transfusion. 2011;51(1):92–6.
20. Fontaine MJ, Mills AM, Weiss S, Hong WJ, Viele M, Goodnough LT. How we treat: risk mitigation for ABO-incompatible plasma in plateletpheresis products. Transfusion. 2012;52(10):2081–5.
21. Tynuv M, Flegel WA. Quality improvement with platelet additive solution for safer out-of-group platelet transfusions. Immunohematology. 2019;35(3):108–15.
22. Qureshi H, Massey E, Kirwan D, Davies T, Robson S, White J, et al. BCSH guideline for the use of anti-D immunoglobulin for the prevention of hemolytic

disease of the fetus and newborn. Transfus Med. 2014;24(1):8–20.

23. Ayache S, Herman JH. Prevention of D sensitization after mismatched transfusion of blood components: toward optimal use of RhIG. Transfusion. 2008;48(9):1990–9.

24. Weinstein R, Simard A, Ferschke J, Vauthrin M, Bailey JA, Greene M. Prospective surveillance of D- recipients of D+ apheresis platelets: alloimmunization against D is not detected. Transfusion. 2015;55(6):1327–30.

25. O'Brien KL, Haspel RL, Uhl L. Anti-D alloimmunization after D-incompatible platelet transfusions: a 14-year single-institution retrospective review. Transfusion. 2014;54(3):650–4.

26. Murphy MF. Managing the platelet refractory patient. ISBT Sci Ser. 2014;9(1):234–8.

27. Hod E, Schwartz J. Platelet transfusion refractoriness. Br J Hematol. 2008;142(3):348–60.

28. Slichter SJ, Davis K, Enright H, Braine H, Gernsheimer T, Kao KJ, et al. Factors affecting posttransfusion platelet increments, platelet refractoriness, and platelet transfusion intervals in thrombocytopenic patients. Blood. 2005;105(10):4106–14.

29. Murphy MF, Waters AH. Platelet transfusions: the problem of refractoriness. Blood Rev. 1990;4(1):16–24.

30. Slichter SJ. Transfusion and bone marrow transplantation. Transfus Med Rev. 1988;2(1):1–17.

31. Li G, Liu F, Mao X, Hu L. The investigation of platelet transfusion refractory in 69 malignant patients undergoing hematopoietic stem cell transplantation. Transfus Apher Sci. 2011;45(1):21–4.

32. Leukocyte reduction and ultraviolet B irradiation of platelets to prevent Alloimmunization and refractoriness to platelet transfusions. The Trial to Reduce Alloimmunization to Platelets Study Group. New Engl J Med. 1997;337(26):1861–70.

33. Hagino T, Sato T, Tsuno NH, Tasaki T. Incidence and management of non-immune platelet transfusion refractoriness: a narrative review. Ann Blood. 2021;6:28.

34. Doughty HA, Murphy MF, Metcalfe P, Rohatiner AZ, Lister TA, Waters AH. Relative importance of immune and non-immune causes of platelet refractoriness. Vox Sang. 1994;66(3):200–5.

35. Howard JE, Perkins HA. The natural history of alloimmunization to platelets. Transfusion. 1978;18(4):496–503.

36. Saris A, Pavenski K. Human leukocyte antigen alloimmunization and alloimmune platelet refractoriness. Transfus Med Rev. 2020;34(4):250–7.

37. Hunt BJ, Allard S, Keeling D, et al. A practical guideline for the hematological management of major hemorrhage. Br J Hematol. 2015;170(6):788–803.

38. Kerkhoffs JL, Eikenboom JC, van de Watering LM, van Wordragen-Vlaswinkel RJ, Wijermans PW, Brand A. The clinical impact of platelet refractoriness: correlation with bleeding and survival. Transfusion. 2008;48(9):1959–65.

39. Meehan KR, Matias CO, Rathore SS, et al. Platelet transfusions: utilization and associated costs in a tertiary care hospital. Am J Hematol. 2000;64(4):251–6.

40. Forest SK, Hod EA. Management of the platelet refractory patient. Hematol Oncol Clin North Am. 2016;30(3):665–77.

41. Triyono T, Vrielink H. Therapeutic apheresis in Asia: an Indonesia single center experience. J Clin Apher. 2015;30(3):139–40.

42. Wandt H, Schaefer-Eckart K, Wendelin K, et al. Therapeutic platelet transfusion versus routine prophylactic transfusion in patients with hematological malignancies: an open-label, multicentre, randomised study. Lancet. 2012;380(9850):1309–16.

43. Stanworth SJ, Estcourt LJ, Llewelyn CA, Murphy MF, Wood EM, Investigators TS. Impact of prophylactic platelet transfusions on bleeding events in patients with hematologic malignancies: a subgroup analysis of a randomized trial. Transfusion. 2014;54(10):2385–93.

44. Stanworth SJ, Estcourt LJ, Powter G, et al. A no-prophylaxis platelet-transfusion strategy for hematologic cancers. N Engl J Med. 2013;368(19):1771–80.

45. Kumar A, Mhaskar R, Grossman BJ, et al. Platelet transfusion: a systematic review of the clinical evidence. Transfusion. 2015;55(5):1116–27.

46. Anthon CT, Granholm A, Sivapalan P, et al. Prophylactic platelet transfusions versus no prophylaxis in hospitalized patients with thrombocytopenia: a systematic review with meta-analysis. Transfusion. 2022;62(10):2117–36.

47. Lye DC, Archuleta S, Syed-Omar SF, Low JG, Oh HM, Wei Y, et al. Prophylactic platelet transfusion plus supportive care versus supportive care alone in adults with dengue and thrombocytopenia: a multicentre, open-label, randomised, superiority trial. Lancet. 2017;389(10079):1611–8.

48. Khan Assir MZ, Kamran U, Ahmad HI, et al. Effectiveness of platelet transfusion in dengue fever: a randomized controlled trial. Transfus Med Hemother. 2013;40(5):362–8.

49. Murphy S, Litwin S, Herring LM, et al. Indications for platelet transfusion in children with acute leukemia. Am J Hematol. 1982;12(4):347–56.

50. Solomon J, Bofenkamp T, Fahey JL, Chillar RK, Beutel E. Platelet prophylaxis in acute non-lymphoblastic leukaemia. Lancet. 1978;1(8058):267.

51. Takami A, Matsushita T, Ogata M, Fet al. Guideline for the use of platelet transfusion concentrates based on scientific evidence. Jpn J Transfus Cell Ther. 2017;63(4):569–84. https://doi.org/10.3925/jjtc.63.569.

52. Slichter SJ. Relationship between platelet count and bleeding risk in thrombocytopenic patients. Transfus Med Rev. 2004;18(3):153–67.

53. Djerassi I, Farber S, Evans AE. Transfusions of fresh platelet concentrates to patients with secondary thrombocytopenia. N Engl J Med. 1963;268:221–6.

54. Schiffer CA, Anderson KC, Bennett CL, et al. Platelet transfusion for patients with cancer: clinical practice guidelines of the American Society of Clinical Oncology. J Clin Oncol. 2001;19(5):1519–38.

55. Murphy MF, Brozovic B, Murphy W, Ouwehand W, Waters AH. Guidelines for platelet transfusions. British Committee for Standards in Hematology, Working Party of the Blood Transfusion Task Force. Transfus Med. 1992;2(4):311–8.

56. Schiffer CA, Bohlke K, Anderson KC. Platelet transfusion for patients with cancer: American Society of Clinical Oncology clinical practice guideline update summary. J Oncol Pract. 2018;14(2):129–33.

57. Estcourt LJ, Birchall J, Allard S, Bassey SJ, Hersey P, Kerr JP, et al. Guidelines for the use of platelet transfusions. Br J Hematol. 2017;176(3):365–94.

58. Killick SB, Bown N, Cavenagh J, et al. Guidelines for the diagnosis and management of adult aplastic anaemia. Br J Hematol. 2016;172(2):187–207.

59. Nahirniak S, Slichter SJ, Tanael S, et al. Guidance on platelet transfusion for patients with hypoproliferative thrombocytopenia. Transfus Med Rev. 2015;29(1):3–13.

60. Kaufman RM, Djulbegovic B, Gernsheimer T, et al. Platelet transfusion: a clinical practice guideline from the AABB. Ann Intern Med. 2015;162(3):205–13.

61. Al-Riyami AZ, Jug R, La Rocca U, et al. Quality of evidence-based guidelines for platelet transfusion and use: a systematic review. Transfusion. 2021;61(3):948–58.

62. Schiffer CA, Bohlke K, Delaney M, et al. Platelet transfusion for patients with cancer: American Society of Clinical Oncology clinical practice guideline update. J Clin Oncol. 2018;36(3):283–99.

63. Liumbruno G, Bennardello F, Lattanzio A, Piccoli P, Rossetti G. Recommendations for the transfusion of plasma and platelets. Blood Transfus. 2009;7(2):132–50.

64. Slichter SJ, Kaufman RM, Assmann SF, et al. Dose of prophylactic platelet transfusions and prevention of hemorrhage. N Engl J Med. 2010;362(7):600–13.

65. Heddle NM, Cook RJ, Tinmouth A, et al. A randomized controlled trial comparing standard- and low-dose strategies for transfusion of platelets (SToP) to patients with thrombocytopenia. Blood. 2009;113(7):1564–73.

66. Solves Alcaina P. Platelet transfusion: and update on challenges and outcomes. J Blood Med. 2020;11:19–26.

67. Storch EK, Custer BS, Jacobs MR, Menitove JE, Mintz PD. Review of current transfusion therapy and blood banking practices. Blood Rev. 2019;38:100593.

68. Newland A, Bentley R, Jakubowska A, et al. A systematic literature review on the use of platelet transfusions in patients with thrombocytopenia. Hematology. 2019;24(1):679–719.

69. Tallman MS, Altman JK. How I treat acute promyelocytic leukemia. Blood. 2009;114(25):5126–35.

70. Sanz MA, Tallman MS, Lo-Coco F. Tricks of the trade for the appropriate management of newly diagnosed acute promyelocytic leukemia. Blood. 2005;105(8):3019–25.

71. Lee RH, Kasthuri RS, Bergmeier W. Platelet transfusion for patients with platelet dysfunction: effectiveness, mechanisms, and unanswered questions. Curr Opin Hematol. 2020;27(6):378–85.

72. Pagano D, Milojevic M, Meesters MI, et al. 2017 EACTS/EACTA guidelines on patient blood management for adult cardiac surgery. Eur J Cardiothorac Surg. 2018;53(1):79–111.

73. Siller-Matula JM, Petre A, Delle-Karth G, et al. Impact of preoperative use of P2Y12 receptor inhibitors on clinical outcomes in cardiac and non-cardiac surgery: a systematic review and meta-analysis. Eur Heart J Acute Cardiovasc Care. 2017;6(8):753–70.

74. Kwak YL, Kim JC, Choi YS, Yoo KJ, Song Y, Shim JK. Clopidogrel responsiveness regardless of the discontinuation date predicts increased blood loss and transfusion requirement after off-pump coronary artery bypass graft surgery. J Am Coll Cardiol. 2010;56(24):1994–2002.

75. Ferraris VA, Saha SP, Oestreich JH, et al. 2012 update to the Society of Thoracic Surgeons guideline on use of antiplatelet drugs in patients having cardiac and noncardiac operations. Ann Thorac Surg. 2012;94(5):1761–81.

76. Zakko L, Rustagi T, Douglas M, Laine L. No benefit from platelet transfusion for gastrointestinal bleeding in patients taking antiplatelet agents. Clin Gastroenterol Hepatol. 2017;15(1):46–52.

77. Baharoglu MI, Cordonnier C, Al-Shahi Salman R, det al. Platelet transfusion versus standard care after acute stroke due to spontaneous cerebral hemorrhage associated with antiplatelet therapy (PATCH): a randomised, open-label, phase 3 trial. Lancet. 2016;387(10038):2605–13.

78. Holcomb JB, del Junco DJ, Fox EE, et al. The prospective, observational, multicenter, major trauma transfusion (PROMMTT) study: comparative effectiveness of a time-varying treatment with competing risks. JAMA Surg. 2013;148(2):127–36.

79. Holcomb JB, Tilley BC, Baraniuk S, et al. Transfusion of plasma, platelets, and red blood cells in a 1:1:1 vs a 1:1:2 ratio and mortality in patients with severe trauma: the PROPPR randomized clinical trial. JAMA. 2015;313(5):471–82.

80. Cardenas JC, Zhang X, Fox EE, Cotton BA, Hess JR, Schreiber MA, t al. Platelet transfusions improve hemostasis and survival in a substudy of the prospective, randomized PROPPR trial. Blood Adv. 2018;2(14):1696–704.

81. Hess AS, Ramamoorthy J, Hess JR. Perioperative platelet transfusions. Anesthesiology. 2021;134(3):471–9.

82. Hayakawa M, Gando S, Ono Y, Wada T, Yanagida Y, Sawamura A. Fibrinogen level deteriorates before other routine coagulation parameters and massive transfusion in the early phase of severe trauma: a retrospective observational study. Semin Thromb Hemost. 2015;41(1):35–42.

83. Practice Bulletin No. 183: Postpartum Hemorrhage. Obstet Gynecol. 2017;130(4):e168–e86.

84. Villalba A, Santiago M, Freiria C, et al. Anti-D Alloimmunization after RhD-positive platelet transfusion in RhD-negative women under 55 years diagnosed with acute leukemia: results of a retrospective study. Transfus Med Hemother. 2018;45(3):162–6.

85. Veen J, Nokes T, Makris M. The risk of spinal hematoma following neuraxial anaesthesia or lumbar puncture in thrombocytopenic individuals. Br J Hematol. 2009;148:15–25.

86. Estcourt LJ, Malouf R, Doree C, Trivella M, Hopewell S, Birchall J. Prophylactic platelet transfusions prior to surgery for people with a low platelet count. Cochrane Database Syst Rev. 2017;2017(9).

87. Practice guidelines for perioperative blood transfusion and adjuvant therapies: an updated report by the American Society of Anesthesiologists Task Force on perioperative blood transfusion and adjuvant therapies. Anesthesiology. 2006;105(1):198–208.

88. Webert KE, Mittal R, Sigouin C, Heddle NM, Kelton JG. A retrospective 11-year analysis of obstetric patients with idiopathic thrombocytopenic purpura. Blood. 2003;102(13):4306–11.

89. Abebe Gebreselassie H, Getachew H, et al. Incidence and risk factors of thrombocytopenia in neonates admitted with surgical disorders to neonatal intensive care unit of Tikur Anbessa specialized hospital: a one-year observational prospective cohort study from a low-income country. J Blood Med. 2021;12:691–7.

90. Ferrer-Marin F, Liu ZJ, Gutti R, Sola-Visner M. Neonatal thrombocytopenia and megakaryocytopoiesis. Semin Hematol. 2010;47(3):281–8.

91. Dreyfus M, Kaplan C, Verdy E, Schlegel N, Durand-Zaleski I, Tchernia G. Frequency of immune thrombocytopenia in newborns: a prospective study. Immune Thrombocytopenia Working Group. Blood. 1997;89(12):4402–6.

92. Elmoneim AA, Zolaly M, El-Moneim EA, Sultan E. Prognostic significance of early platelet count decline in preterm newborns. Indian J Crit Care Med. 2015;19(8):456–61.

93. Sillers L, Van Slambrouck C, Lapping-Carr G. Neonatal thrombocytopenia: etiology and diagnosis. Pediatr Ann. 2015;44(7):e175–80.

94. Zerra PE, Josephson CD. Transfusion in neonatal patients: review of evidence-based guidelines. Clin Lab Med. 2021;41(1):15–34.

95. Curley A, Stanworth SJ, Willoughby K, et al. Randomized trial of platelet-transfusion thresholds in neonates. N Engl J Med. 2019;380(3):242–51.

96. Fustolo-Gunnink SF, Fijnvandraat K, van Klaveren D, et al. Preterm neonates benefit from low prophylactic platelet transfusion threshold despite varying risk of bleeding or death. Blood. 2019;134(26):2354–60.

97. Moore CM, D'Amore A, Fustolo-Gunnink S, Hudson C, Newton A, Santamaria BL, et al. Two-year outcomes following a randomised platelet transfusion trial in preterm infants. Arch Dis Child Fetal Neonatal Ed. 2023;108(5):452–7.

98. Patel RM, Josephson C. Neonatal and pediatric platelet transfusions: current concepts and controversies. Curr Opin Hematol. 2019;26(6):466–72.

99. Sola-Visner M, Leeman KT, Stanworth SJ. Neonatal platelet transfusions: new evidence and the challenges of translating evidence-based recommendations into clinical practice. J Thromb Hemost. 2022;20(3):556–64.

100. Kelly AM, Garner SF, Foukaneli T, et al. The effect of variation in donor platelet function on transfusion outcome: a semirandomized controlled trial. Blood. 2017;130(2):214–20.

101. Magid-Bernstein J, Beaman CB, Carvalho-Poyraz F, et al. Impacts of ABO-incompatible platelet transfusions on platelet recovery and outcomes after intracerebral hemorrhage. Blood. 2021;137(19):2699–703.

102. Sparger KA, Assmann SF, Granger S, Winston A, Christensen RD, Widness JA, et al. Platelet transfusion practices among very-low-birth-weight infants. JAMA Pediatr. 2016;170(7):687–94.

103. Baer VL, Lambert DK, Henry E, Christensen RD. Severe thrombocytopenia in the NICU. Pediatrics. 2009;124(6):e1095–100.

104. Roschitz B, Sudi K, Kostenberger M, Muntean W. Shorter PFA-100 closure times in neonates than in adults: role of red cells, white cells, platelets and von Willebrand factor. Acta Paediatr. 2001;90(6):664–70.

105. Gerrard JM, Docherty JC, Israels SJ, et al. A reassessment of the bleeding time: association of age, hematocrit, platelet function, von Willebrand factor, and bleeding time thromboxane B2 with the length of the bleeding time. Clin Invest Med. 1989;12(3):165–71.

106. Cetinkaya M, Atasay B. Editorial: transfusions in the neonatal period. Front Pediatr. 2022;10:982918.

107. Sallmon H, Weimann A, Buhrer C, Metze B, Dame C, Cremer M. Immature platelet counts and thrombopoietin plasma concentrations in thrombocytopenic and non-thrombocytopenic preterm infants. Front Pediatr. 2021;9:685643.

108. Kahn S, Chegondi M, Nellis ME, Karam O. Overview of plasma and platelet transfusions in critically ill children. Front Pediatr. 2020;8:601659.

109. Davoren A, Curtis BR, Aster RH, McFarland JG. Human platelet antigen-specific alloantibodies implicated in 1162 cases of neonatal alloimmune thrombocytopenia. Transfusion. 2004;44(8):1220–5.

110. Winkelhorst D, Kamphuis MM, de Kloet LC, Zwaginga JJ, Oepkes D, Lopriore E. Severe bleeding complications other than intracranial hemorrhage in neonatal alloimmune thrombocytopenia: a case series and review of the literature. Transfusion. 2016;56(5):1230–5.

111. Baker JM, Shehata N, Bussel J, Murphy MF, Greinacher A, Bakchoul T, et al. Postnatal intervention for the treatment of FNAIT: a systematic review. J Perinatol. 2019;39(10):1329–39.

112. Lieberman L, Greinacher A, Murphy MF, et al. Fetal and neonatal alloimmune thrombocytopenia: recommendations for evidence-based practice, an international approach. Br J Hematol. 2019;185(3):549–62.

113. Liley AW. Intrauterine transfusion of foetus in hemolytic disease. Br Med J. 1963;2(5365):1107–9.

114. Mo YD, Bahar B, Jacquot C. Intrauterine, neonatal and pediatric transfusion therapy. Ann Blood. 2022;7:13.

Red Blood Cell Transfusion

9

Richard R. Gammon, Naomi Rahimi-Levene,
Flavia M. Bandeira, and Arwa Z. Al-Riyami

9.1 Red Blood Cell Transfusion

9.1.1 Indications for Red Cell Transfusion

Red cell transfusion is a widespread medical intervention. In the United States (US), in 2021, 11,784,000 red blood cell (RBC) units were collected, and 10,764,000 RBC units were transfused [1]. As of 2018, an estimated 3.8% of hospitalizations in the US included a RBC transfusion [2]. In Northern England, about 50% of units are given to medical and 40% to surgical patients; hip replacement and coronary artery bypass graft procedures were the most common surgical indications [3]. RBC units are also frequently administered to critically ill patients as supportive therapy to patients receiving chemotherapy and marrow transplants, and patients with blood loss from medical conditions such as gastrointestinal bleeding [4]. Approximately 25% of all RBCs transfused are given to patients with a primary diagnosis of cardiac disease [5], and 8% of all cardiology admissions are transfused with RBCs [5]. In recent years, blood use has declined as clinicians adopt a more restrictive approach to transfusion [6].

While most patients can increase tissue oxygen delivery and the extraction of oxygen from the RBCs over a range of hemoglobin concentrations [7], RBCs are transfused to increase oxygen-carrying capacity in patients with anemia whose physiologic compensatory mechanisms are inadequate to maintain normal tissue. There are many causes of anemia (Table 9.1).

In patients with chronic stable anemia, RBC transfusion is often unnecessary. For example, replacing iron is the appropriate maneuver to correct the anemia in a patient with well-compensated anemia from iron deficiency. RBC transfusion may also be lifesaving in individuals with anemia, where physiologic compensatory mechanisms are inadequate to maintain tissue oxygenation, such as in individuals with trauma-induced hemorrhage. In nonbleeding patients, the hemoglobin concentration is used to help guide RBC transfusion decisions because 98% of blood oxygen is hemoglobin bound, the hemoglobin is easy to measure, and no better physiologic measurements

R. R. Gammon
OneBlood, Orlando, FL, USA

N. Rahimi-Levene
Blood Bank, Shamir (Assaf Harofeh) Medical Center, Zerifin, delson School of Medicine, Ariel Universtiy, Ariel, Israel
e-mail: nrlevene@shamir.gov.il

F. M. Bandeira
Blood Bank and Transfusion Medicine Department, Rio de Janeiro State University, Pedro Ernesto University Hospital, Rio de Janeiro, Brazil

A. Z. Al-Riyami (✉)
Department of Haematology, Sultan Qaboos University Hospital, Sultan Qaboos University, Muscat, Oman
e-mail: arwa@squ.edu.om

© The Author(s), under exclusive license to Springer Nature Switzerland AG 2024
C. T. Smit Sibinga, Y. E. Abdella (eds.), *Clinical Use of Blood*,
https://doi.org/10.1007/978-3-031-67332-0_9

Table 9.1 Causes of anemia

Common causes of anemia	
Hypoplastic	Iron deficiency
	B12 deficiency
	Folate deficiency
	Anemia of inflammation (anemia of chronic disease)
	Drugs
	Toxins
	Pure red blood cell aplasia (viral or idiopathic)
	Myelodysplastic syndrome
	Marrow replacement caused by malignancy
Hemolytic	Inherited hemoglobinopathies
	Inherited membrane disorders
	Glucose 6 phosphate deficiency (G6PD)
	Autoimmune hemolytic anemia
	Microangiopathic hemolytic anemia

Adapted from Chapter 35, Approach to anemia in the adult and the child, JC Linn and EJ Benz. In: Hematology, Basic Principles and Practice, editors Hoffman et al., Elsevier 2023

to support RBC transfusion are currently available. As will be discussed, the hemoglobin thresholds where transfusions are recommended are lower than those used previously [8].

9.1.2 Donor Characteristics and Transfusion Recipient Outcomes

The quality of RBC can be significantly affected by the characteristics of blood donors (e.g., health status, various phenotypes-antigens present on RBCs), and an important aim of current measures in reducing risks for recipients is to better select blood donors [9]. Relevant transfusion-transmitted infections (RTTIs) can potentially affect recipients' long-term outcome. Such is the case of human immunodeficiency virus (HIV) and other pathogens. These risks can be reduced by a variety of measures, including donor questionnaires that assess infectious risk, RTTI blood screening, and other quality measures, many of which are already implemented by blood centers. Other characteristics have been suggested to affect the outcome of transfusion recipients, notably in plasma transfusion [10, 11]. For example, the female sex, a history of pregnancy, and the presence of anti-leukocytes antibodies in blood products have been associated with the risk

of transfusion-related acute lung injury (TRALI), which is the second most common cause of mortality after blood transfusion [12, 13]. These findings have led to potentially successful interventions (transfusion of predominantly male plasma), with the subsequent decrease in the occurrence of TRALI [9].

Although one could easily draw comparisons between RBC transfusions and solid organ or bone marrow transplantation, there needs to be more data regarding the impact of donor characteristics on transfusion outcomes. Identifying donor characteristics associated with transfusion recipient outcomes may lead to the optimal selection of blood donors and donor–recipient matching. For example, findings suggesting that donations from donors with specific characteristics (age, sex, blood groups, comorbidities, etc.) negatively affect transfusion outcomes may lead to revised donation practices with the exclusion of such donors from the donor pool [9].

A systematic review was conducted to assess the association between blood donor characteristics and RBC transfusion outcomes. From 6121 citations identified by the literature search, 59 studies met eligibility criteria (50 observational and 9 interventional). The study involved the evaluation of the potential association of 17 donor characteristics on RBC transfusion recipient outcome (Table 9.2).

Table 9.2 List of donor characteristics evaluated for their effect on blood transfusion recipients

Age
Gender
Cancer history
Human leukocyte antigen (HLA) selection
White blood cell (WBC) antibody status
RBC antigen selection
Previously pregnant or transfused
Walking donor program
Parental donor
Babesiosis
Cytomegalovirus
Hepatitis B virus
Hepatitis C virus
Human herpes virus-8
Human T-lymphotropic virus
Liver biochemistry test status
Human parvovirus B19
Travel to West Nile endemic area
Travel of malaria-endemic area
Human immunodeficiency virus

9.1.2.1 Donor Gender

Potential associations were observed for donor gender with reduced survival at 90 days and 6 months in male recipients that receive donated blood from females (hazard ratio [HR] 2.60 [1.09, 6.20] and HR 2.40 [1.10, 5.24], respectively; $n = 1$), human leukocyte antigen-antigen D related (HLA-DR) selected transfusions (odds ratio [OR] 0.39 [0.15, 0.99] for the risk of transplant alloimmunization, $n = 9$), presence of antileukocyte antibodies (OR 5.84 [1.66, 20.59] for risk of TRALI, $n = 4$), and donor RBC antigens selection (OR 0.20 [0.08, 0.52] for risk of alloimmunization, $n = 4$) [9]. The study concluded that, based on very low to low-quality evidence, some donor characteristics may affect RBC transfusion outcomes. Notably, the authors stated that the evidence is insufficient to draw definitive conclusions about any donor characteristics [9].

Another study used survival analysis to compare four groups: female-to-female, female-to-male, male-to-female, and male-to-male transfusion. A multivariate logistic model was used to evaluate the association between donor gender and intensive care unit (ICU) mortality. Associations between transfusion and acute kid-

ney injury (AKI), acute respiratory distress syndrome (ARDS), and nosocomial infections were assessed [14].

Of the 6992 patients included in the original cohort study, 403 patients received a unisex transfusion. Survival analysis and the logistic model showed that transfusion of female RBCs to male patients was associated with an increased ICU mortality compared with transfusion of female RBCs to female patients (odds ratio, 2.43; 95% CI, 1.02–5.77; $P < 0.05$). There was also a trend toward increased ARDS in patients receiving RBC from female donors compared with those receiving blood from males ($P = 0.06$), whereas AKI was higher in donor–recipient sex-matched transfusion groups compared with sex-mismatched groups ($P = 0.05$). The study concluded that there were significant associations between male patients who received RBCs from female donors and ICU mortality, which may in part be due to ARDS, although other, as yet undetermined, factors, they stated, are likely to be present. It was emphasized that this was an exploratory study with potential uncontrolled confounders that limited the broad generalization of the findings [14].

A third study evaluated the concern that transfusion of RBCs from female donors has been associated with increased mortality in male recipients. This was a retrospective cohort study of first-time transfusion recipients at six major Dutch hospitals enrolled over a 10-year period. The primary analysis was the no-donor-mixture cohort (i.e., either all RBC transfusions exclusively from male donors or all exclusively from female donors without a history of pregnancy or all exclusively from female donors with a history of pregnancy). The association between mortality and exposure to transfusions from ever-pregnant or never-pregnant female donors was analyzed.

The cohort for the primary analyses consisted of 31,118 patients (median age, 65 [interquartile range, 42–77] years; 52% female) who received 59,320 RBC transfusions exclusively from 1 of 3 types of donors (88% male, 6% ever-pregnant female, and 6% never-pregnant female). The number of deaths in this cohort was 3969 (13% mortality). For male recipients of RBC transfusions, all-cause mortality rates after a RBC transfusion from an ever-pregnant female donor vs. male donor were 101 vs. 80 deaths per 1000 person-years (time-dependent "per transfusion" HR for death, 1.13 [95%CI, 1.01–1.26]). For receipt of transfusion from a never-pregnant female donor vs. male donor, mortality rates were 78 vs. 80 deaths per 1000 person-years (HR, 0.93 [95%CI, 0.81–1.06]). Among female recipients of RBC transfusions, mortality rates for an ever-pregnant female donor vs. male donor were 74 vs. 62 per 1000 person-years (HR, 0.99 [15]); for a never-pregnant female donor vs. male donor, mortality rates were 74 vs. 62 per 1000 person-years (HR, 1.01 [95%CI, 0.88–1.15]). The study concluded that among patients who received RBC transfusions, receipt of a transfusion from an ever-pregnant female donor, compared with a male donor, was associated with increased all-cause mortality among male recipients but not among female recipients. It also noted that transfusions from never-pregnant female donors were not associated with increased mortality among male or female recipients [15].

The final study was a retrospective analysis of all neonates receiving one or more RBC transfusion during a 12-year period at one US hospital system, matching mortality and specific morbidities of each transfusion recipient with the gender and age of each donor. There were 6396 RBC transfusions administered to 2086 infants in 15 hospitals. A total of 825 infants were transfused exclusively with RBC from female donors, 935 infants were transfused exclusively with RBC from male donors, and 326 infants were transfused with RBC from both female and male donors. Infants who received blood from both male and female donors had more RBC transfusions (5.3 ± 2.9 transfusions if received both male and female donor blood vs. 2.6 ± 2.2 if received blood from only one sex, mean $\pm$ SD, $p < 0.001$). The study identified no significant differences in mortality or morbidities associated with the sex or age of blood donors. Similarly, an analysis of matched vs. mismatched donor/recipient sex revealed no associations with death or neonatal morbidities. The study concluded that these data support the practice of transfusing newborn infants with RBC obtained from donors of either gender and regardless of donor age [16]. Other studies have evaluated specific medications, foods, or substances.

9.1.2.2 Peanut Allergies

A 6-year-old boy with acute lymphoblastic leukemia had an anaphylactic reaction while receiving a leukocyte reduced pooled buffy-coat product with ABO-identical platelets. The patient's mother stated that her son had a similar reaction after eating peanuts at the age of 1 year. Three of the five blood donors, contacted shortly after the transfusion reaction, recalled eating several handfuls of peanuts the evening before donation. The digestion-resistant peptide from *Arachis hypogea* (*Ara h2*) can be detected in serum for up to 24 h after ingestion. The authors corroborated the recipient's peanut allergy with an ImmunoCAP assay (Phadia) that revealed a serum level of peanut-specific IgE of 72.5 kU/L (normal level, <0.35). These data are consistent with the hypothesis that the consumption of peanuts by the donors before blood donation provided the trigger for this patient's transfusion reaction [17].

A second case involved a 4-year-old male with acute lymphocytic leukemia who was transfused a unit of RBCs and platelets. Reflex enzyme-linked immunosorbent assay identified *Ara h1, h2, and h3*: 0.38, 3.71, and 0.22 kU of antibody per liter (kU/L; reference range, ≤ 0.1 kU/L), respectively. The blood product donors were contacted for pre-donation peanut intake, and while the RBC donor did not recall ingesting peanuts, the platelet donor recalled eating peanut butter for breakfast the morning of the donation [18].

9.1.2.3 Lead Levels

A study ascertained if hazardous concentrations of blood lead levels (BLL) are still present in transfused blood. The study measured the BLL of 100 units of blood by atomic absorption spectroscopy. The mean BLL was 0.11 9 µmol/L (SD 0.17), and the median was 0.07 umol/L (range 0.02–1.37). Two units had BLL of 0.99 µmol/L and 1.37 µmol/L, respectively, representing, per the authors, an unacceptable hazard of lead exposure, particularly for extremely low birthweight (ELBW) infants, who often receive multiple transfusions from the same donor [19]. The authors stated that to limit the dose of a premature infant receiving a 20 mL/kg blood transfusion to less than 0.36 ug/kg (and assuming blood transfusion is the only route of exposure to lead), the donor unit must have a lead concentration of less than 0.09 µmol/L. It was noted that 64% of the measured units in this study fit these criteria [19].

Another study conducted in Quebec had as an objective to determine BLLs in a representative sample of blood donors and to identify risk factors associated with BLLs of 0.15 mmol/L or more [20]. This number was determined by a health risk assessment performed by Institute National de Santé Publique du Quebec, the maximum level of lead in a blood donation that could safely be given to vulnerable patients, infants, and children less than 2 years of age [21]. The study was conducted from 2006 to 2007 in blood drive sites in Quebec. Lead analysis was performed by inductively coupled plasma mass spectrometry. Data on Quebec blood donors from 2003 to 2006 were used to establish a reference population. Of eligible individuals, 3490 participated (1392 women and 2098 men). Their mean age was 46.5 years. Results were weighted for region, sex, and age. The mean of BLLs was 0.082 mmol/L (95%CI, 0.027–0.247; range, 0.011–2.90 mmol/L). BLLs of more than 0.15 mmol/L were found in 15.5% of participants. In multivariate analysis, BLLs were mainly explained by the age and sex of participants ($p < 0.001$). A significant association was also found between BLLs and the region of residence, education level, dwelling age, and occupational and leisure activities at high risk for lead exposure, smoking, and alcohol intake ($p < 0.001$). The authors concluded that BLL in blood donors is strongly explained by sex and age, a fact that can be taken into consideration when transfusing neonates [20].

A recent study from China found similar results to the study by Bearer et al. of 2142 blood donors, 1434 were male and 708 were female, with an average age of 34.8 years. The mean of BLL was 26.03 µg/L (95% CI 25.52–26.56), and donors in the high blood lead group (≥ 35 µg/L) accounted for 25.6% of the study population [22]. Multivariate logistic regression analysis showed that males, increasing age, living in certain regions of China, duration of residence ≥ 30 years, and smoking were risk factors for high BLL, with odds ratios (95% CI) being 2.10 (1.61–2.73), 1.03 (1.01–1.04), 3.89 (1.09–13.86), 1.64 (1.22–2.20), and 1.76 (1.40–2.22), respectively. The study concluded that there are a number of risk factors associated with higher BLL.

Whether or not to establish a policy of transfusing RBCs containing only low lead levels in vulnerable populations, namely neonates and young children, remains a controversial issue. Implementing such a policy necessarily involves consultation with physicians transfusing susceptible patient populations, due consideration for the logistics involved and the impact of such a policy on product availability, and a study of the distribution of lead levels in the donor population if the policy decision is to supply "low-risk" units based on epidemiologic characteristics of the donor [20].

9.1.2.4 Nicotine

A US-based study examined segments from 105 RBC units that were tested for the presence of nicotine, cotinine, or trans-3′-hydroxy cotinine by liquid chromatography–tandem mass spectrometry. Of the 20 (19%) units that contained detectable concentrations of nicotine, cotinine, or trans-3′-hydroxy cotinine, 19 (18.1%) contained concentrations consistent with the use of a nicotine-containing product within 48 h of specimen collection. One RBC unit contained nicotine concentrations consistent with passive exposure. The study conclusion was that chemicals from nicotine-containing products are detectable within the US RBC supply. There were limitations of this study that included reported concentrations of nicotine and the metabolites in the RBC units may or may not represent a clinically significant amount, and it was not designed to establish an association between nicotine concentrations and clinical outcomes. The authors recommended further investigation to determine the risks of transfusion-associated exposure to nicotine and other tobacco-associated chemicals among vulnerable patient populations such as neonates [23].

9.1.2.5 Testosterone Therapy

Testosterone prescribing practices have significantly increased over the past 10 years in the US and Canada [24]. In response to a growing number of prospective blood donors on prescription testosterone, the US Food and Drug Administration (FDA) and Association for Advancement of Blood & Biotherapies (AABB) developed policies and procedures to address the safety of blood components collected through therapeutic phlebotomy of individuals with testosterone-induced erythrocytosis. Minutes from a 2014 meeting recommended that in order to decrease the risk of exposure to recipients, only RBCs may be distributed for transfusion, whereas the plasma and platelets should be discarded [25].

A study at a US-based blood center was conducted that quantified the concentrations of free (bioavailable; pg/mL) and total (protein-bound and free; ng/dL) testosterone in plasma (frozen within 24 h) and supernatants from 42-day stored leukocyte-reduced RBC units from 17 testosterone replacement therapy (TRT) male donors and 17 matched controls (no TRT). Plasma-free and total testosterone concentrations in TRT donors were 2.9 and 1.8 times higher than that of controls. Total testosterone concentrations in RBC supernatants were about 30% of that of plasma. In contrast, free testosterone concentrations in RBC supernatants were 80–100% of that of plasma and were significantly ($p = 0.005$) higher in TRT compared with controls (252.3 ± 245.3 vs. 103.4 ± 88.2 pg/mL). Supraphysiological free testosterone concentrations (>244 pg/mL) in RBC supernatants were observed in five TRT donors and two control donors.

Do supraphysiological concentrations of free testosterone in RBC pose a risk to transfusion recipients? There is no definitive answer to this question, given the absence of controlled clinical trials that would determine the impact of supra-

physiological testosterone in RBC units on transfusion outcomes. However, current knowledge suggests that the supraphysiological levels of free testosterone measured in this study were not likely to promote adverse events in most transfused patients.

While likely innocuous to most patients, there are cases in which patient exposure to testosterone may be unfavorable. Such cases include androgen-sensitive patients or patients with liver failure whose body may not be able to efficiently convert free testosterone to its inactive metabolites. One group, which was discussed during the 2014 FDA and AABB meeting, is neonates who may be subjected to multiple transfusions from a dedicated RBC unit.

The authors did suggest expanding the screening of blood donors with prescription testosterone to include more information about the type of testosterone medication and dose, side effects (erythrocytosis), and timing of the last dose taken prior to blood collection. It was noted that a significant spike in blood testosterone levels is likely to occur within the first 24 h after dosing; therefore, avoiding blood collection soon after testosterone therapy may reduce the chance of issuing blood products with supraphysiological testosterone levels [26].

9.1.2.6 Marijuana

Despite the fact that recreational marijuana consumption is legal in several countries around the world, there is a paucity of international literature on marijuana use, specifically among blood donors. A survey was conducted at a US-based blood center to define and quantify both the perspectives regarding and actual usage of marijuana in proximity to blood product donation.

The overall response rate was 8.03% (12,186 surveys sent with 979 responses). Of responding donors, 23.5% indicated that they felt that consuming various forms of marijuana was acceptable prior to blood donation. Marijuana use <72 h prior to blood donation was reported in all demographic groups surveyed except age 18–24 years. Of donors who reported daily marijuana use, 47.4% indicated >20 donations and 52.6% indicated apheresis platelet donations. The study concluded that nearly one-quarter of responding blood donors feel that marijuana use is acceptable prior to blood donation, and nearly every demographic group surveyed indicated the use of marijuana <72 h prior to donation.

The potential impact of Δ9-tetrahydrocannabinol (THC), the psychoactive component of marijuana, or its metabolites in donated blood products on a recipient is currently unknown. THC has been found in plasma products [27], and approximately 10% is bound to red cells [28]. While the large volume of distribution of THC would seem to make significant transfusion-associated marijuana exposure seem less likely in adults, the potential impact of THC on vulnerable populations through a blood transfusion, such as pregnant women, premature infants, or the fetus during intrauterine transfusion, has not been established and for which only future studies can determine [29].

A mention needs to be made of synthetic cannabinoids (SCs) that can either be used as spray-on agents to plant material or be combined in other ways for recreational use and are now classified as controlled substances by the US Drug Enforcement Administration. As such, the chemical formula of these compounds is changed frequently to avoid detection and legal regulation, explaining the startling evolution in toxicologic presentations [30].

In 2018, 94 individuals with "serious unexplained bleeding" presented to emergency departments; and there were two deaths. Illinois public health epidemiologists found reports of SCs use among all 63 patients interviewed. Of interest, three patients were discovered to have donated plasma before admission for coagulopathy management [31]; however, the final disposition of these units and the outcome of potential lookback studies were not reported. Treatment responses were noted to fresh-frozen plasma and high-dose vitamin K, and, in at least 18 patients, brodifacoum exposure was confirmed (despite a negative history of exposure to rodenticides containing this agent).

Brodifacoum is the most commonly encountered long-acting anticoagulant rodenticide (LAAR) in the US and has a half-life of 16–34 days. Since ingestion would affect blood products collected, some blood centers imposed a 6-month deferral period (i.e., five half-lives) from the date of last known SC use as a precaution [32].

9.1.3 Transfusion Guidelines and Clinical Decision Support

A method of improving compliance with hospital transfusion guidelines is the Computerized Provider Order Entry (CPOE) system with clinical decision support (CDS) through Best Practice Advisories (BPAs) [33]. BPAs appear when triggered by the most recent laboratory values if they fall outside institutional guidelines or reach a predetermined level [34].

A common concern raised by providers is that they are not aware of the institutional guidelines or do not have ready access to them. One format in the CPOE that has been helpful in addressing these concerns provides (1) the first line of the procedure for the relevant component (e.g., RBCs), with threshold values, (2) a hyperlink to the entire procedure that lists the guidelines, and (3) the most recent relevant laboratory values of the specific patient for which a transfusion is being ordered. The latter can include the three most recent values in case of concern about the validity of the most recent value. It should be noted that the laboratory values are helpful with the stable, and not acutely bleeding patient. While the provider's attention is engaged with the CDS tools, it is also beneficial to promote the use of single-unit transfusions. Once the clinician has the opportunity to review all the information provided, a clinical decision can then be made to continue with the transfusion or to cancel it. Figure 9.1 shows the first line of the relevant procedure; a link to the entire procedure; the three most recent relevant laboratory values; and finally, the option to continue or cancel the transfusion. In this case, while the laboratory values

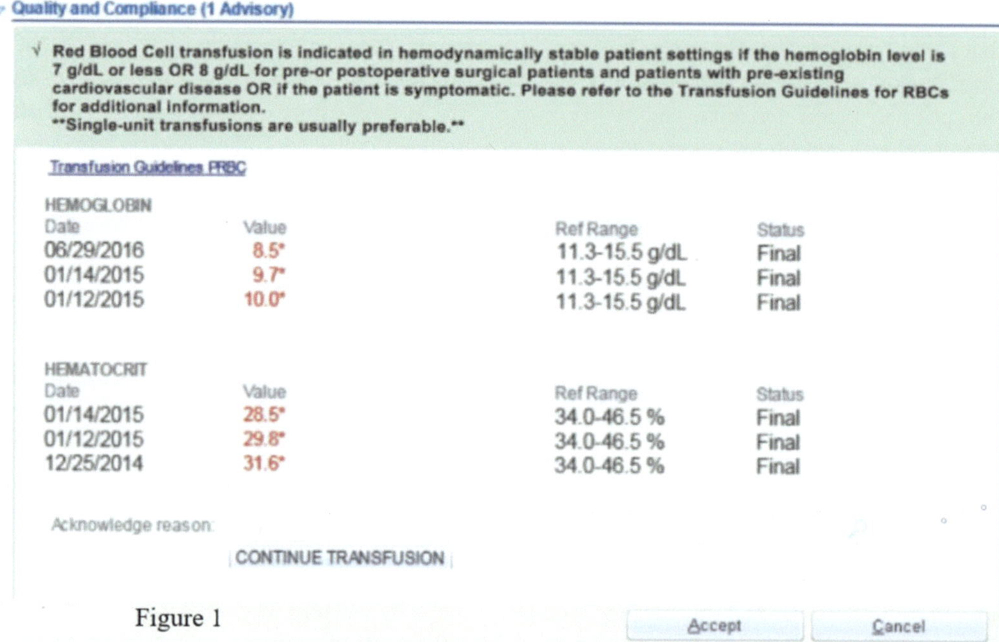

Fig. 9.1 Example of a Clinical Decision Support (CDS) system. A screenshot from an electronic RBC transfusion order with recommendations on a transfusion trigger for an adult patient with a Hb of >7 g/dL or > 8 g/dL with cardiovascular disease

are above the hospital's transfusion thresholds, the ordering provider makes the final decision on how to proceed.

The BPA serves two purposes. First, it prevents unnecessary transfusions that may expose the patient to both infectious and noninfectious risks. Second, it provides substantial cost savings. It has been demonstrated that the cost of a transfused unit is 3.2–4.8 times higher than blood acquisition costs [35]. With the cost of leukocyte-reduced RBCs averaging $223 in the United States in 2021, two units administered to a patient unnecessarily can result in over $2000 in additional patient care costs (*unpublished data provided by American's Blood Centers, May 2023*).

One US-based three-hospital system with an active patient blood management (PBM) program reviewed BPA data from 2016 through 2022. It found total unit orders cancelled and the cost avoidance was the following: RBC 1045/$209,159.43, platelets 120/$53,898.48, and plasma 76/$4276.16 for a total of $267,334.07. It was concluded that PBM achieved both of its goals by preventing unnecessary transfusions through the use of the BPA and providing cost avoidance. In this hospital system, the implementation of a transfusion threshold BPA was helpful (*unpublished data, abstract submitted to AABB2023*). From a hospital administration perspective, these numbers can be used to support the continuation of a PBM program and at least part of the salary of a transfusion safety officer [36].

CPOE with BPAs can result in alarm fatigue, in which clinicians get tired of or annoyed by computer messages telling them how to practice. While one study showed that after a successful educational campaign resulting in a reduction of red cell usage, the implementation of CPOE with BPAs had no significant additional effects on reducing blood use; however, this cannot be generalized. Each institution, with differences in provider training, provider backgrounds, PBM education and feedback, and patient populations, may have a different experience [34, 37].

9.2 Adult Red Blood Cell Transfusions

9.2.1 Liberal vs. Restrictive Strategies

Hebert et al., in the Transfusion Requirements in Critical Care (TRICC) trial (1999) [38], randomly assigned 838 critically ill euvolemic patients in the ICU with hemoglobin (Hgb) <9 g/dL within 72 h after admission to a restrictive strategy of transfusion, in which RBCs were transfused if the Hgb <7 g/dL (Hgb was maintained at 7–9 g/dL), and to a liberal strategy, in which transfusions were given if Hgb < 10 g/dL (Hgb was maintained at 10–12 g/dL). Overall, 30-day mortality was similar in both groups. There were statistically significantly lower rates with the restrictive transfusion strategy among patients who were less acutely in the restrictive-strategy group than in the liberal-strategy group (8.7% and 16.1% respectively; $P = 0.03$) and among patients aged <55 years of age (5.7% and 13%, respectively; $P = 0.02$), but not among patients who had clinically significant cardiac disease. The mortality rate was significantly lower among the patients in the restrictive arm (22.% vs. 28.2%, $P = 0.05$). They concluded that a restrictive strategy of RBC transfusion was at least as effective as and possibly superior to a liberal transfusion strategy in critically ill patients, with the possible exception of patients with acute myocardial infarction and unstable angina. This landmark study was the first to change the paradigm of requiring a high Hgb (10 g/dL) in acutely ill patients.

The Functional Outcomes in Cardiovascular Patients Undergoing Surgical Hip Fracture Repair (FOCUS) study [39] addressed the question of restrictive versus liberal transfusion thresholds in high-risk patients after elective hip surgery. They enrolled 2016 patients of ≥50 years of age with either a history of or risk factors for cardiovascular disease, with Hgb < 10 g/dL after hip-fracture surgery. The patients were randomly assigned to a liberal transfusion strategy (Hgb < 10 g/dL) or a restrictive transfusion strategy (symptoms of anemia or at physician discre-

tion for Hgb <8 g/dL). A median of two units of RBCs was transfused in the liberal group and none in the restrictive one. The rates of in-hospital acute coronary syndrome or death were 4.3% and 5.2%, respectively (absolute risk difference, −0.9%; 99% CI, −3.3 to 1.6), and rates of death on 60-day follow-up were 7.6% and 6.6%, respectively (absolute risk difference, 1.0%; 99% CI, −1.9 to 4.0). It should be noted that the liberal-transfusion strategy compared to the restrictive one, did not reduce rates of death or inability to walk independently on 60-day follow-up or reduce in-hospital morbidity in elderly patients at high cardiovascular risk. A strength of this study was that the mean age of the study population was 81.6 years (range 51–103) and mirrored that of most hospitalized patients.

Villanueva et al. studied transfusion strategies for acute upper gastrointestinal (UGI) bleeding [40]. A total of 921 patients with acute UGI bleeding were randomly assigned a restrictive strategy (transfusion when Hgb < 7 g/dL) and a liberal strategy (transfusion when Hgb < 9 g/dL). Approximately 50% in the restrictive arm did not receive RBC transfusions vs. 15% in the liberal arm ($P < 0.001$). The probability of survival at 6 weeks was higher in the restrictive-strategy group than in the liberal one, 95% vs. 91% (hazard ratio for death with a restrictive strategy, 0.55; 95% CI, 0.33–0.92; $P = 0.02$). There was significantly less bleeding in the restrictive group (10%) compared to the liberal one (16%) ($P = 0.01$) and significantly fewer adverse events in the restrictive group (40%) vs. the liberal group (48%) ($P = 0.02$). The probability of survival was slightly higher with the restrictive strategy than with the liberal strategy in the subgroup of patients who had bleeding associated with a peptic ulcer (HR, 0.70; 95% CI, 0.26–1.25) and was significantly higher in the subgroup of patients with cirrhosis and Child–Pugh class A or B disease (HR, 0.30; 95% CI, 0.11–0.85), but not in those with cirrhosis and Child–Pugh class C disease (HR, 1.04; 95% CI, 0.45–2.37).

Guidelines for RBC transfusion were published by the AABB in 2012 [41], updated in 2016, and again in 2023 [42]. The latest guidelines include four recommendations. The first is to transfuse hemodynamically stable hospitalized adult patients when the Hgb is less than 7 g/dL (including critically ill patients. This was a strong recommendation of moderate certainty evidence. It also stated that in accordance with the restrictive strategy threshold used in most trials, clinicians may choose a threshold Hgb of 7.5 g/dL for patients undergoing cardiac surgery and an Hgb of 8.0 g/dL for those undergoing orthopedic surgery or those with preexisting cardiovascular disease. The second recommendation was that for hemodynamically stable adult patients with hematologic and oncologic disorders, a restrictive transfusion strategy should be considered when the hemoglobin concentration is less than 7.0 g/dL. The authors noted this was a conditional recommendation of low certainty evidence. Two additional recommendations were made for pediatric patients. Recommendation three stated that in critically ill children and those at risk of critical illnesses who are hemodynamically stable and without hemoglobinopathies, cyanotic cardiac conditions, or severe hypoxemia, a restrictive transfusion strategy can be considered when the Hgb concentration is less than 7.0 g/dL. This was a strong recommendation of moderate certainty evidence. The final recommendation addressed hemodynamically stable children with congenital heart disease. The transfusion thresholds were based on the cardiac abnormality and stage of surgical repair (Table 9.3). This was a

conditional recommendation of low certainty evidence. While a specific recommendation on the shelf-life of red blood cells was removed from the 2023 update, the authors did state that given that the randomized clinical trials demonstrated no effect on mortality, the storage age of transfused red blood cells need not be considered in transfusion conditions. The authors concluded by stating that it is good practice to consider the overall clinical context and alternate therapies when making transfusion decisions about individual patients (Table 9.3).

In 2013 a guideline for the treatment of anemia in cardiac patients was published by the American College of Physicians [43]. They recommended using a restrictive RBC transfusion strategy (Hgb threshold 7–8 g/dL compared with higher Hgb levels) in hospitalized patients with coronary heart disease.

The Cochrane review from 2021 compared 30-day mortality for Hgb transfusion triggers in various clinical conditions. A total of 48 trials, involving data from 21,433 participants (at baseline) across a range of clinical contexts (e.g., orthopedic, cardiac, or vascular surgery; critical care; acute blood loss (including gastrointestinal bleeding); acute coronary syndrome; cancer; leukemia; hematological malignancies), met the eligibility criteria. The Hgb concentration used to define the restrictive transfusion group in most trials [36] was between 7 and 8 g/dL. The liberal

Table 9.3 Hemoglobin transfusion practice

Hemoglobin threshold ≤ (g/dL)	Patient population
Adults	
7.0	Hospitalized hemodynamically stable patients
7.0	Hematologic and oncologic disorders
7.5	Cardiac surgery
8.0	Orthopedic surgery
8.0	Preexisting cardiovascular disease
Children	
7.0	Critically ill and those at risk of critical illness who are hemodynamically stable and without hemoglobinopathies, cyanotic cardiac conditions or severe hypoxemia
7.0	Biventricular repair
7.0	Single-ventricle palliation
7.0–9.0	Uncorrected congenital heart disease

Adapted from: Carson JL, Stanworth SJ, Guyatt G, et al. Red Blood Cell Transfusion, 2023 AABB International Guidelines. JAMA. 2023;330(19):1892–1902. https://doi.org/10.1001/jama.2023.12914

threshold was 9–10 g/dL. They concluded that transfusion at a restrictive Hgb concentration decreased the proportion of patients exposed to RBC transfusion by 41%. The study found no evidence to suggest that a restrictive transfusion strategy impacted mortality or morbidity (i.e., cardiac events, myocardial infarction, stroke, pneumonia, thromboembolism, infection) compared with a liberal transfusion strategy.

The Myocardial Ischemia and Transfusion (MINT) trial randomly assigned patients with myocardial infarction and an Hgb level of less than 10 g/dL to either a restrictive transfusion strategy (Hgb cutoff of 7–8 g/dL) or a liberal transfusion strategy (Hgb cutoff less than 10 g/dL). The primary outcome was a composite of myocardial infarction or death at 30 days. There was a statistically significant higher incidence of myocardial infarction and death in the restrictive-strategy group compared with the liberal-strategy group. The authors observed that the results suggest a clinical benefit for the liberal transfusion strategy and do not suggest a benefit for the more restrictive transfusion strategy [103]. They also noted that these findings differed from the 2021 Cochrane review [36].

Yang et al. addressed the subject of the number of RBC units transfused. In their study, they demonstrated that a campaign of giving only one unit of RBC at a time succeeded in reducing RBC transfusions [44]. Entzel et al. combined a single unit order default setting with a restrictive transfusion trigger and reduced RBC transfusion ordering practices variation [45]. Today common practice in stable patients is to transfuse one RBC unit, and only if there is a specific need is another unit administered.

9.2.2 Red Blood Cell Transfusions in Specific Clinical Situations

9.2.2.1 Thalassemia

Thalassemia is among the most commonly inherited Hgb disorders. Individuals have reduced production of α- or β-globin chains. β-thalassemia, with reduced β globin chain production, and it is a multiorgan disease and is associated with considerable morbidity and mortality. Thalassemia's are inherited recessively; both α-thalassemia and β-thalassemia can cause anemias necessitating chronic RBC transfusions, depending on the specific type of mutation involved. Transfusion dependency is tied to the imbalance between α and β globin chains [46]. Anemia in thalassemia is secondary to both hemolysis and ineffective erythropoiesis [47]. Patients suffering from β-thalassemia major will require regular RBC transfusion, often beginning in childhood. The goal is to maintain a Hgb of 9–10 g/dL [48], and twice monthly transfusions may be needed. Chronic RBC transfusion exposes patients to many donors, eventually causing alloimmunization in 20–30% of patients. Phenotyping of common antigens causing alloimmunization can be performed prior to transfusion in order to minimize alloimmunization. Genotyping of the patients and the donors is also an option.

Multiple transfusions also lead to severe iron overload, which can be reduced with appropriate treatment by iron chelation. This can be achieved with oral or subcutaneous iron chelators, including deferoxamine, deferiprone, or deferasirox. The latter is the only chelator specifically approved for thalassemic patients on the basis of data from a randomized, phase 2 trial showing significant reductions in serum ferritin and liver iron concentrations over a 2-year period of therapy [49].

Luspatercept, a recombinant fusion protein comprising a modified extracellular domain of the human activin receptor type IIB fused to the Fc domain of human IgG1, is approved in the US and Europe for transfusion-dependent β-thalassemia. It has been shown to reduce the transfusion burden by 33% compared to a placebo over a fixed 12-week period. Serum ferritin levels were also reduced. However, clinically meaningful changes in liver or myocardial iron concentrations were not observed [50].

Hematopoietic stem cell transplantation is a definitive treatment in children with favorable risk profiles and matched sibling donors [46]. Gene therapy is a treatment option under investigation [51]. There are also ongoing studies investigating the correction of genetic mutations or disrupting specific DNA sequences using ZINC finger and CRISPR nucleases [52, 53].

9.2.2.2 Sickle Cell Disease

A missense point mutation in the β-globin gene causes a change in the hemoglobin A (HgbA) to become hemoglobin S (HgbS). HgbS, in circumstances where the availability of oxygen is decreased, can polymerize into intracellular fibers that, along with the inflammatory status in sickle cell disease (SCD), is responsible for a myriad of clinical symptoms such as symptomatic anemia, ischemic stroke, multiple organ failure, etc.

In SCD, RBC transfusion is still, along with hydroxyurea, a primary therapeutic option [46, 54, 55]. RBC transfusion, besides improving oxygen delivery, reduces the percentage of HgbS relative to HgbA (56), thus decreasing blood viscosity [56, 57]. Simple transfusion and red blood cell exchange (RCE) are the common ways of infusing RBC in SCD patients. Both have limitations, advantages, and disadvantages and will be defined based on the indication, venous access, availability of trained personnel, iron overload, and iron chelation therapy, amongst others [57]. The lack of randomized controlled clinical trials (RCT) on transfusion in SCD imposes different clinical practices amongst institutions; however, several guidelines and reviews have been published elsewhere [46, 55]. New disease modifier agents like L-glutamine, voxelotor, and crizanlizumab are not yet available on a large scale and are not accessible to all.

A common complication of transfusion in SCD is alloimmunization when patients develop antibodies against transfused RBC antigens resulting in a delayed hemolytic transfusion reaction [58]. Therefore, there is a need to include Rh and Kell phenotyping at diagnosis and subsequent matching for at least C, E, K or C/c, E/e, K antigens [59–62]. Most alloimmunization cases are due to C, E, and Kell alloantibodies following transfusion in SCD patients [63, 64]. If possible, extended phenotyping should be conducted, including common red cell antigens like D, C, c, E, e, M, N, S, s, P1, Le[a], Le[b], K, k, Jk[a], Jk[b], Fy[a], and Fy[b]. Another complication of transfusion is

iron overload; hence, ferritin levels should be monitored and iron chelation therapy made available.

According to Davis et al. 2017 [65], RBC for SCD patients should be HgbS-free and preferably should be <10 days old for simple transfusion and <7 days old for exchange transfusion. The older RBCs may also be washed to remove excess potassium. Also, one should consider older RBC in the case of alloimmunized patients, where a delay in finding the perfect phenotyped blood may place the patient at risk of additional complications of the disease. It is essential to register the baseline Hgb and reticulocyte count, as an acute drop in Hgb >2 g/dL and an increase in reticulocyte count could be a sign of hemolysis, thus a possible indication for transfusion.

9.2.2.2.1 Acute Indications for Transfusion in Sickle Cell Disease

Emergency situations that may require increasing the oxygen-carrying capacity and decreasing vaso-occlusive complications are indications for blood transfusion, such as acute anemia, acute ischemic stroke, multiorgan failure, acute sickle hepatopathy, and severe sepsis. Acute pain, priapism, and acute chest syndrome do not require transfusion unless there are additional complications and an increase in severity or no response to the initial treatment [56].

9.2.2.2.2 Preoperative Blood Transfusion in SCD

Morbidity due to operations in SCD patients is not uncommon; therefore, it has been advocated that transfusions may be required to prevent complications, where the most feared are pain crisis and acute chest syndrome. One randomized trial evaluated 604 surgical procedures in SCD patients who were randomly assigned to receive either an "aggressive transfusion regimen" designed to decrease the HgbS level to less than 30% (group 1) or a "conservative regimen" designed to increase the Hgb level to 10 g/dL (group 2)(66). The conservative transfusion regimen was as effective as an aggressive regimen in preventing perioperative complications in patients with SCD, and the conservative approach resulted in only half as many transfusion-associated complications [66].

There is very low evidence regarding the need for transfusion in surgeries lasting longer than 1 h and under general anesthesia. However, a guideline published in 2020 suggests that the decision to transfuse should be made individually considering disease genotype, level of surgery, total baseline hemoglobin, complications with prior transfusions, and disease severity [59]. Hgb less than 9 g/dL should be considered for simple transfusion, and those with baseline Hgb > 9 g/dL should be considered for red cell exchange (RCE). Hgb should not exceed 11 g/dL due to the risk of hyper viscosity.

9.2.2.2.3 Transfusion and Pregnancy in SCD

According to what is currently available in the literature, it seems that there is a potential benefit of chronic transfusions for pregnant women with SCD, namely those with twin pregnancies, fetal or obstetric complications, and recurrent severe and prolonged vaso-occlusive crisis. There is still a lack of evidence supporting the routine use of prophylactic transfusions during pregnancy and what would be the best modality regarding whether it should be simple or exchange transfusion. A Hgb threshold for transfusion during pregnancy is not yet defined, but it would be recommended to transfuse when Hgb is below 7 g/dL or when there is a reduction of 2 g/dL from the baseline [54, 59].

9.2.2.3 Transfusions in Autoimmune Hemolytic Anemia

Autoimmune hemolytic anemia (AIHA) involves the destruction of autologous RBCs caused by autoantibodies against erythrocyte surface antigens [67]. Transfusion can be challenging in these patients. The antibody screen is positive, and the autoantibody may interfere with crossmatching RBC units for these patients. Hemolysis of transfused RBCs can occur; however, in life-threatening conditions, this risk should be considered. As in thalassemia, If possible, phenotyping of Rh subgroups and Kell, MNS,

Kidd, S/s, and Duffy antigens can be performed prior to transfusion in order to minimize alloimmunization from transfusions; genotyping is also an option if time permits. Transfusion must be given slowly at first with an observation of the patient for signs of hemolysis; if none are seen, the transfusion can be completed at a regular rate.

9.2.2.4 Patients Treated with Anti-CD38 Antibodies

The first anti-CD38 antibody given to multiple myeloma (MM) patients in daratumumab caused an interference with antibody screening [68]. A second antibody, Isatuximab [69], has been approved for the treatment of MM, and a third, felzartamab (MOR202), is being developed; more antibodies will probably follow. CD38 is a transmembrane glycoprotein of the RBC as well as the MM cells. Treatment with the anti-CD38 antibody is very effective but also binds in vitro to RBCs and interferes with antibody screening and RBC crossmatching, thus delaying or even preventing the timely transfusion of RBCs. There are ways to mitigate this interference, including dithiothreitol (DTT) treatment of RBCs [70]. The problem with the DTT treatment is that it denatures certain RBC antigens other than CD38, the most important among them is K, necessitating transfusion of compatible blood. A new reagent, DaraEx plus (Inno-Train) [71], has been developed and can inhibit the interference of anti-CD38 antibodies, including daratumumab, felzartamab, and rituximab treatment with antibody screening and crossmatching RBC units [71]. Further monoclonal antibody treatments are being developed, and transfusion medicine will have to deal with the mitigation of those that interfere with RBC antigens.

9.2.2.5 Massive Transfusion and Emergency Release of Blood

In patients admitted with severe anemia or massive bleeding, emergency transfusion of RBC is sometimes necessary. Massive bleeding is defined as the loss of more than one blood volume within 24 h, 50% of the patient's total blood volume lost in less than 3 h, or bleeding in excess of 150 mL/min [72]. According to the clinical presentation of the patient, a decision must be made to release one or more units of RBCs prior to performing a blood type and an antibody screen. There are protocols for massive bleeding in order to avoid transfusion delay in this life-threatening emergency; Fig. 9.2, a flowchart for massive bleeding, and Table 9.4, an example of a massive bleeding packs program. The protocols provide a framework for preparing blood components during massive bleeding, enabling continuous transfusion until the patient stabilizes [73].There are protocols for postpartum hemorrhage, specially adapted, as these patients require more fibrinogen/cryoprecipitate than trauma patients.

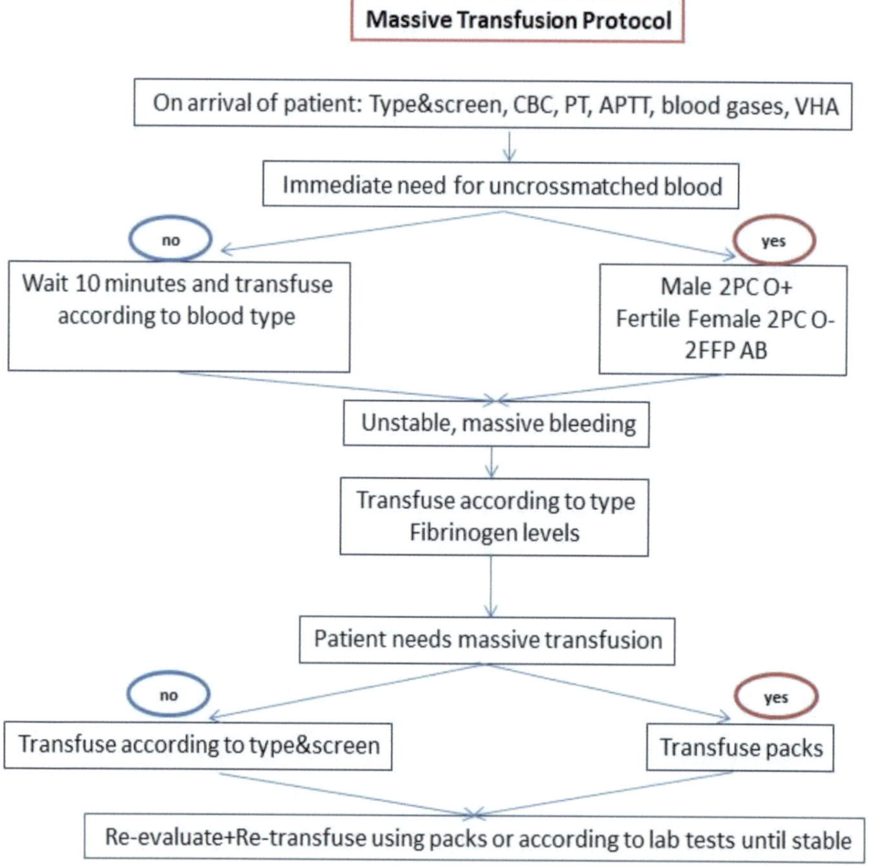

Fig. 9.2 An example of a massive transfusion protocol flowchart

Table 9.4 An example of a massive transfusion packs program (73)

Pack number	Components
1	4 RBC + 3 FFP
2	3 RBC + 2 FFP
3	3 RBC + 2 FFP + 5 RDP or 1 SDP + 10 units cryoprecipitate (or fibrinogen concentrate 2 gm[a])
4	3 RBC + 2 FFP

RBC packed red blood cells; *FFP* frozen fresh plasma; *RDP* random donor platelets; *SDP* single donor apheresis platelets
[a] In countries where cryoprecipitate is not available

Viscoelastic testing with thromboelastography (TEG) or rotational thromboelastometry (ROTEM) can help guide the transfusion of components until the patient is stabilized. The transfusion service is often geographically far from the emergency room, the operating room, and the intensive care units (ICUs). Remote storage of RBCs is an option to enable immediate transfusion, avoiding delays. The blood storage units must have temperature control as required in the transfusion service, with automatic notification when conditions are not according to the requirements. There has to be someone responsible for monitoring and replacing the inventory in order to save blood components on the one hand, and transfusion of outdated components on the other hand. There must be clear guidelines covering all these issues and defining the indications for the transfusion of blood components from the remote storage units. All the disciplines of the medical staff have to be familiar with them.

9.2.2.6 Transfusion Practices with Extracorporeal Membrane Oxygenation

Extracorporeal membrane oxygenation (ECMO) is an essential treatment option for critically ill patients with acute cardiopulmonary collapse [74]. This technology permits temporary extracorporeal blood flow and gas exchange, thereby supporting damaged organs until they recover or receive definitive corrective treatments.

ECMO systems operate using two general configurations: veno-venous (VV-ECMO), in which venous return receives enhanced oxygenation prior to returning to the right heart via the vena cava and/or right atrium, or veno-arterial (VA-ECMO), which facilitates direct arterial reinfusion via the femoral artery (peripheral cannulation) or aorta (central cannulation) after the extracorporeal gas exchange is complete. Due to their precarious clinical status, ECMO patients frequently require numerous transfusions of blood components, typically during the initial phase of ECMO management; however, there is no specific guidance on this issue [75, 76].

The foundation of successful ECMO outcomes is the cooperation between medical specialties, and blood component administration is an indispensable aspect of the overall management of these patients. Traditional treatment of patients on ECMO aims for a hemoglobin level of 7 g/dL or higher, similar to that of other intensive care patients. Studies examining more conservative versus liberal hematocrit thresholds for transfusion of ECMO-supported patients are ongoing. Ultimately, the decision of what Hgb threshold to transfuse the patient depends on the specific case and available resources, requiring individual evaluation of the patient.

There are hospitals all over the world, including the Shamir Medical Center in Israel, that have specialized transport vehicles outfitted with ECMO machines that are fully functional (Fig. 9.3a and b). The remote inventory of RBCs in the ICU of this medical center also includes two units of O RhD-positive RBCs for patients with life-threatening bleeding on ECMO and readily available for use on board, to be transported in a temperature-monitored cooler. If not transfused and out of the ICU for ≤2 h or less, in the monitored cooler, these RBC units are returned to the ICU remote supply. If out for >2 h, they are returned to the blood bank and discarded.

These vehicles help to expedite the delivery of rescue services to sites outside of the hospital involving other healthcare facilities through partnerships with specialized ambulance providers. In this case, this partnership was formed with Magen David Adom, the national organization responsible for emergency pre-hospital medical care and blood services, which provides pre-hospital ECMO Cardio Pulmonary Resuscitation for cases of Out-of-Hospital Cardiac Arrest. The ambulance with the ECMO is kept connected to electricity in order to maintain the equipment at a compatible temperature all the time (Personal Communication: Eduard Ilgiyaev M.D., Director of Intensive Care Unit, Shamir Medical Center Zerifin, Israel).

Fig. 9.3 An extracorporeal membrane oxygenation unit in a mobile intensive care unit (ICU) (**a**). Note the blue box in the center where blood is stored (**b**). (**c**) The ECMO mobile unit, plugged in to maintain a compatible temperature

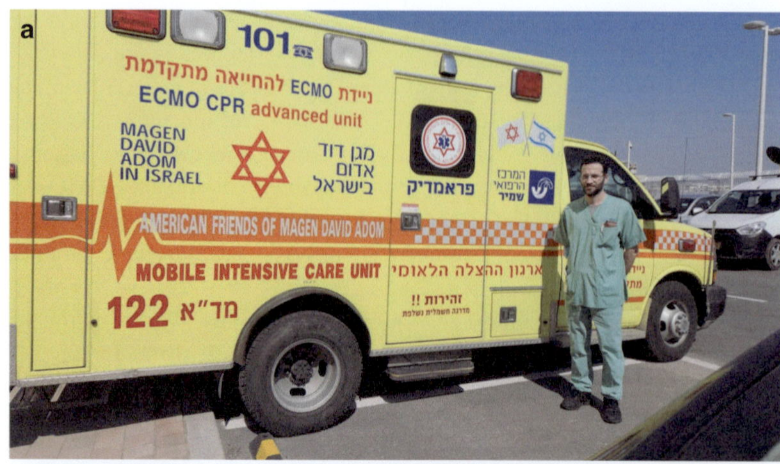

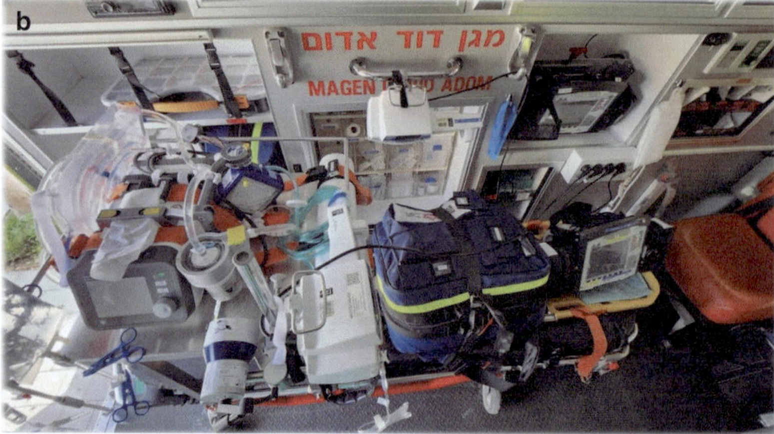

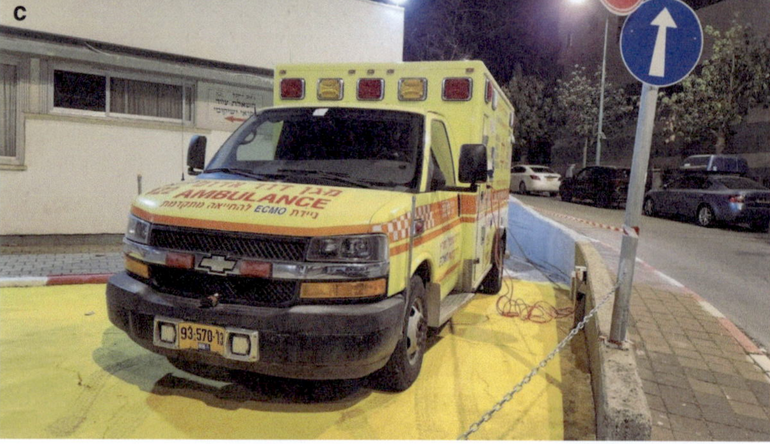

9.3 Neonatal and Pediatric Red Cell Transfusion

Different body volumes and responses to hypoxia and hypovolemia make transfusion practice in pediatrics continue to be a challenge. The blood volume of a full-term newborn is 85 mL/kg, whereas in preterm, it is approximately 100 mL/kg; however, because of their specific physiology, iatrogenic blood loss during hospital stay should be considered as a risk factor for RBC transfusion. Several studies have been conducted to measure the impact of blood sample collection on total body volume, and according to the child's general state of health. Caution is warranted in children with depleted blood volume or Hgb or who are not able to replenish the amount of blood drawn [77].

According to Goel R et al. 2020 [78], data from the Kids' Inpatient Database among 5,604,984 total hospitalizations showed an overall prevalence of RBC transfusions of 1.07% (95% CI, 0.94–1.22%) in 2016 in the US, making it a relevant subject for health practitioners globally [78]. Premature neonates, namely low birth weight neonates (40%) and extreme low birth weight (ELBW) neonates (90%), require RBC transfusion, although there is variability in current practices worldwide [79].

9.3.1 Thresholds for RBC Transfusion

The primary objective of RBC transfusion is to ensure the delivery of oxygen and promote oxygen consumption [80] thus reducing the risk of complications associated with anemia. To optimize the use of transfusion and minimize the negative impact on morbidity and mortality, it is crucial to avoid unnecessary transfusions [81]. The appropriate thresholds for RBC transfusion in neonates and pediatric populations are still under debate, and more RCTs are needed to establish evidence-based guidelines regarding Hgb level [82].

The decision-making process for RBC transfusion should take into account various factors, including clinical symptoms, particularly cardiopulmonary, Hgb levels, the timing of onset of anemia, underlying conditions (such as infections and malignancies), and the blood loss. Restrictive strategy suggests transfusion when Hgb level falls below 7 g/dL, whereas the liberal strategy recommends transfusion when Hgb levels drop below 10 g/dL. Similar strategies have been advocated for other patients groups as well. In critically ill children or those at risk for critical illness, a panel of experts recommended RBC transfusion if the Hgb concentration is <5 g/dL [80, 83].

However, transfusion decisions should not rely solely on the Hgb level. For example, different medical conditions associated with chronic anemia may require a lower Hgb level as an indication for transfusion, while ongoing bleeding, cardiopulmonary distress, or infection may require a lower threshold. In the case of stable infants with anemia of prematurity, a blood transfusion may be necessary to mitigate the harmful effects of anemia-induced hypoxia during development [84].

Unnecessary transfusions have been associated with unfavorable outcomes [85]; hence, it is important to define RBC transfusion thresholds in pediatric patients. For infants younger than 4 months, Roseff SD, et al. [86] provide a guideline for RBC transfusion in children. Table 9.5 summarizes indications of RBC transfusion in children below 4 months of age.

9.3.2 Administration in Neonate and Pediatric Recipients

The volume used for RBC transfusion of neonates and infants is usually 10–15 mL/kg, and the increment in Hgb will vary from 2 to 3 g/dL based on the hematocrit of the selected RBC. Preterm neonates could necessitate a very small volume of transfusion; hence one should take into account the use of equipment such as infusion pumps for RBC administration, and to consider when preparing the transfusion aliquots for this group of patients the lost volume of blood in the transfusion sets with extracorporeal plastic tubing.

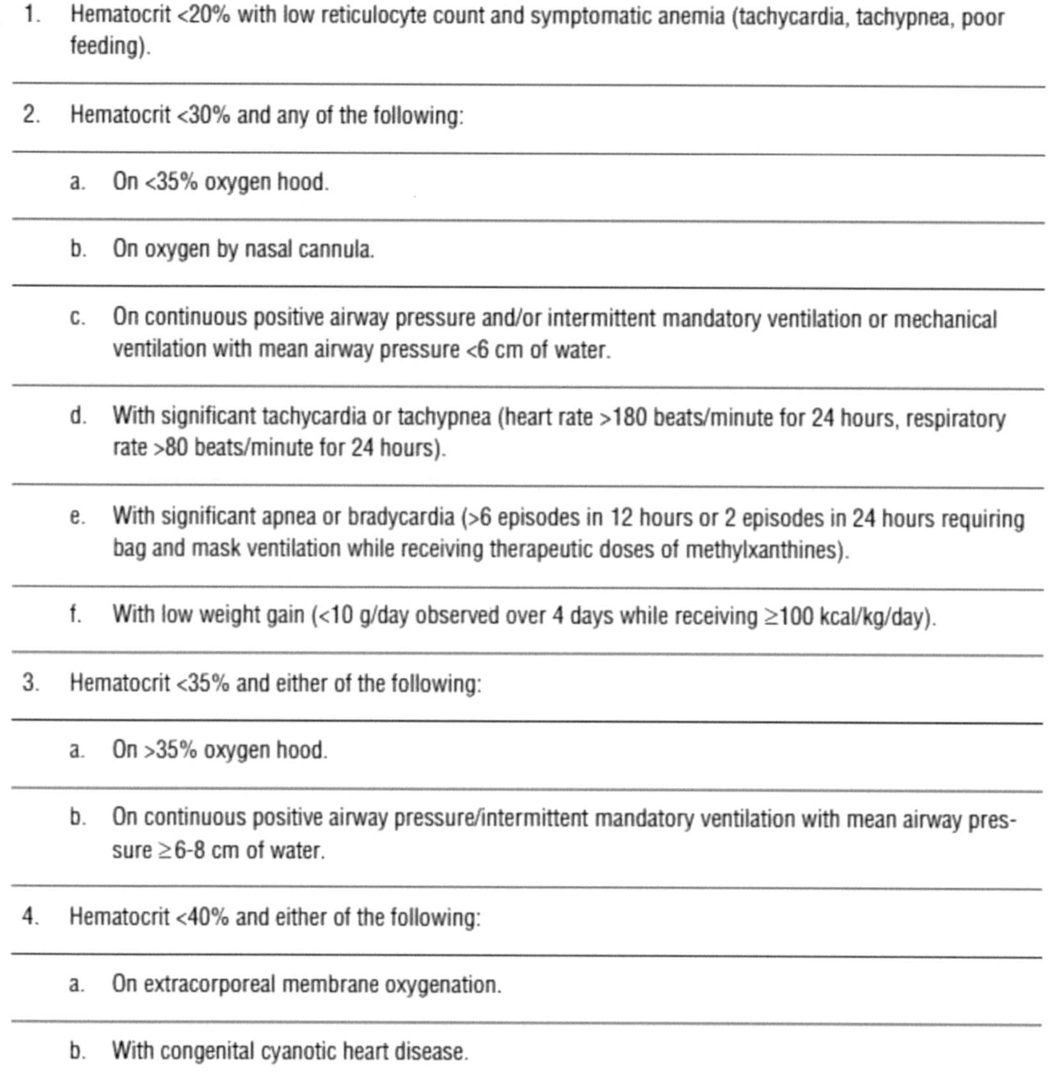

1.		Hematocrit <20% with low reticulocyte count and symptomatic anemia (tachycardia, tachypnea, poor feeding).
2.		Hematocrit <30% and any of the following:
	a.	On <35% oxygen hood.
	b.	On oxygen by nasal cannula.
	c.	On continuous positive airway pressure and/or intermittent mandatory ventilation or mechanical ventilation with mean airway pressure <6 cm of water.
	d.	With significant tachycardia or tachypnea (heart rate >180 beats/minute for 24 hours, respiratory rate >80 beats/minute for 24 hours).
	e.	With significant apnea or bradycardia (>6 episodes in 12 hours or 2 episodes in 24 hours requiring bag and mask ventilation while receiving therapeutic doses of methylxanthines).
	f.	With low weight gain (<10 g/day observed over 4 days while receiving ≥100 kcal/kg/day).
3.		Hematocrit <35% and either of the following:
	a.	On >35% oxygen hood.
	b.	On continuous positive airway pressure/intermittent mandatory ventilation with mean airway pressure ≥6-8 cm of water.
4.		Hematocrit <40% and either of the following:
	a.	On extracorporeal membrane oxygenation.
	b.	With congenital cyanotic heart disease.

Table 9.5 Guideline for red cell transfusion in children <4 months of age). (Goel R, Punzalan RC, Wong ECC. Neonatal and Pediatric Transfusion Practice. In: Cohn C, et al. eds. Technical Manual. 21st ed. Bethesda, MD: AABB Press, 2023:736)

Ensuring appropriate vascular access is a crucial consideration for infants who require long-term infusions, such as extremely premature infants, critically ill children, and trauma patients. In a prospective cohort study conducted in an Australian quaternary-referral neonatal ICU, peripheral intravenous catheters were the most commonly used vascular devices ($n = 186$; 62%), followed by umbilical venous catheters ($n = 52$; 17%) [87]. Umbilical venous catheters are typically the first choice for transfusion and fluid administration soon after birth. When using vascular catheters and small needles such as 24-gauge (G) and 25G, respectively, maintaining a constant flow can help prevent/avoid hemolysis [88]. An intro non-inferiority study evaluated the safety of transfusing RBC over 4 h at a rate of 4 mL/h through 24G silicone and 28G polyurethane peripherally inserted central catheter (PICC) lines, compared to a peripheral 24G short catheter. The study found that RBC transfusion through 24G silicone and 28G polyurethane PICC lines was feasible without any detectable hemolysis or concerns about pressures. However, the authors emphasized the need for prospective assessment in preterm infants [89].

Routine transfusions should not exceed 4 h, and the transfusion service should be able to provide small aliquots to ensure the recommended infusion time, aiming to prevent circulatory overload and limit donor exposures. In some cases, using blood warmers may be necessary considering the transfusion indication [90], patients' clinical condition, and required volume Hospital transfusion services may have syringe sets that are more accurate when the volume to be transfused is based on volume-per-weight. Although trauma is a significant cause of death in the pediatric population, there is still a lack of evidence on massive transfusion for this population.

9.3.3 Special Considerations

9.3.3.1 Indications for Irradiation

Irradiation of red blood cells (RBCs) for immunocompromised recipients using gamma or x-ray radiation performed to prevent viable T-lymphocytes from replicating thus preventing transfusion-associated graft-versus-host disease (TA-GVHD), a rare but life-threatening condition. One trial (NIMO-Rad trial) compared the impact of transfusing freshly irradiated RBCs versus irradiated and stored RBC components on, cerebral oxygen delivery in preterm infants with anemia. The study found that the infusion of freshly irradiated RBCs resulted in a small improvement in cerebral oxygenation that lasted for at least 5 days after transfusion, compared to transfusion of irradiated and stored RBC components. It seems that infusion of freshly irradiated RBCs conferred a "small benefit in cerebral oxygenation that persisted for at least 5 days after transfusion compared with transfusion of irradiated and stored RBC components" [79, 91].

TA-GVHD is a rare adverse event that has been reported primarily through case reports, most commonly observed after intrauterine transfusion following maternal donation. In these cases, the recipient and donor may share an HLA-haplotype and this complication can also occur in extremely premature infants. The AABB provides guidelines for irradiation of cellular components considering prematurity and birth weight less than 1200 g, clinical conditions such as immune deficiency and immunosuppression due to chemotherapy and irradiation treatment, as well as patients receiving components from relatives/family, HLA-matched or crossmatched platelet components, and granulocyte transfusion [88].

9.3.3.2 Anticoagulants

The use of anticoagulant-preservative solutions in young children has always raised concern due to their potential harm to renal function and interference in coagulation. These concerns primarily arise from the use of citrate-phosphate-dextrose-adenine (CPDA-1) and additive solutions (AS) such as AS-3, AS-1 and saline-adenine-glucose-mannitol (SAGM), These solutions are utilized to extend the shelf life of RBC components. AS contains adenine and mannitol, and the diuretic effect of these may cause cerebral blood flow fluctuations in preterm infants. However, the literature has demonstrated the safety and effectiveness of blood components stored in AS for small-volume transfusions in neonates [92]. If large-volume transfusions are necessary, it is recommended to monitor ionized calcium and potassium levels. For neonates with renal insufficiency, the additive solution should be removed through the washing process to mitigate any potential complications [93].

9.3.3.3 Age of Units

The term "RBC storage lesion" is used to refer to a series of changes in the RBC, including biochemical, metabolic, and structural alternations. These changes can affect the stability of the red cell membrane leading to hemolysis. The extracellular K+ is one of the known biomarkers used to evaluate storage lesions and could be associated with transfusion complications, especially in the pediatric group [94]. Some authors refer to this adverse event as transfusion-associated hyperkalemia (TAH), which can cause cardiac implications, including arrhythmia, impaired cardiac contraction and cardiac arrest. Critically ill children, neonates, and those requiring high-volume transfusion are at increased risk for developing TAH.

In a recently published retrospective study, the authors investigated the occurrence of hyperkalemia during or within12 h after RBC transfusion over a 1-year period. They concluded that while the prevalence of TAH in children was low, the 1-day mortality after TAH was high (20%). However, it was noted that other comorbidities might have influenced the mortality rate. The study also concluded that the irradiation status and storage age of the RBC units did not have an impact on the occurrence of TAH, contrary to the expectations [95]. Another source suggests that if RBCs have been irradiated and stored for more than 24 h, it is advisable to consider washing the units. Additionally, when transfusing neonates and children, it is important to consider the risk of hypothermia (cold stress), as it can trigger severe responses such as increased metabolic rate, hypoglycemia, metabolic acidosis, and apneic events.

9.3.4 Special Indications in Pediatrics and Neonatology

9.3.4.1 Sickle Cell Disease

When administering RBC transfusions to pediatric patients, it is important to consider their unique blood volume, which differs from the adults. The RBC dosing is 10–15 mL/kg and not exceeding 4-h infusion time. There is currently no evidence suggesting a clear benefit from using fresher RBCs (<10 days old). Venous access can be a concern in pediatric patients with SCD when considering RBC exchange transfusion [96]. There is no indication for transfusion during uncomplicated pain crises, priapism, asymptomatic anemia, or acute kidney injury when not

associated with multiple organ failure and recurrent splenic sequestration [96].

9.3.4.2 Intrauterine Red Blood Cell Transfusions

Intrauterine fetal red blood cell transfusion (IUT) was first introduced in the 1960s for the treatment of anemia caused by red cell immunization. The current technique, involves intravascular IUT into the umbilical cord [97], first described by Rodeck et al. (97). IUT is also used to treat non-immune conditions, such as human parvovirus B19 infection, fetomaternal hemorrhage, twin-twin transfusion syndrome, and placental/fetal tumors, among others. RBC for IUT should be leukocyte depleted and irradiated.

9.3.4.3 Neonatal Exchange Transfusions

Neonatal exchange transfusion (NET) is a procedure in which the infant's blood is removed and replaced with "fresh" donor blood and/or plasma. The most frequent indication is hemolytic disease of the newborn when intensive phototherapy is either lacking or ineffective in reducing bilirubin levels. It is also indicated in infants with severe neonatal hyperbilirubinemia or symptoms of acute bilirubin encephalopathy. An observational multicenter prospective cohort study in Turkey, conducted between September 2015 and September 2016 at 50 neonatal intensive care units (NICUs), evaluated neonatal jaundice and reported the underlying causes such as hemolytic jaundice were ABO incompatibility, Rh incompatibility, minor blood group incompatibility, and G6PD [98]. Other indications for NET are sepsis, metabolic disorders, severe fluid or electrolyte imbalance, disorder requiring complement, opsonin, or gamma globulin, and polycythemia.

The types of exchange transfusion can be based on the volume exchanged and the indications as summarized in Table 9.6.

The choice of blood for NET should be CMV-safe/leukocyte depleted, irradiated, and lacking HgbS. While choosing the blood type and degree of crossmatch, the cause for NET should be considered.

Table 9.6 Types of exchange transfusion

Type of exchange transfusion	Estimated blood volume	Indications
Single-volume exchange blood transfusion	Refers to one times the estimated blood volume at ⁓60% of the infant's blood volume	Severe hyperbilirubinemia, for alloimmune hemolytic disease of newborns, to remove antibodies and abnormal proteins, and for idiopathic severe hypermagnesemia, disseminated intravascular coagulation (DIC), congenital leukemia, neonatal sepsis, malaria, malignant pertussis, drug overdose, and metabolic toxin removal (hyperammonemia, organic academia, lead poisoning)
Double-volume exchange blood transfusion	Refers to two times the estimated blood volume at ⁓85% of the infant's blood volume	
Isovolumetric double-volume exchange blood transfusion	Exchange is done simultaneously by pulling blood out of the umbilical artery and pushing blood into the umbilical vein.	Indicated in sick and unstable neonates because of less fluctuation of blood pressure and cerebral hemodynamics (e.g., hydrops fetal
Partial-volume exchange (<2 volumes) transfusion	This type of exchange is indicated in neonates with polycythemia (to decrease the hematocrit and whole blood viscosity) or to correct severe anemia (usually associated with congestive cardiac failure or hypervolemia)	

Adapted from "Exchange Transfusion." *Neonatology: Management, Procedures, On Call Problems, Diseases, and Drugs, 7e* Eds. Tricia Lacy Gomella, et al. McGraw Hill,2013,https://accesspediatrics.mhmedical.com/content.aspx?bookid=1303§ionid=79661818

9.3.4.4 RBC Transfusion for Pediatric ECMO Patients

ECMO aims to provide adequate oxygen delivery to meet the body's oxygen consumption. The risk of bleeding and thrombosis is high during the use of this device, and it is always used in very sick children. Patients on ECMO are usually transfused with large volumes of RBCs. Observational studies have shown that less than 5% of the transfusions actually increase O_2 delivery, and some other studies indicate that the more RBC units transfused, the longer the time on the ventilator, the higher the in-hospital mortality. RBC transfusions have been independently associated with increased odds of mortality. There is no strong evidence advocating for Hct level or any biomarker to guide RBC transfusion during ECMO for pediatric patients. However, a consensus guideline suggested using physiologic measures and biomarkers of oxygen delivery, in addition to Hgb concentration (and not Hct), to guide RBC transfusion [80].

A retrospective study [99] was conducted to evaluate a restrictive transfusion policy of RBC and platelets in pediatric patients submitted to ECMO [99]. The study reported that a restrictive RBC and platelet transfusion policy was safe and allowed a good outcome, although active bleeding was a surrogate marker for liberal transfusion (Hgb >7 g/dL).

9.3.5 Considerations for Transfusion in Preterm Infants

9.3.5.1 Preterm Anemia

The hypoxic intrauterine environment contributes to a decreased erythropoietin (EPO) level, thus preventing polycythemia. Premature infants produce smaller amounts of EPO at any level of anemia, as they still maintain a liver-based EPO production, unlike kidney-based EPO production, which occurs after term delivery and is regulated based on pO_2 level [88].

Another contributing factor to anemia of prematurity is the amount of blood loss due to repeated blood sampling for laboratory tests. The use of erythropoiesis-stimulating agents (ESA) such as darbepoetin and EPO are currently available pharmaceuticals. For neonates, namely preterm, it has contributed to a reduction in RBC transfusion in that population but has not reduced the exposure to different blood donors. As per a Cochrane Review from 2020, the use of EPO reduced the incidence of intraventricular hemorrhage, periventricular leukomalacia, and necrotizing enterocolitis (NEC), although it showed no significant difference in risk of stage ≥3 retinopathy of prematurity. Administration of EPO is not currently recommended because limited benefits have been identified to date. The use of darbepoetin requires further study. More recently, PBM strategies such as strict transfusion thresholds, the use of point-of-care testing, and decreased phlebotomy rates have all contributed to the reduction of blood transfusions [100].

9.3.5.2 Necrotizing Enterocolitis

Despite RBC transfusion being considered a risk factor for NEC, the precise etiology is still not clear and is most likely multifactorial [79]. There is no robust evidence associating NEC in preterm infants with transfusion. A few observational studies and multivariable analysis studies have associated NEC with anemia, although it is still uncertain whether anemia impacts NEC's development. The Effects of Transfusion Thresholds on Neurocognitive Outcomes of Extremely Low-Birth-Weight Infants (ETTNO) and the Premature Infants in Need of Transfusion (PINT) studies also did not find an association between pretransfusion Hgb level and NEC [101, 102]. Studies have shown a trend in reducing NEC in preterm infants using recombinant human erythropoietin (rEpo), or its derivative darbepoetin, as it may reduce anemia and the need for RBC transfusions.

Key Points

- Due to strict regulatory requirements in most jurisdictions, the blood collected is safe for the recipients. Questions remain regarding the gender of the donor and recipient, lead, nicotine, and marijuana and their effects on vulnerable populations. Further studies may help to determine if any of these factors pose a clinical concern and if practical mitigation strategies can be achieved that do not unnecessarily defer too many donors and maintain an adequate blood supply.
- The BPA serves two purposes. First, it prevents unnecessary transfusions that may expose the patient to both infectious and noninfectious risks. Second, it provides substantial cost savings.
- Most stable hospitalized patients can be transfused using a restrictive transfusion threshold <7 g/dL and stable patients can receive one unit of red blood cells (RBC) at a time to bridge sufficient hematopoiesis.
- Chronic transfusions can cause alloimmunization secondary to exposure to many donors; phenotyping of common antigen using alloimmunization can be performed prior to transfusion in order to minimize alloimmunization; genotyping of the patients and the donors is also an option. Multiple transfusions can also lead to severe iron overload, which may be reduced by iron chelation.
- Massive transfusion protocols were established in order to avoid transfusion delay in a life-threatening emergency. The protocols provide a framework for preparing blood components during massive bleeding, enabling continuous transfusion until the patient's condition has stabilized.
- The pediatric group of patients has different body volumes and responses to hypoxia and hypovolemia; hence transfusion indications, thresholds, and volume may take this into account.
- This is a variation with the laboratory thresholds for RBC transfusion in neonates and pediatric populations; hence, randomized controlled trials are warranted.
- Transfusion-associated hyperkalemia in neonates is a matter of concern regarding the age/shelf life of units.
- Preterm neonates are at risk of anemia due to phlebotomies and iatrogenic causes.

9.4 Conclusions

The quality of RBCs can be significantly affected by the characteristics of blood donors (e.g., health status, phenotypes), and an important aim of current measures in reducing risks for recipients is to better select blood donors. Due to the strict regulatory requirements in most jurisdictions, the blood collected is safe for the recipients. Questions remain regarding the sex of donor and recipient, lead, nicotine, and marijuana and their effects on vulnerable populations. Further studies may help to determine if any of these factors pose a clinical concern and if practical mitigation strategies can be achieved that do not unnecessarily defer too many donors and maintain an adequate blood supply. The BPA serves two purposes. First, it prevents unnecessary transfusions that may expose the patient to both infectious and noninfectious risks. Second, it provides substantial cost savings.

Guidelines from AABB [42] summarize the literature and state that most stable hospitalized patients can be transfused using a restrictive transfusion threshold <7 g/dL and can receive one unit of RBCs at a time with an evaluation of the Hgb between units and signs of organ failure. Chronic transfusions can cause alloimmunization secondary to exposure to many donors; phenotyping of common antigens causing alloimmunization can be performed prior to transfusion in order to minimize alloimmunization; genotyping of the patients and the donors is also an option. Multiple transfusions can lead to severe iron overload, which may be reduced by iron chelation.

Massive transfusion protocols were established in order to avoid transfusion delay in a life-threatening emergency. The protocols provide a framework for preparing blood components during massive bleeding, enabling continuous transfusion until the patient stabilizes. When the transfusion service is situated geographically far away from the emergency room, the operating theatre, and the ICU, remote supervised storage of RBCs may be necessary.

The pediatric group of patients has different body volumes and responses to hypoxia and hypovolemia; hence transfusion indications, thresholds, and volume must take this into account. There is variation in the laboratory thresholds for RBC transfusion in neonates and pediatric populations; hence, randomized controlled trials are warranted. Transfusion-associated hyperkalemia in neonates is a matter of concern regarding the age of units. Preterm neonates are at risk of anemia due to phlebotomies and iatrogenic causes, and this must be considered when treating this special population.

This section of the chapter ends in some ways with more questions than answers. Future studies are needed to determine the best marker for transfusion thresholds, clinical effects on the recipient, if any, of sex and substances found in the donor, and the best strategy to address the massively hemorrhaging patient.

References

1. Free RJ, Sapiano MRP, Chavez Ortiz JL, Stewart P, Berger J, Basavaraju SV. Continued stabilization of blood collections and transfusions in the United States: findings from the 2021 National Blood Collection and Utilization Survey. Transfusion. 2023;63 Suppl 4(Suppl 4):S8–S18.
2. Goel R, Zhu X, Patel EU, et al. Blood transfusion trends in the United States: national inpatient sample, 2015 to 2018. Blood Adv. 2021;5(20):4179–84.
3. Wells W, Mounter PJ, Chapman CE, Stainsby D, Wallis JP. Where does blood go? Prospective observational study of red cell transfusion in North England. BMJ. 2002;325(7368):803.
4. Goodnough LT, Brecher ME, Kanter MH, AuBuchon JP. Transfusion medicine. Second of two parts—blood conservation. N Engl J Med. 1999;340(7):525–33.
5. Carson JL MA, Hebert PC. Anemia and red blood cell transfusion. In: Simon TL GE, McCullough J, Roback JD, Snyder E, editor. Rossi's principles of transfusion medicine. 6th ed. 2022. pp. 25–36.
6. Roubinian NH, Escobar GJ, Liu V, Swain BE, Gardner MN, Kipnis P, et al. Trends in red blood cell transfusion and 30-day mortality among hospitalized patients. Transfusion. 2014;54(10 Pt 2):2678–86.

7. Carson JL, Kleinman S. Indications and hemoglobin thresholds for red blood cell transfusion in the adult. In: Tobial A, Tirnajuer J. eds. Update. 2023. https://www.uptodate.com/contents/indications-and-hemoglobin-thresholds-fro-red-blood-cell-transfusion-in-the-adult?search=indications%20and%haemoglobin%20thresholds%20for%20red%20blood%20cell%20transfusion%20in%20adult%20&source=search_results&selectedTitle=1~150&usage_type=default&display_rank=1. Accessed 26 Oct 2023.

8. Shehata N, M D. Hemotherapy decisions and their outcomes. In: Cohn CSDM, Johnson ST, Katz LM, editors. AABB technical manual. Bethesda: AABB; 2020. p. 553–6.

9. Chassé M, McIntyre L, English SW, et al. Effect of blood donor characteristics on transfusion outcomes: a systematic review and meta-analysis. Transfus Med Rev. 2016;30(2):69–80.

10. Gilliss BM, Looney MR, Gropper MA. Reducing noninfectious risks of blood transfusion. Anesthesiology. 2011;115(3):635–49.

11. Vamvakas EC, Blajchman MA. Transfusion-related mortality: the ongoing risks of allogeneic blood transfusion and the available strategies for their prevention. Blood. 2009;113(15):3406–17.

12. Toy P, Gajic O, Bacchetti P, et al. Transfusion-related acute lung injury: incidence and risk factors. Blood. 2012;119(7):1757–67.

13. Fatalities reported to FDA following blood collection and transfusion annual summary for fiscal year 2020. FDA; 2020.

14. Alshalani A, Uhel F, Cremer OL, et al. Donor-recipient sex is associated with transfusion-related outcomes in critically ill patients. Blood Adv. 2022;6(11):3260–7.

15. Caram-Deelder C, Kreuger AL, Evers D, et al. Association of blood transfusion from female donors with and without a history of pregnancy with mortality among male and female transfusion recipients. JAMA. 2017;318(15):1471–8.

16. Bahr TM, Christensen TR, Tweddell SM, Henry E, Rees T, Astin ME, et al. Associations between blood donor sex and age, and outcomes of transfused newborn infants. Transfusion. 2023;63:1290–7.

17. Jacobs JF, Baumert JL, Brons PP, Joosten I, Koppelman SJ, van Pampus EC. Anaphylaxis from passive transfer of peanut allergen in a blood product. N Engl J Med. 2011;364(20):1981–2.

18. Anani W, Dobrozsi S, Punzalan R. Identification of Peanut allergen in a transfused blood product causing transfusion associated anaphylaxis. Transfusion. 2020;60(5):1108–9.

19. Bearer CF, Linsalata N, Yomtovian R, Walsh M, Singer L. Blood transfusions: a hidden source of lead exposure. Lancet. 2003;362:332.

20. Delage G, Gingras S, Rhainds M. A population-based study on blood lead levels in blood donors. Transfusion. 2015;55(11):2633–40.

21. Rhainds M, Delage G. Health risk assessment of lead exposure from blood transfusion. Epidemiology. 2006;17(6):S492.

22. Qi B, Wang B, Zhang Z, Li Y, Feng Z, Pang S. A survey study of factors influencing elevated blood lead levels in donors from Qingdao. China Blood Transfus. 2023;21(3):193–201.

23. Wiencek JR, Gehrie EA, Keiser AM, Szklarski PC, Johnson-Davis KL, Booth GS. Detection of nicotine and nicotine metabolites in units of banked blood. Am J Clin Pathol. 2019;151(5):516–21.

24. Chin-Yee B, Lazo-Langner A, Butler-Foster T, Hsia C, Chin-Yee I. Blood donation and testosterone replacement therapy. Transfusion. 2017;57(3):578–81.

25. FDA liaison meeting. FDA; 2014.

26. Hazegh K, Anawalt BD, Dumont LJ, Kanias T. Toxic masculinity in red blood cell units? Testosterone therapy in blood donors revisited. Transfusion. 2021;61(11):3174–80.

27. Kraemer M, Madea B, Hess C. Detectability of various cannabinoids in plasma samples of cannabis users: indicators of recent cannabis use? Drug Test Anal. 2019;211(10):1498–506.

28. Widman M, Agurell S, Ehrnebo M, Jones G. Binding of (+)- and (minus)-delta-1-tetrahydrocannabinols and (minus)-7-hydroxy-delta-1-tetrahydrocannabinol to blood cells and plasma proteins in man. J Pharm Pharmacol. 1974;26(11):914–6.

29. Annen K, DomBourian MG. Perceptions on acceptability and reported consumption of marijuana by blood donors prior to donation in the recreational use state of Colorado, USA. Vox Sang. 2022;117(2):177–84.

30. Pressroom. Alexandria, VA. American Association of Poison Control Center (AAPCC); 2017.

31. Outbreak alert: potential life-threatening vitamin K-dependent antagonist coagulopathy associated with synthetic cannabinoids use. Center for Disease Control and Prevention; 2018.

32. Tran MH, Perez-Alvarez I, Swaroop B. Synthetic cannabinoid: an unexpected cause of coagulopathy. Transfusion. 2018;58(11):2743–4.

33. Gammon RR, Blanton K, Gilstad C, et al. How do we obtain and maintain patient blood management certification? Transfusion. 2022;62(8):1483–94.

34. Frank SMJD, Resar LMS. Development of a patient blood management program. Patient blood management: multidisciplinary approaches to optimizing care. Bethesda: AABB Press; 2016. p. 13–38.

35. Shander A, Hofmann A, Ozawa S, Theusinger OM, Gombotz H, Spahn DR. Activity-based costs of blood transfusions in surgical patients at four hospitals. Transfusion. 2010;50(4):753–65.

36. RR G. (2019) Best practice advisories. In: Fredrich N GR, Richards CA, Tauer R., editor. PBM metrics. Bethesda: AABB Press.

37. Zuckerberg GS, Scott AV, Wasey JO, et al. Efficacy of education followed by computerized pro-

vider order entry with clinician decision support to reduce red blood cell utilization. Transfusion. 2015;55(7):1628–36.

38. Hébert PC, Wells G, Blajchman MA, et al. (1999)A Multicenter, randomized, controlled clinical trial of transfusion requirements in critical care. Transfusion Requirements in Critical Care Investigators, Canadian Critical Care Trials Group. N Engl J Med 340(6):409–417.

39. Carson JL, Terrin ML, Noveck H, et al. Liberal or restrictive transfusion in high-risk patients after hip surgery. N Engl J Med. 2011;365(26):2453–62.

40. Villanueva C, Colomo A, Bosch A, et al. Transfusion strategies for acute upper gastrointestinal bleeding. N Engl J Med. 2013;368(1):11–21.

41. Carson JL, Grossman BJ, Kleinman S, et al. Red blood cell transfusion: a clinical practice guideline from the AABB*. Ann Intern Med. 2012;157(1):49–58.

42. Carson JL, Guyatt G, Heddle NM, Grossman BJ, Cohn CS, Fung MK, et al. Clinical practice guidelines from the AABB: red blood cell transfusion thresholds and storage. JAMA. 2016;316(19):2025–35.

43. Qaseem A, Humphrey LL, Fitterman N, Starkey M, Shekelle P. Treatment of anemia in patients with heart disease: a clinical practice guideline from the American College of Physicians. Ann Intern Med. 2013;159(11):770–9.

44. Yang WW, Thakkar RN, Gehrie EA, Chen W, Frank SM. Single-unit transfusions and hemoglobin trigger: relative impact on red cell utilization. Transfusion. 2017;57(5):1163–70.

45. Entzel P, Nielsen M, Weiss S, et al. How do I reduce variation in red blood cell transfusion practices in a large integrated health care system? Transfusion. 2023;63(6):1113–21.

46. Taher AT, Musallam KM, Cappellini MD. β-Thalassemias. N Engl J Med. 2021;384(8):727–43.47.

47. Rund D, Rachmilewitz E. Beta-thalassemia. N Engl J Med. 2005;353(11):1135–46.

48. Cohn CS, Johnson ST, Katz LM. AABB technical manual. 20th ed. AABB; 2020.

49. Taher AT, Porter JB, Viprakasit V, et al. Deferasirox effectively reduces iron overload in non-transfusion-dependent thalassemia (NTDT) patients: 1-year extension results from the THALASSA study. Ann Hematol. 2013;92(11):1485–93.

50. Cappellini MD, Viprakasit V, Taher AT, et al. A phase 3 trial of Luspatercept in patients with transfusion-dependent β-thalassemia. N Engl J Med. 2020;382(13):1219–31.

51. Thompson AA, Walters MC, Kwiatkowski J, et al. Gene therapy in patients with transfusion-dependent β-thalassemia. N Engl J Med. 2018;378(16):1479–93.

52. Psatha N, Reik A, Phelps S, et al. Disruption of the BCL11A erythroid enhancer reactivates fetal hemoglobin in erythroid cells of patients with β-thalassemia major. Mol Ther Methods Clin Dev. 2018;10:313–26.

53. Antoniani C, Meneghini V, Lattanzi A, et al. Induction of fetal hemoglobin synthesis by CRISPR/Cas9-mediated editing of the human β-globin locus. Blood. 2018;131(17):1960–73.

54. Sharma D, Ogbenna AA, Kassim A, Andrews J. Transfusion support in patients with sickle cell disease. Semin Hematol. 2020;57(2):39–50.

55. Han H, Hensch L, Tubman VN. (2021) indications for transfusion in the management of sickle cell disease. Hematology Am Soc Hematol Educ Program. 2021;1:696–703.

56. Howard J. (2016) sickle cell disease: when and how to transfuse. Hematol Am Soc Hematol Educ Program. 2016;1:625–31.

57. Zheng Y, Chou ST. Transfusion and cellular therapy in pediatric sickle cell disease. Clin Lab Med. 2021;41(1):101–19.

58. Pirenne F, Yazdanbakhsh K. How I safely transfuse patients with sickle-cell disease and manage delayed hemolytic transfusion reactions. Blood. 2018;131(25):2773–81.

59. Chou ST, Alsawas M, Fasano RM, et al. American Society of Hematology 2020 guidelines for sickle cell disease: transfusion support. Blood Adv. 2020;4(2):327–55.

60. Madu AJ, Ugwu AO, Efobi C. Hyperhemolytic syndrome in sickle cell disease: clearing the cobwebs. Med Princ Pract. 2021;30(3):236–43.

61. Linder GE, Chou ST. Red cell transfusion and alloimmunization in sickle cell disease. Hema. 2021;106(7):1805–15.

62. Zheng Y, Gossett JM, Chen PL, et al. Proinflammatory state promotes red blood cell alloimmunization in pediatric patients with sickle cell disease. Blood Adv. 2023;7(17):4799–08.

63. Vichinsky EP. Current issues with blood transfusions in sickle cell disease. Semin Hematol. 2021;38(1 Suppl 1):14–22.

64. Wahl S, Quirolo KC. Current issues in blood transfusion for sickle cell disease. Curr Opin Pediatr. 2009;21(1):15–21.

65. Davis BA, Allard S, Qureshi A, Pet al. Guidelines on red cell transfusion in sickle cell disease. Part I: principles and laboratory aspects. Br J Hematol. 2017;176(2):179–91.

66. Vichinsky EP, Haberkern CM, Neumayr L, Earles AN, Black D, Koshy M, et al. A comparison of conservative and aggressive transfusion regimens in the perioperative management of sickle cell disease. N Engl J Med. 1995;333(4):206–14.

67. Berentsen S, Barcellini W. Autoimmune hemolytic anemias. N Engl J Med. 2021;385(15):1407–19.

68. Chapuy CI, Nicholson RT, Aguad MD, et al. Resolving the daratumumab interference with blood compatibility testing. Transfusion. 2015;55(6 Pt 2):1545–54.

69. Martin TG, Corzo K, Chiron M, Velde HV, Abbadessa G, Campana F, et al. Therapeutic opportunities with pharmacological inhibition of CD38 with Isatuximab. Cells. 2019;8(12):1522.

70. Treating Red Cells: 0.2 M DTT Procedure. In: Judd WJ JS, Storry J, editor. Judd's methods in immmunohematology. AABB; 2022. p. 287.

71. Habicht CP, Ridders M, Grueger D, Adolph S, Immenschuh S, Schneeweiss C. Mitigation of therapeutic anti-CD38 antibody interference with fab fragments: how well does it perform? Transfusion. 2023;63(4):808–16.

72. Handbook of transfusion medicine. In: Norfolk, D, editor. Handbook of transfusion medicine. 5th ed. 2013. p. 82.

73. Rahimi-Levene N, Dann E. Massive bleeding protocols—the transfusion service perspective. https://www.isbtweb.org/isbt-working-parties/clinical-transfusion/resources/patient-blood-management-resources/massive-bleeding-protocols.html. Accessed 7 June 2023.

74. Kelly DP, Grandin EW, O'Brien KL. How we manage blood product support and coagulation in the adult patient requiring extracorporeal membrane oxygenation. Transfusion. 2022;62(4):741–50.

75. Abbasciano RG, Yusuff H, Vlaar APJ, Lai F, Murphy GJ. Blood transfusion threshold in patients receiving extracorporeal membrane oxygenation support for cardiac and respiratory failure-a systematic review and meta-analysis. J Cardiothorac Vasc Anesth. 2021;35(4):1192–202.

76. Worku ET, Win AM, Parmar D, Anstey C, Shekar K. Hematological trends and transfusion during adult extracorporeal membrane oxygenation: a single Centre study. J Clin Med. 2023;12(7):2629.

77. Howie SR. Blood sample volumes in child health research: review of safe limits. Bull. 2011;89(1):46–53.

78. Goel R, Josephson CD, Patel EU, et al. Individual- and hospital-level correlates of red blood cell, platelet, and plasma transfusions among hospitalized children and neonates: a nationally representative study in the United States. Transfusion. 2020;60(8):1700–12.

79. Villeneuve A, Arsenault V, Lacroix J, Tucci M. Neonatal red blood cell transfusion. Vox Sang. 2021;116(4):366–78.

80. Valentine SL, Bembea MM, Muszynski JA, et al. Consensus recommendations for RBC transfusion practice in critically ill children from the pediatric critical care transfusion and anemia expertise initiative. Pediatr Crit Care Med. 2018;19(9):884–98.

81. Teruya J, Tobian A, Armsby C. Red blood cell transfusion in infants and children: administration and complications. UpToDate. https://www.uptodate.com/contents/red-blood-cell-transfusion-in-infants-and-children-administration-and-complications?search=Red%20blood%20cell%20transfusion%20in%20infants%20and%20children:%20Administration%20and%20complications&source=search_result&selectedTitle=1~150&usage_type=default&display_rank=1. Accessed 11 July 2023.

82. Luban NL. Neonatal red blood cell transfusions. Curr Opin Hematol. 2002;9(6):533–6.

83. Lacroix J, Hébert PC, Hutchison JS, et al. Transfusion strategies for patients in pediatric intensive care units. N Engl J Med. 2007;356(16):1609–19.

84. Saito-Benz M, Flanagan P, Berry MJ. Management of anaemia in pre-term infants. Br J Hematol. 2020;188(3):354–66.

85. Sohail H, Ahmed SA, Usman P, Khalid F, Haque AU, Abbas Q. Red blood cell transfusion in critically-ill children and its association with outcome. J Pak Med Assoc. 2021;71(8):1967.

86. Roseff SD, Luban NL, Manno CS. Guidelines for assessing appropriateness of pediatric transfusion. Transfusion. 2002;42(11):1398–413.

87. McIntyre C, August D, Li C, et al. Neonatal vascular access practice and complications: an observational study of 1,375 catheter days. J Perinat Neonat Nursing. 2022;37(4):332–9. https://doi.org/10.1097/JPN.0000000000000589.

88. Edward CC. Wong M, Rowena C, Punzalan, MD. Therapeutic apheresis. In: Cohn C, Delaney M, Johnson ST, Katz LM, editors. AABB Technical manual. 20th ed. 2020. p. 689.

89. Rosa-Mangeret F, Waldvogel-Abramowski S, Pfister RE, Baud O, Fau S. Safety of red blood cell transfusion using small central lines in neonates: an in vitro non-inferiority study. Front Pediatr. 2021;9:606611.

90. Teruya J. Red blood cell transfusion in infants and children: administration and complications. 2023. https://docs.google.com/document/d/1I-z0pgVHyighACwCNsZ8iwF_q8vXq-quQ8KE7NcSUHk/edit#.

91. Saito-Benz M, Bennington K, Gray CL, et al. Effects of freshly irradiated vs irradiated and stored red blood cell transfusion on cerebral oxygenation in preterm infants: a randomized clinical trial. JAMA Pediatr. 2022;176(5):e220152.

92. Luban NL, Strauss RG, Hume HA. Commentary on the safety of red cells preserved in extended-storage media for neonatal transfusions. Transfusion. 1991;31(3):229–35.

93. Lau W. Neonatal and pediatric transfusion. Canadian Blood Services; 2017.

94. Burke M, Sinha P, Luban NLC, Posnack NG. Transfusion-associated hyperkalemic cardiac arrest in neonatal, infant, and pediatric patients. Front Pediatr. 2021;9:765306.

95. Yamada C, Edelson M, Lee A, Saifee NH, Bahar B, Delaney M. Transfusion-associated hyperkalemia in pediatric population: prevalence, risk factors, survival, infusion rate, and RBC unit features. Transfusion. 2021;61(4):1093–101.

96. Sannon C. Walker aDS. Transfusion approaches and controversies. In: Andrews J MM, editor.

Transfusion support for patients with sickle cell disease. 2nd ed. AABB; 2022.

97. Rodeck C, Nicolaides K, Warsof S, Fysh W, Gamsu H, Kemp J. The management of severe rhesus isoimmunization by fetoscopic intravascular transfusions. Am J Obstet Gynecol. 1984;150(6): 769–74.

98. Okulu E, Erdeve Ö, Tuncer O, et al. Exchange transfusion for neonatal hyperbilirubinemia: a multicenter, prospective study of Turkish Neonatal Society. Turk Arch Pediatr. 2021;56(2):121–6.

99. Duarte CM, Lopes MI, Abecasis F. Transfusion policy in pediatric extracor2021poreal membrane oxygenation patients: less could be more. Perfusion. 2022; 2676591221105610

100. Ohlsson A, Aher SM. Early erythropoiesis-stimulating agents in preterm or low birth weight infants. Cochrane Database Syst Rev. 2017;11:CD004863.

101. Kirpalani H, Whyte RK, Andersen C, et al. The Premature Infants in Need of Transfusion (PINT) study: a randomized, controlled trial of a restrictive (low) versus liberal (high) transfusion threshold for extremely low birth weight infants. J Pediatr. 2006;149(3):301–7.

102. Franz AR, Engel C, Bassler D, et al. Effects of Liberal vs restrictive transfusion thresholds on survival and neurocognitive outcomes in extremely low-birth-weight infants: the ETTNO randomized clinical trial. JAMA. 2020;324(6):560–70.

103. Carson JL, Brooks MM, Hébert PC, et al. Restrictive or Liberal transfusion strategy in myocardial infarction and anemia. N Engl J Med. 2023;389(26):2446–56. https://doi.org/10.1056/NEJMoa2307983.

Part IV

Quality Management in Clinical Transfusion Medicine

Yetmgeta E. Abdella

Need for a Quality System and Quality System Management in Clinical Transfusion Medicine

Cees Th. Smit Sibinga, Mohammed Farouk, and Yetmgeta E. Abdella

10.1 Introduction

Globally there are many guidelines circulating on clinical use of blood; regulatory and peer composed and distributed. However, they are all technical and performance oriented, but none guides the broad transfusion medicine concept for blood prescribing clinicians. Blood transfusion is a supportive transplantation practice or hemotherapy, which needs a well-designed and understood environment and clinical climate to the benefit of the recipients or patients [1]. Blood transfusion serves a manifold of clinical blood prescribing disciplines like internal medicine, hematology and oncology, surgery and anesthesiology, traumatology and intensive care, pediatrics and neonatology, and obstetrics and gynecology. Consequently, the practice needs uniformity through harmonization and a strong and well-

C. T. Smit Sibinga (✉)
International Development of Transfusion Medicine, University of Groningen and IQM Consulting, Zuidhorn, Netherlands

M. Farouk
Africa Society for Blood Transfusion, Pinetown, South Africa
e-mail: mohammed.farouk@adsbt.org

Y. E. Abdella
Self-employed, Freelance Consultant in Blood and other Products of Human Origin, Addis Ababa, Ethiopia

developed clinical interface of the healthcare facility and the manufacturing establishment. As the starting point of the vein-to-vein blood and transfusion chain, it needs a quality system and system management to flourish as a fully respected and developed clinical overarching and cohesive supportive discipline.

10.2 Need for Quality and Its Management

Blood components are living elements of the donated human blood and have been processed or manufactured under strict quality and pharmaceutical conditions by the supplying blood establishment [2]. The manufacturing process or procurement of blood follows the principles of quality through a quality system and its system management. The quality system (QS) usually applied is Good Manufacturing Practice (GMP), which needs management to become operational. It should extend into the health care institution to protect from untoward, use and handling conditions as Good Clinical Practice (GCP). However, it is of paramount importance to manage along the three major principles:

- Know and understand what needs to be managed;
- Document what you do;
- Do what you have documented.

Evidently, blood components or products as living and functional elements of human blood need to be preserved while entering a new life in the healthcare facility destined to be transfused into patients in need. Analyzing the clinical process of patient transfusion with a specific blood component brings to light three different processes (see Chap. 4, Fig. 4.2) [3].

1. **Bedside**: Diagnosis, indication setting, and decision-making with informed consent and the ordering of what is wanted and needed together with a patient blood sample for immunohematology and compatibility testing (Fig. 10.1); this happens mostly at the bedside, but sometimes at the outpatient department (OPD) in anticipation of a medical intervention. Order or request should be done through a standardized blood request form (see Chap. 4) in triplicate of which one is archived in the patient file as an evidence document of the request.

2. **Transfusion service laboratory**: Reception of the order and blood sample at the transfusion service laboratory, testing and selection of the wanted/needed blood component, administration of the data, and cold chain transport to the ward, OR of ICU. One completed copy of the request form remains in the transfusion service laboratory archive.

   A flow chart of this blood component selection process is in Fig. 10.2.

3. **Bedside**: Reception by the attending nurse of the requested unit(s) of blood component(s) and the comparison with the original first part of the request form to identify both the right patient and the right blood component unit. Patient preparation, with vital signs, venous insertion of a needle or catheter to which the administration set is connected, primed with 0.9% NaCl. Then the blood component unit is connected, and a slow drip is started to observe for immediate adverse events to happen.

During the transfusion episode the patient shall be observed regularly (every half an hour) by the attending nurse and vital signs taken and

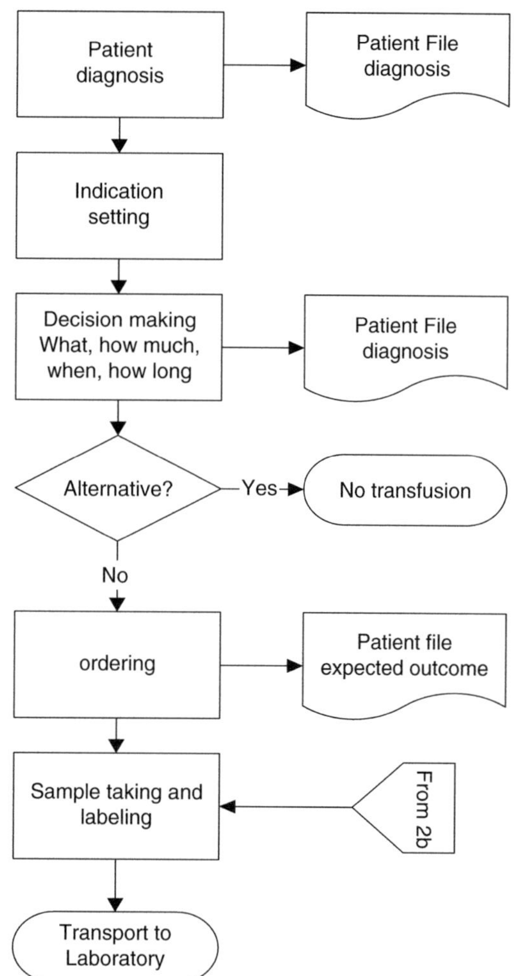

Fig. 10.1 Blood request process

documented in the patient file. Of all small steps evidence (data) shall be documented in the patient file and on the transfusion report form (hemovigilance) to be sent to the healthcare facility hemovigilance officer.

The steps in this third process are depicted in Fig. 10.3a and b.

These three distinctly different but interrelated processes with the 17 composing procedures need professional management by competent personnel, working together as a team—medical specialist, nursing staff, and transfusion service laboratory professionals. Only then quality can be guaranteed as a preferred outcome of these clinical processes, evidenced by transparency and clear and complete documentation.

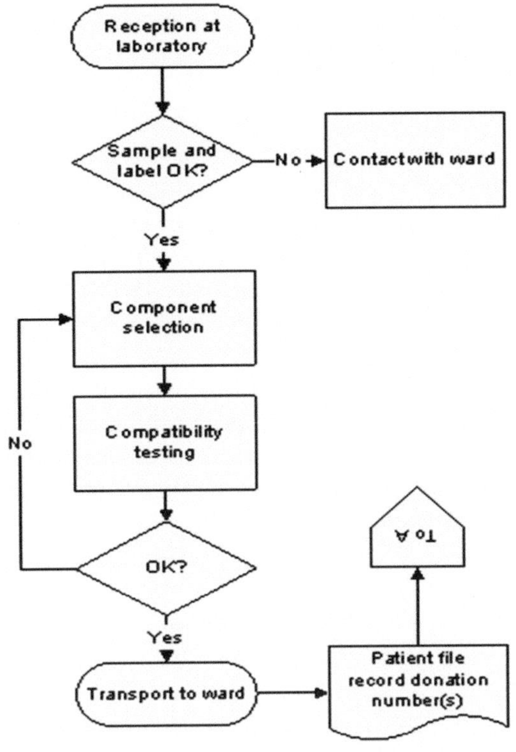

Fig. 10.2 Blood component selection process

10.3 Existing Clinical Quality Systems

There are a limited number of clinical quality systems focused on Good Clinical Practice. Most are clinical research oriented and find their origin in a series of unsuccessful and ineffective clinical trials in the past. Discussions led to the development of certain regulations, WHO Guidance and guidelines, which evolved into the "code of practice" for international consistency of quality research, e.g., EU Directive 2001/20/EC [4] and ISO 14155 [5].

However, none of these touches upon the need to develop standardized transfusion practices to support safe patient care and treatment, eliminating avoidable harm.

An important initiative is with the International Society for Quality in Health Care (ISQua) [6], which believes that person-centeredness is an important aspect of safe and quality health care. The movement towards patient-centered care has been developed over the past two decades, and ISQua has a vibrant community who are invested

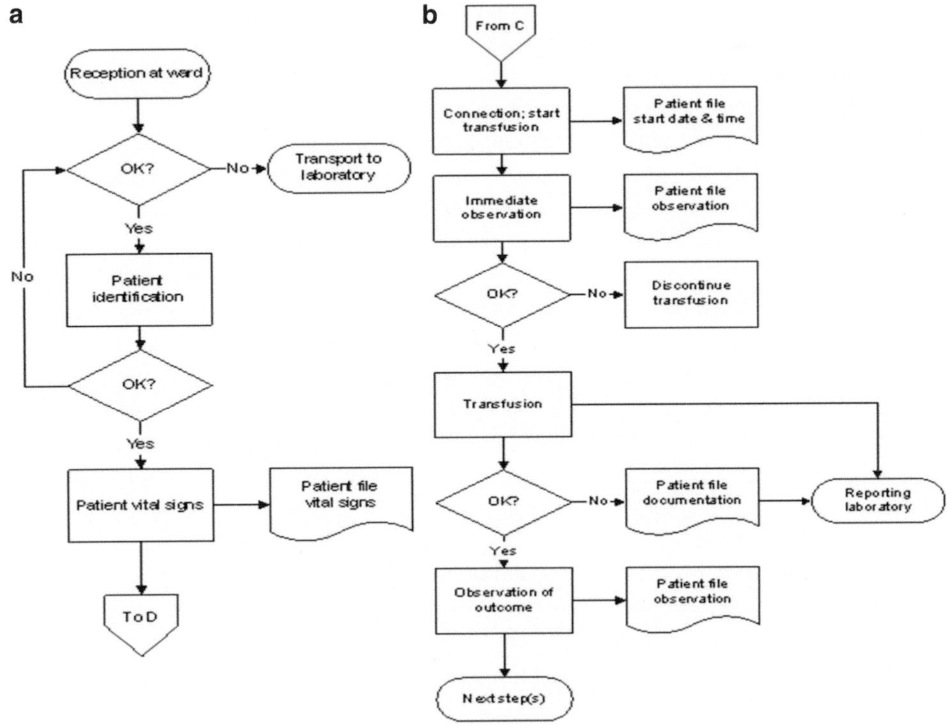

Fig. 10.3 (**a**) Reception of blood component at the ward and patient preparation. (**b**) Ultimate patient transfusion

in making patient-centered care a core element in healthcare systems globally. However, it does not relate to or include clinical transfusion medicine as an overarching supportive intervention in blood prescribing disciplines. Like ISO it is patient/customer-oriented and results in certification or accreditation of a healthcare institute. The International Society for Quality in Health Care External Evaluation Association (IEEA) was established as a separate legal entity by the International Society for Quality in Health Care in 2018 to deliver external evaluation services.

The IEEA, based in Geneva, Switzerland, commenced operations in January 2019. The IEEA provides third-party external evaluation services to health and social care facilities and health care standards developing bodies around the globe [7].

WHO launched in 2021 a Global Patient Safety Action Plan 2021–2030 [8] focusing on elimination of avoidable harm in health care, improving on quality of care in a patient-centered way engaging patients and families in safe care.

Patient safety is defined as "A framework of organized activities that creates cultures, processes, procedures, behaviors, technologies and environments in health care that consistently and sustainably lower risks, reduce the occurrence of avoidable harm, make errors less likely and reduce the impact of harm when it does occur."

Guiding principles of this clinically oriented quality of care plan establish underpinning values to shape the development and implementation of the action plan are the following:

1. Engage patients and families as partners in safe care (patient-centered);
2. Achieve results through collaborative working (clinical teams and interfaces);
3. Analyze and share data to generate learning (documentation);
4. Translate evidence into actionable and measurable improvement (safety);
5. Base policies and action on the nature of the care setting (supportive blood transfusion);
6. Use both scientific expertise and patient experience to improve safety (knowledge economy);

7. Instill a safety culture in the design and delivery of health care (quality culture).

These principles should translate into a quality system and system management especially for the overarching and medical discipline of supporting clinical transfusion practice. The implementing and controlling authority usually is the Hospital Transfusion Committee (HTC), which oversees the transfusion practice in the healthcare facilities.

Despite all these initiatives there is an increasing need for a universal quality system and system management in clinical transfusion medicine with set standards, documentation, education, and assessment.

10.4 Quality and Clinical Transfusion Practice

In the largely supply-driven transfusion chain, the quality of bedside transfusion practice is affected by a number of factors which may be intrinsic to the prescribing clinician like prior medical school training and working experiences or can be external like availability of continuing medical education, peer recommendations, feedbacks from hemovigilance teams, administrative support from hospital governance, financial incentives, and patient attitudes and desires [9]. However, the most prominent factor is the continued shortage of supply of quality blood components caused by an absence of well-functioning interfaces in particular between the hospital and its blood supplier: the clinical interface.

Blood transfusion is an essential part of modern healthcare. However, like most therapeutic interventions, it is also associated with significant clinical risks. Minimizing the risks and optimizing the benefits of transfusion depend on close collaboration vice versa throughout the "transfusion chain" from the clinical prescribers of blood, nursing staff, and blood transfusion service laboratory professionals, and patients to the suppliers of the blood and blood components. The two main elements for safe, effective, and quality transfusion are current good clinical practice (cGCP) and a sufficient supply of safe and efficacious blood and blood components. In developed countries, there is generally a sufficient supply of blood although motivation, retention and aging of donors are significant challenges.

Good transfusion practice (GTP) requires the avoidance of clinical and laboratory errors leading to "wrong blood transfusion," "wrong name on tube," appropriate decision-making about the evidence-based rational use of blood based on assessment of clinical findings and laboratory parameters, and the monitoring of patients for adverse effects of transfusion and their management if they occur. Unfortunately, there is evidence of sub-optimal practice in all these aspects of transfusion. The main themes underlying this poor practice are typically very similar, and have been described in detail elsewhere along with interventions to improve practice [10]. The key clinical (in-hospital) transfusion medicine interfaces in the "advanced" transfusion chain in advanced situations are the HTC and clinical teams, clinicians and patients, clinicians and hospital blood bank, the hospital blood bank and the blood supplier, and the blood supplier and the HTC as well as the potential donors (external). To be effective, these clinical transfusion medicine interfaces should operate bidirectionally; for example, clinicians make requests (demand) for blood to the hospital blood bank, and hospital blood banks provide ad hoc advice to clinicians and draw attention to local and national guidelines for good practice.

Clinicians clearly have a key role in the safety and quality of the transfusion process, decision-making about the use of blood and alternatives to blood, providing information to patients (informed consent), and monitoring patients during and after transfusions. The key interfaces of clinicians are with patients, the hospital blood bank, and the HTC. Many patients, and indeed the public, have a very limited understanding of the true benefits and risks of transfusion, and may consequently have considerable fears and anxieties about transfusion. Patients who have received a transfusion often do not recall the consent process, either because they were not given full information or because they rapidly forgot it.

However, communication by clinicians with transfusion recipients needs to be improved. There is considerable variation in the methods used for obtaining and documenting consent to transfusion as a proposed supportive intervention. Involvement of patients in decision-making about the use of blood and the safety of transfusion procedures such as blood sample collection and the administration of blood are potentially important interventions to improve the quality and safety of blood transfusion and increase blood avoidance where this is appropriate [11]. However, it is yet unclear how willing patients and healthcare staff would be to engage more robustly in these activities.

There is clearly a variable emphasis on good transfusion practice by clinical teams. Some teams carry out even major procedures without blood transfusion by intensive attention to patient care throughout the perioperative period. It is the role of the HTC and the hospital blood bank or transfusion service laboratory to encourage clinicians to use restrictive transfusion thresholds and other good blood management practices. As well as providing ad hoc advice, drawing attention to local and national guidelines and the WHO guidance for good transfusion practice, the HTC and hospital blood bank can encourage clinicians and clinical teams to participate in local, regional, and national audits of transfusion practice, for example, on the usage of blood and blood components.

In recent years, blood suppliers/establishments in many advanced countries have promoted better blood management and safe transfusion practice through national initiatives involving the creation of hemovigilance schemes for adverse event reporting, and the establishment of national and regional committees to improve the clinical transfusion medicine education and training of clinical staff prescribing blood, developing guidelines on blood usage, and providing the mechanism for reviewing blood use in local, regional and/or national audits with feedback of data to clinicians. That is only possible if a transparent and clear documentation system is in place and adhered to. Evidently, the introduction of artificial intelligence (AI), radiofrequency identification (RFID), and clinical transfusion medicine digital foot printing will contribute to strengthening these aspects [12] (see also Chaps. 5 and 6).

10.5 How to Manage Quality and Ensure Patient Satisfaction?

In a patient-centered system patient blood management (PBM) plays an important role in achieving quality of the transfusion and creating customer or patient satisfaction. This is a holistic outcome depending on a manifold of healthcare institution aspects, e.g., environment and clinical climate, attitude of healthcare workers, open and transparent involvement of the patient, explanation in simple and understandable language avoiding unnecessary medical terminology and jargon, quality of the transfusion process including the quality of the components to be transfused, sincere and human interest in the patient and the medical problem, following strictly Standard Operation Procedures (SOPs) and Equipment Operating Procedures (EOPs), and the facilities policies and strategies for a safe and quality transfusion medicine practice, whether bedside or transfusion service laboratory and the cold chain during transport. There are at least seven interfaces in the patient-centered process of blood transfusion and management. PBM is a patient-centered and patient-driven initiative that focuses on an evidence-based, multidisciplinary approach to optimizing the care of patients who might need transfusion support. As described in a recently published report on best practices, a PBM program needs a clearly defined structure and resources allocated to manage it, monitor, and evaluate its effectiveness [13]. To be successful, these programs require collaboration among different clinical specialties, each treating the patient as a member of the healthcare team. This results in multiple interfaces between the patient and various medical and surgical specialists and ancillary staff (Fig. 10.4).

In most healthcare institutions, the HTC (or a similar committee) offers a perfect opportunity to bring all stakeholders on board to initiate a PBM program [13, 14]. PBM programs are aimed at treating the reason for transfusion support and avoiding transfusion in the first place, if possible.

The AABB (former American Association of Blood Banks) has created and made available in 2016 Standards for a PBM program which need to be adhered to by all AABB accredited Blood Banks and Transfusion Services [15]. However, they are stand-alone and not embedded in a quality system and system management structure. Several strategies can be employed to achieve that goal, e.g., in a typical surgical PBM program, patients undergo medical evaluation by an anesthetist. A part of that evaluation includes screening for anemia. Where the hemoglobin concentration is low, the patient is treated by the clinical team using an agreed algorithm for anemia management or referred to a hematologist for evaluation and correction of anemia before the surgery is scheduled.

To ensure that the transfusion service laboratory will have compatible blood available should the patient need a transfusion for surgery, a blood sample for type and screen (T&S) testing is drawn on all patients who are scheduled to undergo surgical procedures that have a reasonable likelihood of requiring the support of a transfusion [15].

In the hospital setting, care is typically provided by a team of experts. As a result, patient and providers must navigate multiple interfaces to ensure that optimal care is delivered. Minimizing blood losses due to phlebotomy is an important part of any PBM program. Since diagnostic testing can contribute to anemia among the hospitalized patients, only the tests that are medically justified and necessary should be ordered and the volume of blood sample collected should be reduced to the minimum needed for testing [16]. If transfusion is needed, exposure to allogeneic blood can be prevented by the use of autologous blood and implementing auto-transfusion techniques, such as acute normovolemic hemodilution (ANH) or intra- or post-operative red cell recovery or salvage. The application of targeted

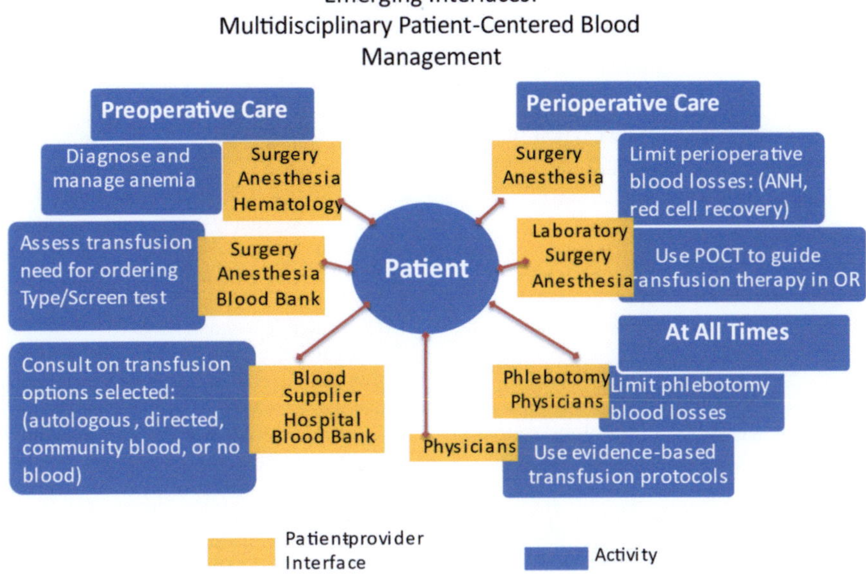

Fig. 10.4 Example of emerging transfusion medicine interfaces: Multidisciplinary Patient-Centered Blood Management, with seven interfaces (yellow); three during the preoperative stage, two during the perioperative intervention stage, and two general (all times) [3]

blood component therapy aided by point-of-care testing (POCT) can also help reduce the exposure to allogeneic blood. Instead of transfusing red cells, plasma, cryoprecipitate, and platelets all at the same time to control the bleeding, POCT can identify the specific component(s) that would be most effective in controlling the bleeding. POCT also offers other advantages, such as a smaller blood volume requirement and rapid turnaround times [17].

PBM programs are applicable to both surgical and nonsurgical patients. Strategies such as limiting blood losses through phlebotomy and use of evidence-based practice guidelines for red cells, platelets, and plasma transfusions should be adhered to for all patients and regularly monitored by appropriate committees, e.g., HTC for all services, multidisciplinary. Finally, modern and advanced healthcare, which includes transfusion practice, needs to adapt to new evidence about optimal patient care [18]. For example in transfusion medicine, blood suppliers are responding to a better understanding of serious complications of transfusion and taking measures to minimize the risk of, e.g., TRALI and bacterial contamination of platelets. However, it may sometimes be difficult to know how to respond to new data, e.g., on restricted versus liberal transfusion strategies in pediatric or adult patients (see Chaps. 7 and 9).

10.6 Conclusion and Recommendations

Clinical transfusion medicine as a multidisciplinary supportive specialty needs a uniform practice based on standards and a quality system and system management to warrant safety and efficiency of blood transfusion. The implementation of patient blood management (PBM) could prevent or at least mitigate the occurrence of adverse transfusion events, where standardized documentation will provide the evidence of good clinical transfusion practice.

A clinical transfusion medicine quality system and quality system management, together with outcome defined education of transfusion involved clinical personnel—clinicians, nurses, and transfusion service laboratory professionals is paramount in improving quality of clinical transfusion medicine and ensure patient satisfaction.

Interfaces form the quality connections between the patient and the multidisciplinary clinical approach and environment when managing a patient-centered optimal and safe clinical transfusion practice.

10.6.1 Recommendations

1. Clinical transfusion practice should be patient centered supported by quality;
2. Where not yet existing, patient blood management should be implemented to improve on healthcare;
3. Tangible references or clinical standards need to be implemented and adhered to;
4. Existing guidelines and WHO Guidance should change into clinical standards of transfusion medicine practice.

Key Points

- Patient rights protection is not only an ethical and legal principle but also a basic clinical quality principle;
- Quality needs a structured system and system management;
- Documentation, hemovigilance, and patient blood management are quality tools in clinical transfusion medicine;
- Patient-centered blood management is a multidisciplinary transfusion medicine approach with many interfaces important for the quality of the care.
- There is a need for a quality system and system management in clinical transfusion medicine.
- There is a distinct difference between the supportive and interactive role of the hospital transfusion laboratory and the transfusion medicine bedside practice.

References

1. Holmberg JA, Rosin N. Chapter II. Need for quality management in transfusion medicine. In: Smit Sibinga CT, editor. Quality management in transfusion medicine. New York: Nova Scientific Publ. Inc.; 2013. p. 35–53.
2. Smit Sibinga CT, Jansen van Galen JP. Chapter 8. The blood supply—a special manufacturing process. In: Mellal MH, editor. Manufacturing systems. New York: Nova Scientific Publ Inc.; 2020. p. 165–86.
3. Murphy MF, Saxena S, Smit Sibinga CT. Chapter IX. Patient safety and quality management. In: Smit Sibinga CT, editor. Quality management in transfusion medicine. New York: Nova Scientific Publ. Inc.; 2013. p. 283–314.
4. EU Directive 2001/20/EC on the approximation of the laws, regulations and administrative provisions of the Member States relating to the implementation of good clinical practice in the conduct of clinical trials on medicinal products for human use. 2001L0020 - EN - 07.08.2009–002.001-1. 2001. https://health.ec.europa.eu/system/files/2016-11/dir_2001_20_en_0.pdf.
5. ISO14155 clinical investigation of medical devices for human subjects—good clinical practice. 3rd ed. 2020. accessible as PDF at https://health.ec.europa.eu/system/files/2016-11/dir_2001_20_en_0.pdf.
6. ISQua Inspiring & driving Improvements in the Quality and Safety in Health Care Worldwide. www.isqua.org.
7. ISQua IEEA International Society for Quality in Health Care External Evaluation Association. https://isqua.org/external-evaluation.html.
8. WHO Action framework to advance universal access to safe, effective and quality-assured blood products 2020–2023. Licence: CC BY-NC-SA 3.0 IGO. Geneva: World Health Organization; 2020. p. 17.
9. Donahue JG, Munoz A, Ness PM, et al. The declining risk of post transfusion hepatitis C infection. N Engl I Med. 1992;327:367–73.
10. Murphy MF, Stanworth SJ, Yazer M. Transfusion practice and safety: current status and possibilities for improvement. Vox Sang. 2011;100:46–59.
11. Davis RE, Vincent CA, Murphy MF. Blood transfusion safety: the potential role of the patient. Transfus Med Rev. 2011;25:12–23.
12. Smit Sibinga CT. Will digital foot printing change the future of transfusion medicine? Int J Clin Studies Med Care Rep. 2022:1–7. https://doi.org/10.46998/IJCMCR.2021.17.000412.
13. Aubuchon JP, Puca K, Saxena S, et al. Getting started in patient blood management. Bethesda, MA: AABB Press; 2011.

14. Becker J, Shaz B. Guidelines for patient blood management and blood utilization. In: AABB clinical transfusion medicine CTTEE and transfusion medicine section coordinating committee. Bethesda, MA: AABB Press; 2011.
15. Standards for a patient management program. 1st ed. Bethesda MA: AABB Press; 2016.
16. Saxena S, Nelson JM, Osby M, Shah M, Kempff M, Shulman IR. Ensuring timely completion of type and screen testing and the verification of ABO/Rh status for elective surgical patients. Arch Path Lab Med. 2007;131:576–81.
17. Saxena S, Belzberg H, Chogyoyi M, Wilcox S, Shulman IR. Reducing phlebotomy losses by streamlining laboratory test ordering in a surgical intensive care unit. Lab Med. 2003;34:728–32.
18. Global Patient Safety Action Plan 2021–2023. Towards eliminating avoidable harm in health care. Licence: CC BY-NC-SA 3.0 IGO. Geneva: World Health Organization; 2021.

The Effect of Standards and Guidelines in Clinical Practice

Mohammed Farouk, Cees Th. Smit Sibinga, and Yetmgeta E. Abdella

11.1 Introduction

Over the last decades, healthcare financial constraints, varied patient outcomes, inconsistent medical practices, tremendous advances in treatment as a result of medical research, and medico-legal concerns associated with providing care to patients made it more complex for clinicians and created a great deal of subjectivity and inconsistency of medical care outcomes. This made it necessary to find ways to overcome all these challenges while ensuring best possible patient outcomes. Adopting clinical practice guidelines and clinical practice standards was one of the tools the medical communities, and other healthcare stakeholders, adopted to deal with these challenges.

Although the terms "clinical practice guidelines" and "clinical practice standards" sometimes are being used interchangeably, they are different. In general, practice standards are authoritative, and they may be used as the basis for accreditation, whereas practice guidelines are mostly recommendations. In this chapter, we are more oriented to clinical practice guidelines in the field of blood transfusion.

Clinical practice guidelines draw on synthesized research findings to set forth recommendations for state-of-the-art care. Trustworthy clinical practice guidelines are critical to improving quality of care [1]. This is fully applicable on blood transfusion clinical practice guidelines.

The process of developing clinical practice standards and guidelines is quite complicated and needed to be standardized itself to avoid subjectivity and reliance on mere personal experience rather than objective-based medicine [2].

This chapter focuses on a variety of topics related to clinical practice guidelines and guidances in the blood transfusion field, starting with positioning of clinical practice guidelines in the healthcare field, then converging to clinical practice guidelines in the blood transfusion field including their impact on improving patient outcomes and different strategies to promote adoption of clinical practice guidelines by healthcare organizations and individual clinicians.

M. Farouk
Africa Society for Blood Transfusion,
Pinetown, South Africa
e-mail: mohammed.farouk@adsbt.org

C. T. Smit Sibinga (✉)
International Development of Transfusion Medicine,
University of Groningen and IQM Consulting,
Zuidhorn, Netherlands

Y. E. Abdella
Self-employed, Freelance Consultant in Blood and
other Products of Human Origin,
Addis Ababa, Ethiopia

11.2　Clinical Practice Guidelines

The United States Institute of Medicine (IOM) defined clinical practice guidelines as "statements that include recommendations intended to optimize patient care that are informed by a systematic review of evidence and an assessment of the benefits and harms of alternative care options" [1]. The term "evidence-based" in relation to healthcare practices found its first use in the early 1990s as one of the possible bases for the development of clinical guidelines [3]. The past 30 years have seen a major expansion of evidence-based medicine that assumed an increasingly important role in the work of all health care professionals. Evidence-based medicine itself is defined as "integrating individual clinical expertise with the best available external clinical evidence from systematic research" [4, 5].

Historically, until the 1970s, medical actions were indirectly regulated through the training and credentials guaranteed by both the organized profession and government authorities. Armed with these credentials, individual physicians were assumed to be competent enough to determine the appropriate medical procedures. Although the opinions of experts, expressed informally or formally, supplemented educational credentials, and provided some guidance for practice, they were either diffused narrowly or had little formal status. However, this proved not to be enough to standardize and improve medical procedures (in terms of efficiency and patient outcomes) as the results of medical research vastly complicated the world of medical practice and its regulation. Starting in the early twentieth century and accelerating after World War II, the expansion of research created new problems in translating this knowledge into better health care [6]. Coupling this with the soaring costs of healthcare and the need of physicians to protect their collective professional autonomy, clinical guidelines and evidence-based medicine emerged as the toll to address these concerns.

In arguing for the development of evidence-based medicine and clinical guidelines, Sackett et al. point to the substantial variation in clinical practice that exists in all healthcare systems and the considerable difficulties clinicians face in keeping pace with the relevant research from scientific and medical journals. For example, consultant physicians might be expected to read approximately 19 articles per day, 365 days/year to keep pace with relevant primary research in their field [5].

In clinical practice, there are different types of guidance that vary in complexity and scope. For example, guidance can be a comprehensive overarching clinical practice guideline or a more specific clinical protocol. Regardless of the variation in scope and focus, it is important that the development of all clinical guidance is underpinned by core standards using an evidence-based approach, to assist clinician and patient decisions about appropriate healthcare for specific clinical circumstances. Through consistency in approach and reduction in duplication, variation in practice can be reduced. Sharing of best practice can optimize use of health service resources and expertise [7].

In all cases, it remains important for good practice guidelines to be evaluated fully for their effectiveness in improving health, and to be rigorously developed so that they have the power to translate the complexity of scientific research findings into recommendations for clinical practice and potentially enhance healthcare quality and outcomes. However, the current state of good practice guidelines development has yet to meet this potential [8].

Apart from the US formal IOM definition highlighted at the beginning of this section, the clinical practice guidelines can be simply defined as recommendations on how to diagnose and treat a medical condition, mainly written for doctors, but also for nurses and other health care professionals. Clinical practice guidelines and guidance are meant to help ensure that patients receive appropriate treatment and care. They summarize the current medical knowledge, weigh the benefits and harms of diagnostic procedures and treatments, and give specific recommendations based on this information. They should also provide scientific information about the supporting evidence for those recommendations. Clinical practice guidelines must be updated regularly [9]. Clinical practice guidelines can be used to inform individual clinical decision-making, provide best practice recommendations for the treatment and care of people by health professionals, develop standards to guide and assess the clinical practice of individual health professionals and healthcare organizations, help educate and train health professionals, and help patients make informed decisions [10].

Clinical practice guidelines differ from standard literature reviews and textbooks in the explicit methods used in their construction, which usually involve a representative guideline development group of professionals, (and increasingly patients and care providers), who use a systematic approach to identify and evaluate the evidence [11]. Evidence from secondary research, usually in the form of systematic reviews, is used in combination with the expertise of the guideline and WHO guidance development group to arrive at a set of recommendations for clinical practice. Guideline and WHO guidance development groups increasingly follow standard methods for development of recommendations including, where appropriate, formal, and informal consensus methods. An important characteristic of high-quality clinical guidelines is that the method is transparent and well described so that the evidence supporting each recommendation is clearly identifiable. Although interest in clinical guidelines has never been greater, uncertainty persists about whether they are effective. The debate has been hampered by the lack of a rigorous overview. Among 59 published evaluations of clinical guidelines that met defined criteria for scientific rigor (24 investigated guidelines for specific clinical conditions, 27 studied preventive care, and eight looked at guidelines for prescribing or for support services), all but four of these studies detected significant improvements in the process of care after the introduction of guidelines and all but 2 of the 11 studies that assessed the outcome of care reported significant improvements. Accordingly, it can be concluded that explicit guidelines do improve clinical practice, when introduced in the context of rigorous

evaluations. However, the size of the improvements in performance varied considerably [12].

Nowadays, clinical practice guidelines are ubiquitous in our healthcare system. The Guidelines International Network database currently lists around 3315 guidelines from 27 countries [13]. Its US counterpart, the National Guideline Clearinghouse (NGC), accepted 722 guidelines to its database in 2008 alone, so that its total collection is nearly 2700 [1].

Guidelines and WHO guidances have largely focused on the effectiveness of interventions. Over time, however, they have paid more attention to the size of the effect and the balance between effects on the one hand and harms and costs on the other as well as on the feasibility of following guidelines. Another emerging development is the concept of individualized guidelines and guidance, whereby risk factors specific to the individual patient, rather than population-based risk factors, are incorporated into tools weighing risks and benefits to guide treatment decisions.

11.3 Standards and Guidelines in Transfusion Medicine

Blood transfusion is one of the most frequently performed therapeutic procedures; it occurs in more than 10% of all hospital stays that include a procedure and was itself the most frequently performed procedure in 2009 [14]. Blood transfusion crosses many medical disciplines, has been identified as one of the top five overused therapies, and is associated with negative patient outcomes and increased costs [15].

Transfusion of blood products is used for patients with a wide range of medical conditions to improve tissue oxygenation, achieve hemostasis, and/or fight infections, and it enables many complex procedures, such as organ transplantation, cardiac and other surgeries, and stem cell transplantation. Yet the curricula of academic medical and nursing programs provide limited exposure and training towards helping providers to understand the attributes of the different types of blood, appreciate the risks of transfusion, and raise awareness of the accumulating body of evidence that is helping to refine the understanding of clinical indications for each type of transfusion [16].

For these reasons and likewise many other medical disciplines that faced the concerns of patients' outcomes, soaring costs and physicians' autonomy, the need emerged to have evidence-based clinical guidelines in the field of blood transfusion. Moreover, the availability of hemovigilance data that document the adverse effects of transfusion, randomized controlled trials demonstrating both the benefits and risks of transfusion, and growing debates regarding alternate therapies provided a good foundation to develop evidence-based resources to aid in transfusion care of today and the future [16].

In the blood transfusion spheres, over the past two or three decades, many blood transfusion professional societies, medical organizations, and government bodies from different countries developed and issued standards and clinical practice guidelines covering different aspects of the clinical use of blood, examples include the UK Blood Transfusion Guidelines published by the National Institute for Health and Care Excellence (NICE) [17], the French guideline on Platelet transfusion: products, indications, 2015 issued by Haute Autorité de santé (HAS) [18], and the US Association for the Advancement in Blood and Biotherapies (AABB) Red Blood Cells Transfusion: Clinical Practice Guidelines [19].

In some other cases, blood transfusion-related clinical practice guidelines were issued also by organizations or professional societies of medical specialties that use blood as one of the lines of treatment, for example, American Society of Hematology 2020 guidelines for sickle cell disease: transfusion support [20].

On the international level, in addition to publishing the WHO "Clinical use of blood in medicine, obstetrics, pediatrics, surgery and anesthesia, trauma and burns" [21], which has been updated in 2021 to the Guidance Education Modules on Clinical Use of Blood [22] and "Clinical Use of Blood Handbook" [23], the World Health Organization (WHO) provided guidance to Member States on developing national blood clinical guidance (Aide Mémoire for National Health Programmes: the clinical use of blood) highlighting that "Transfusion guidelines should represent a consensus by clinical specialists, the blood transfusion services, pharmacists and professional bodies on the most effective treatments for specific conditions. They should be practical, comprehensive, and relevant to local conditions. They should include: Clinical and laboratory indications for the use of blood, blood products and alternatives to transfusion; Information on available blood products and alternatives to transfusion: dosage, storage conditions, risk of transfusion-transmissible infection, means of administration, contraindications and precautions; Standard blood request form to provide full information about the patient and the need for transfusion; Blood ordering schedule, as a guide to the number of units of blood and blood products that should normally be requested for each type of operation, with guidance on its adaptation by each hospital; Instructions for the development of standard operating procedures at hospital level" [24].

The Aide Mémoire from the World Health Organization also encouraged Member States to establish hospital transfusion committees (HTCs) highlighting that "A transfusion committee should be established in each hospital to implement the national policy and guidelines and monitor the use of blood and blood products at the local level. The committee should have authority within the hospital structure to determine hospital policy in relation to transfusion and resolve any identified problems. The main functions of a hospital transfusion committee include: Developing systems for the implementation of the national guidelines within the hospital; Liaison with the blood transfusion services to ensure the availability of required blood and blood products at all times; Liaison with the relevant department to ensure a reliable supply of intravenous replacement fluids and other alternatives to transfusion at all times; Developing a hospital blood ordering schedule" [25].

Another remarkable step in terms of standardizing the clinical practices, improving patient outcomes, and enhancing blood transfusion efficiency was the development of Patient Blood

Management (PBM) (see Chap. 7). Guidelines emphasizing the patient focus in contrast to product focus of transfusion medicine. Patient blood management defined as "patient-centered, systematic, evidence-based approach to improve patient outcomes by managing and preserving a patient's own blood, while promoting patient safety and empowerment" [26] aims to improve clinical outcomes for individual patients by managing the patient's own blood as a standard of clinical care. This is achieved by a multidisciplinary team determining, with a specific personalized patient management plan, which makes every reasonable endeavor to address the three pillars of PBM, that is, optimize the patient's own blood volume, especially red cell mass; minimize the patient's blood loss; and optimize the patient's physiological tolerance of anemia. Allogeneic blood transfusion should only be a therapy when there are no other reasonable alternatives [27]. Patient Blood Management is built on the evidence that allogeneic blood transfusion has always been a potentially hazardous form of therapy and that in spite of the reduction of the risk of transfusion-transmitted infectious agents due to transfusion, still there are numerous other serious reactions reported in hemovigilance programs, and the fact that allogeneic blood transfusion is an independent risk factor contributing to poorer clinical outcomes [28].

An example of such standards is the Association for the Advancement of Blood and Biotherapies (AABB) Patient Blood Management Program standards 2023 that outline requirements for essential activities of a Patient Blood Management program surrounding patient evaluation and clinical management of those who may or may not require a transfusion. Specific topics include the use of appropriate indications for transfusion, minimization of blood loss, and optimization of patient red cell mass [29].

In some countries, Patient Blood Management guidelines are already replacing blood component guidelines. For example, Australia has made this move by developing National PBM guidelines to replace its decade old blood component use guidelines. These PBM guidelines are freely available on the internet from the Australian National Blood Authority [30].

11.4 Effectiveness and Impact of Guidelines on Quality and Patient Outcome

Clinical practice guidelines are a valued resource for clinicians looking for expert recommendations to direct clinical decision-making. However, the reliability and trustworthiness of many clinical practice guidelines were subpar as many guidelines were fraught with expert opinion, conflicts of interest, and bias [31]. This is different with the WHO Guidance which follows an extensive worldwide expert review before being implemented.

The basic elements essential to develop high-quality clinical practice guidelines vary between different professional bodies and healthcare organizations. Paul Shekelle, et al. summarized the Institute of Medicine (IOM, 2011)-recommended best practices to develop trustworthy high-quality clinical practice guidelines. These recommendations indicated that such guidelines should [2]

- have an explicit description of development and funding processes that is publicly accessible;
- follow a transparent process that minimizes bias, distortion, and conflicts of interest;
- be developed by a multidisciplinary panel comprising clinicians, methodological experts, and representatives, including a patient or consumer, of populations expected to be affected by the guideline;
- use rigorous systematic evidence review and consider quality, quantity, and consistency of the aggregate of available evidence;
- summarize evidence (and evidentiary gaps) about potential benefits and harms relevant to each recommendation;
- explain the parts that values, opinion, theory, and clinical experience play in deriving recommendations;
- provide a rating of the level of confidence in the evidence underpinning each recommendation and a rating of the strength of each recommendation;
- undergo extensive external review that includes an open period for public comment; and
- have a mechanism for revision when new evidence becomes available.

Clinical effectiveness is a key component of patient safety and quality. The integration of best evidence in service provision, through clinical effectiveness processes such as clinical practice guidance, promotes healthcare that is up to date, effective, and consistent. The added value of standards for clinical practice guidance for policy, health system, public, and patients can include the following [6]:

- Improving and optimizing patient outcomes;
- Evidence-based practice;
- Standardization of approach to avoid duplication;
- Facilitation of audit: provides parameters for audit;
- Reduction of variation in clinical practice;
- Consistency of nomenclature;
- Improvement of methodological rigor.

It is important to review and revise standards and guidelines at regular intervals, e.g., every 18 months to remain up to date and in line with the developing clinical transfusion medicine science.

Assessing the impact of published guidelines is important for future guideline development as well as assuring policymakers that they are an appropriate tool for enacting change.

It has been always debatable if implementation of clinical practice guidelines and guidance is necessarily associated with improvement of healthcare services utilization and patient outcomes. The European Observatory on Health Systems and Policies (2019) highlighted that clinical guidelines have the potential to reduce unwarranted practice variation and enhance translation of research into practice and highlighted that the overall hypothesis is that a well-developed guideline which is also well implemented will help improve patient outcomes by optimizing the process of care [32]. However, even with a high-quality trustworthy clinical practice guidelines in hand, many factors mediate their effectiveness and impact, including the discipline of users, dissemination, and implementation.

The European Observatory on Health Systems and Policies, 2019, concluded that systematically developed, evidence-based clinical guidelines are being used in many countries as a clinical quality strategy. Their usefulness in knowledge economy and translation, particularly in the context of ever-growing volumes of primary research, is not contested. However, their rigor of development, mode of implementation, and evaluation of impact can be improved in many settings to enable their goal of achieving "best practice" in healthcare and clinical transfusion medicine. One of the most important knowledge gaps in this direction is the extent to which guidelines affect patient outcomes and how this effect can be enhanced to ensure better care. For that purpose, both quantitatively measured parameters and service user experience should be considered [33].

Research findings in the blood transfusion field on effectiveness and impact of clinical practice guidelines on quality and patient outcomes are hovering around the same conclusions above. However, while some available studies indicate that implementation of clinical practice guidelines has a positive impact on patients outcomes and quality of care, there are clearly areas where available data are limited and research is still required.

Balafas et al. evaluated by means of a data-driven approach if and when the guidelines on red blood cell transfusions (RBCTs) issued by Swiss Smarter Medicine in 2016 had an impact on RBCTs practice within a Swiss hospital network, where awareness of guidelines was promoted mainly among internal medicine specialties. Data on RBCTs performed in the Swiss hospital network from January 2014 to April 2021 were analyzed to assess whether guidelines led to a decrease in inappropriate RBCTs. RBCTs were defined as "inappropriate" if patients had a hemoglobin level ≥ 70 g/L without or ≥ 80 g/L with significant cardiovascular comorbidities. Overall, prior to March 2017 there were more inappropriate than appropriate RBCTs, but after October 2017 the opposite could be observed. A change-point in the time trend was estimated from transfusion data to occur in the time interval between March and October 2017. This change was mainly driven by practice changes in the medical wards, while no significant change was observed in the critical care, surgical and oncology wards. In conclusion, the results show that a significant change in the RBCTs practice at the hospital level occurred approximately 18 months after national guidelines were issued [33]. Balafas, S., et al. highlight that in the absence of a targeted interventions, guidelines alone may not contribute efficiently to rapidly influence medical practice [33]. More structured intervention that includes dissemination of awareness, education and training, social interaction, decision support systems, and standing orders may be necessary to influence clinical practice in accordance with the introduction of new guidelines [33].

Another study by Adam H. Irving, et al. assessed how blood transfusions and patient outcomes in cardiac surgery changed after Australia's National Blood Authority published, in March 2012, national patient blood-management guidelines for perioperative care that was developed by a systematic review and clinical expert opinion. This study indicated that following the publication of the guidelines, there was a measurable reduction in perioperative blood transfusions in cardiac surgery with an associated reduction in hospital length of stay but no detectable differences in other patient outcomes [34].

11.5 Promoting Implementation of Clinical Standards and Guidelines

A 2003 study of adults living in 12 metropolitan areas of the United States found that participants received recommended care 54.9% of the time [35]. Another observational study of ten Dutch guidelines concluded that general practitioners followed guideline recommendations in only 61% of relevant situations [36]. Hence it is obvious that promoting uptake and use of clinical practice guidelines at the point of care delivery is as important as developing trustworthy clinical practice guidelines, it represents a final translation hurdle to move scientific findings into practice. Characteristics of the intended users and context of practice are as important as guideline

attributes for promoting adoption of CPG recommendations. Characteristics of a CPG that influence the extent to which it can be implemented to include clarity, specificity, strength of the evidence, perceived importance, relevance to practice, and simplicity versus complexity of the medical condition it is addressing [1].

Pronovost PJ identified five strategies, summarized below, that could help ensure clinical practice guidelines are adopted and used by clinicians. He highlighted that it is unlikely that guideline developers, typically experts in clinical epidemiology, have expertise in implementation science or systems engineering. This expertise is needed to identify and automate the use of guidelines and, by doing so, help reduce the morbidity and mortality associated with preventable harm. The five suggested strategies are the following [37]:

- Guidelines should incorporate a checklist of prioritized specific interventions;
- Identify barriers to adoption, and design supports to address specific barriers;
- Integrate guidelines for common coexistent conditions;
- Identify systems and technological solutions to promote adherence with recommendations;
- Develop transdisciplinary teams (clinical epidemiology, implementation science, systems engineering) to study ways to foster best practices.

The Committee on Standards for Developing Trustworthy Clinical Practice Guidelines of the US Institute of Medicine recommended the following to promote implementation of clinical practice guidelines [1]:

- Pursue effective multifaceted implementation strategies targeting all relevant populations affected by clinical practice guidelines, should be employed by implementers to promote adherence to trustworthy clinical practice guidelines;
- Guideline developers should structure the format, vocabulary, and content of clinical practice guidelines (e.g., specific statements of

evidence, the target population) to facilitate ready implementation of computer-aided Clinical Decision Support by end-users;

- Clinical practice e, g., clinical transfusion medicine guideline developers, implementers, and designers should collaborate to align their needs with one another.

In addition to the above-mentioned strategies, the IOM committee highlighted that according to Greenhalgh et al. the methods of communication and forms of communication channels can indictors fluence adoption of clinical practice guidelines [38] and stressed the role of such communication channels with a special attention to. education and mass media, academic detailing, and opinion leaders.

In consideration of the legal issues affecting implementation of clinical practice guidelines, the IOM committee suggested that clinicians will be more likely to adopt guidelines if they believe they offer malpractice litigation protection. The committee also suggested that courts will be more likely to adopt guidelines that are trustworthy and urged them, given reliance on clinical practice guidelines, to use those deemed trustworthy when available. In other words, clinical practice guidelines could be used as a "liability shield" to define a standard of care, rather than local customary practice, and protect physicians who follow it. On the other hand, they could be used as a "liability sword" against physicians who commit errors of misuse, underuse, or overuse which may result in patient complications, when not following the appropriate clinical practice guidelines and guidance [39].

11.6 Conclusion and Recommendations

Clinical practice guidelines draw on synthesized research findings to set forth recommendations for state-of-the-art care, educate healthcare workers and patients, and assess the performance of healthcare professionals and organizations. The process of developing clinical practice standards and guidelines is quite complicated and needed

to be standardized itself to avoid subjectivity; they also need be evaluated fully for their effectiveness in improving health.

Although blood transfusion is one of the most frequently performed therapeutic procedures and crosses many medical disciplines, the curricula of academic medical and nursing programs provide limited exposure and training towards helping providers to understand the attributes of the different types of blood components and appreciate the risks of transfusion. For these reasons and likewise many other medical disciplines that faced the concerns of patients' outcomes, soaring costs, and physicians' autonomy, the need emerged to have evidence-based clinical guidelines in the field of blood transfusion.

Over the past decades many blood transfusion professional societies and government bodies from different countries developed and issued standards and clinical practice guidelines covering different aspects of the clinical use of blood. In some other cases, such guidelines were issued also by professional societies of medical specialties that use blood as one of the lines of treatment. On the international level, the WHO issued the guidelines on "Clinical use of blood in medicine, obstetrics, pediatrics, surgery and anesthesia, trauma and burns", "Clinical Use of Blood Handbook" and the 2021 "Education Modules on Clinical Use of Blood." Another remarkable step in terms of standardizing the clinical practices, improving patients' outcomes and enhancing blood transfusion efficiency was development of Patient Blood Management (PBM) Guidelines emphasizing the patient focus in contrast to product focus of transfusion medicine.

Although interest in clinical guidelines has never been greater, uncertainty persists about whether they are effective due to lack of a rigorous overview. However, it is suggested that trustworthy evidence-based clinical guidelines, if disseminated and implemented properly, can enhance clinical practices to a great extent. The same applies on clinical guidelines in the blood transfusion field where some studies highlighted that in the absence of targeted interventions, guidelines alone may not contribute efficiently to rapidly influence medical practice and improve patient outcomes. Hence, more structured interventions are required to leverage the full positive potential of clinical guidance and guidelines. These interventions should comprehensively include promotion, dissemination, education, and training on the clinical practice guidelines.

11.6.1 Recommendations

- Follow standardized best practices to develop trustworthy high-quality clinical practice guidelines.
- Well-developed and implemented trustworthy clinical practice guidelines and guidance are highly likely to improve effectiveness of clinical interventions and the patient outcome.
- Transfusion guidelines should be evidence-based and represent a consensus by clinical specialists, the blood transfusion services, pharmacists, and professional bodies.
- Pursue effective multifaceted clinical guidelines implementation strategies targeting all relevant populations affected by clinical practice guidelines.
- Identify systems and technological solutions to promote adherence with guidelines recommendations.
- A transfusion committee should be established in each hospital to implement the guidelines and monitor the use of blood and blood components.
- The patient-centered approach of "Patient Blood Management" is highly recommended to improve clinical outcomes for individual patients by managing the patient's own blood as a standard of clinical care.

References

1. Institute of Medicine (US). Committee on standards for developing trustworthy clinical practice guidelines. In: Graham R, Mancher M, Miller Wolman D, et al., editors. Clinical practice Guidelines we can trust. 6. Promoting adoption of clinical practice guidelines. Washington, DC: National Academies Press (US); 2011. https://www.ncbi.nlm.nih.gov/books/NBK209543/.
2. Shekelle P, Anderson MD, Givens J. UpToDate: overview of clinical practice guidelines. 2022. https://uptodate.com/contents/overview-of-clinical-practice-guidelines#H1152132. Accessed 20 Oct 2023.
3. Eddy DM. Evidence-based medicine: a unified approach. Health Affairs (Millwood). 2005;24(1):9–17.
4. Pilling S. History, context, process, and rationale for the development of clinical guidelines. Psychol Psychother Theory Res Practice. 2008;81:331–50. https://doi.org/10.1348/14760830x324923.
5. Sackett DL, Rosenberg WMC, Gray JAM, Haynes RB. Evidence-based medicine: what is and what isn't. BMJ. 1996;312:71–2.
6. Weisz G, Cambrosio A, Keating P, Knaapen L, Schlich T, Tournay VJ. The emergence of clinical practice Guidelines. Milbank Q. 2007;85:691–727. https://doi.org/10.1111/j.1468-0009.2007.00505.x.
7. Davidoff F, Haynes. Sackett DL, Smith R. Evidence-based medicine: a new journal to help doctors identify the information they need. BMJ. 1995;310:1085–6.
8. Standards for clinical practice guidance. National Clinical Effectiveness Committee; 2015. p. 4. https://www.nmbi.ie/NMBI/media/NMBI/Forms/standards-for-clinical-practice-guidance-ncec.pdf. Accessed 17 Oct 2023.
9. InformedHealth.org. Cologne. What are clinical practice guidelines? Germany: Institute for Quality and efficiency in health care (IQWiG); 2016. https://www.ncbi.nlm.nih.gov/books/NBK390308/.
10. ESF. Implementation of medical research in clinical practice. European Science Foundation; 2011. http://archives.esf.org/fileadmin/Public_documents/Publications/Implem_MedReseach_ClinPractice.pdf. Accessed 18 Oct 2023.
11. WHO GLOBAL PATIENT SAFETY ACTION PLAN 2021–2030 Towards eliminating avoidable harm in health care. https://iris.who.int/bitstream/handle/10665/343477/9789240032705-eng.pdf?sequence=1.
12. Grimshaw JM, Russell IT. Effect of clinical guidelines on medical practice: a systematic review of rigorous evaluations. Lancet. 1993;342(8883):1317–22. https://doi.org/10.1016/0140-6736(93)92244-N.
13. Guidelines International Network (GIN) Library. https://guidelines.ebmportal.com/. Accessed 18 Oct 2023.
14. Eddy DM, Adler J, Patterson B, Lucas D, Smith KA, Morris M. Individualized guidelines: the potential for increasing quality and reducing costs. Ann Intern Med. 2011;154:629–34.
15. Morton J, Anastassopoulos KP, Patel ST, et al. Frequency and outcomes of blood products transfusion across procedures and clinical conditions warranting inpatient care: an analysis of the 2004 healthcare cost and utilization project nationwide inpatient sample database. Am J Med Qual. 2010;25:289–96.
16. Leahy MF, Hofmann A, Towler S, et al. Improved outcomes and reduced costs associated with a health-system-wide patient blood management pro-

gram: a retrospective observational study in four major adult tertiary-care hospitals. Transfusion. 2017;57(6):1347–58. https://doi.org/10.1111/trf.14006. Epub 2017 Feb 2.

17. A Compendium of Transfusion Practice Guidelines Edition 4.0. 2021. https://www.redcross.org/content/dam/redcrossblood/hospital-page-documents/334401_compendium_v04jan2021_book-markedworking_rwv01.pdf. Accessed 18 Oct 2023.

18. Blood transfusion guidelines published by the National Institute for Health and Care Excellence (NICE). https://www.nice.org.uk/guidance/ng24/resources/blood-transfusion-pdf-1837331897029.

19. Guideline on platelet transfusion: products, indications, 2015 issued by Haute Autorité de santé (HAS). https://www.has-sante.fr/jcms/c_2571571/fr/transfusion-de-plaquettes-produits-indications.

20. Carson JL, Guyatt G, Heddle NM, et al. Clinical practice guidelines from the AABB: red blood cell transfusion thresholds and storage. JAMA. 2016;316(19):2025–35. https://doi.org/10.1001/jama.2016.9185.

21. Chou TS, Alsawas M, Fasano RM, et al. American Society of Hematology guidelines for sickle cell disease: transfusion support. Blood Adv. 2020;4(2):327–55. https://doi.org/10.1182/bloodadvances.2019001143.

22. WHO. The Clinical use of blood in medicine, obstetrics, pediatrics, surgery and anesthesia, trauma and burns". 2001. https://iris.who.int/bitstream/handle/10665/42397/a72894.pdf?sequence=1. Accessed 18 Oct 2023.

23. WHO. Clinical use of blood handbook. 2001. https://iris.who.int/bitstream/handle/10665/42396/9241545399.pdf?sequence=1. Accessed 18 Oct 2023.

24. Educational modules on clinical use of blood. License: CC BY-NC-SA 3,0 IGO. Geneva: World Health Organization; 2021.

25. WHO. Aide-mémoire for National Health Programmes: the clinical use of blood. 2001. https://cdn.who.int/media/docsOctober/default-source/searo/blt/aide-memoire0123-3-04.pdf?sfvrsn=e0b00f77_2. Accessed 18 Oct 2023.

26. Shander A, Hardy JF, Ozawa S, et al. A Global definition of patient blood management. Anesth Analg. 2022;135(3):476–88. https://doi.org/10.1213/ANE.0000000000005873. Epub 2022 Feb 10.

27. Isbister JP. The three-pillar matrix of patient blood management. VOXS. 2015;10:286–94. https://doi.org/10.1111/voxs.12135.

28. Bolton-Maggs PHB, Cohen H. Serious hazards of transfusion (SHOT) haemovigilance and progress is improving transfusion safety. Br J Haematol. 2013;163:303–14. https://doi.org/10.1111/bjh.12547.

29. https://www.aabb.org/standards-accreditation/standards/patient-blood-management-program.

30. Patient Blood Management Guidelines. National Blood Authority. http://www.blood.gov.au/pbm-guidelines. Accessed 19 Oct 2023.

31. Czaja MT, Carson JL. Improving clinical practice through the use of clinical practice guidelines. Vox Sang. 2015;10:73–8. https://doi.org/10.1111/voxs.12161.

32. Busse R, Klazinga N, Panteli D, Quentin W, editors. Improving healthcare quality in Europe: characteristics, effectiveness and implementation of different strategies. Copenhagen (Denmark): European Observatory on Health Systems and Policies; (Health Policy Series, No. 53.). 2019. https://www.ncbi.nlm.nih.gov/books/NBK549276/. Accessed 20 Oct 2023.

33. Balafas S, Gagliano V, Di Serio C, et al. Differential impact of transfusion guidelines on blood transfusion practices within a health network. Sci Rep. 2023;13(1):6264. https://doi.org/10.1038/s41598-023-33549-6.

34. Irving AH, Harris A, Petrie D, et al. Impact of patient blood management guidelines on blood transfusions and patient outcomes during cardiac surgery. J Thorac Cardiovasc Surgery. 2020;160:437–45.e20. https://doi.org/10.1016/j.jtcvs.2019.08.102.

35. McGlynn EA, Asch SM, Adams J. The quality of health care delivered to adults in the United States. N Engl J Med. 2003;348(26):2635–45.

36. Grol R, Dalhuijsen J, Thomas S, Veld C, Rutten G. Attributes clinical guidelines that influence use of guidelines in general practice: observational study. BMJ. 1998;317(7162):858–61.

37. Pronovost PJ. Enhancing physicians' use of clinical guidelines. JAMA. 2013;310:2501.

38. Greenhalgh T, Robert G, Bate P, Macfarlane F, Kyriakidou O. Diffusion of innovations in health service organisations: a systematic literature review. Malden, MA: Blackwell Publishing Ltd; 2005.

39. Rosoff AJ. Evidence-based medicine and the law: the courts confront clinical practice guidelines. J Health Politics Policy Law. 2001;26(2):327–68.

Epilogue

Most of the serious hazards and adverse events of blood transfusion occur in the hospitals, the reason why hemovigilance starts at the bedside. Consequently, those who are involved in the clinical application of blood components need to be competent and have sufficient knowledge of the physiology and pathophysiology of blood cells and plasma proteins to be able to decide, indicate, and prescribe blood and blood components to patients and perform safe and effective blood transfusion at the bedside. Most patients in need of supportive blood transfusion only need a blood component transfused to prevent organ failure or protracted bleeding.

So far, the educational and scientific literature has paid an overwhelming amount of interest in direct transfusion practice; guidelines, protocols, and recently Educational Modules on Clinical Use of Blood, published in scientific journals, books, or scientific conference proceedings. Rational use of blood and blood components should be based on scientific evidence and a sound clinical transfusion medicine quality system and system management with up-to-date clinical transfusion standards.

Since the introduction of more vigilant clinical practice of blood transfusion—hemovigilance—those professionals involved in transfusion medicine were urged to document clearly and transparently what is done and why, documenting more accurately the observed clinical outcome of the transfusion intervention. That is more than just performing and documenting vital signs of the recipient in the clinical personal file at the bedside.

However, relatively few scientific attention has been paid to education (knowledge) to understand the principles of clinical transfusion medicine and the accompanying pathophysiology of individual patients in need of a supportive blood component. The question is not just "What is needed?," but more important "Why is there a need?" and "What is needed?", "How much is needed" and "For how long will there be a need?" Additional questions to be answered and understood are "Could the patient produce sufficient volume of what is supposed to be the need?," "How much time would that take?" and "How do I know?." In other words, "Do we always need to replace what was lost?" This translates into the question "Why should we expose patients in need, e.g., threat of organ failure, to a liberal blood prescription practice and not to a more rational restrictive practice?"

Decision-making and indication setting, whether in adult or pediatric practice, could be more accurate and precise, safe, and evidence-based, and personalized medicine by the introduction of artificial intelligence (AI) with its deep and machine learning (DL and ML) algorithms, the use of radiofrequency identification (RFID), footprinting of the clinical transfusion chain, preventing avoidable clerical errors, and improving personalized patient care. The ques-

C. T. Smit Sibinga, Y. E. Abdella (eds.), *Clinical Use of Blood*, https://doi.org/10.1007/978-3-031-67332-0

tions above could be answered faster and more accurately when one follows these seemingly futuristic processes and procedures. However, this will only work when generation of clinical transfusion medicine data collection and use are transparent, standardized, high quality, and accurate.

The ultimate aim as in the Hippocratic Oath is "primum est non nocere," mitigating or even eliminating avoidable harm to patients.